Normal Child and
Adolescent Development

Normal Child and Adolescent Development

Ralph Gemelli, M.D.

Clinical Associate Professor of Psychiatry
George Washington University School of Medicine
Washington, D.C.

Clinical Associate Professor of Psychiatry
Uniformed Services University of the Health Sciences
F. Edward Hébert School of Medicine
Bethesda, Maryland

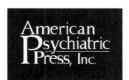

Washington, DC
London, England

Copyright © 1996 American Psychiatric Press, Inc.
ALL RIGHTS RESERVED
Manufactured in the United States of America on acid-free paper
07 06 05 04 03 02   7 6 5 4 3 2

American Psychiatric Press, Inc.
1400 K Street, N.W., Washington, DC   20005

Library of Congress Cataloging-in-Publication Data
Gemelli, Ralph J.
    Normal child and adolescent development / Ralph Gemelli.
        p.   cm.
    Includes bibliographical references and index.
    ISBN 0-88048-258-3
    1. Child psychology.   2. Adolescent psychology.   3. Child development.   4. Adolescence.   I. Title.
    [DNLM: 1. Child Development.   2. Child Psychology.
3. Adolescence.   4. Adolescent Psychology.   WS 105 G3223n 1996]
BF721.G4652   1996
155.4—dc20
DNLM/DLC
For Library of Congress   95-37815
                                                                          CIP

British Library Cataloguing in Publication Data
A CIP record is available from the British Library.

To the family members
who most influenced my development

My grandparents:
Mary (1901–1972) and Michael (1888–1960) Avallone

My parents:
Rose (1922–   ) and Roy (1917–   ) Gemelli

My aunt and uncle:
Nancy (1932–   ) and Eugene (1927–   ) Avallone

Contents

Introduction

This book is intended to be an introduction to normal child and adolescent mental development for mental health professionals enrolled in training programs to prepare for providing services to children, adolescents, and adults with mental and behavioral problems. Throughout this work, I have attempted to provide illustrative examples of both normal and abnormal development. The examples of abnormal development demonstrate the usefulness of normal developmental concepts in understanding the child or adolescent who is struggling with mental problems, behavioral problems, or both.

This book in an attempt to bring many of the partial theories on normal mental development into a reasonably integrated "quilt." It is not intended to be a review of the latest research on normal mental development, nor is it intended for the experienced child or adult psychiatrist. This book is an attempt to interest the beginning mental health professional in acquiring knowledge about the complex maturation and development of the infant's, child's, and adolescent's mind.

In Chapter 2, I outline one possible, and I hope knowledge-enhancing, integrated theoretical model of the mind. This model is based on the theory that the human body is a biological system, of which the brain and mind are a part. I then describe an expanded and revised version of the biopsychosocial integrated theoretical model of mental development. This model is then used throughout the book as a road map or guide for students of development to assist them in beginning to integrate many different facets of mental development from infancy to the end of adolescence.

Major Concepts of This Book

The main message of this book is that the maturation and development of the child's inner mental world is organized and can be studied using the biopsychosocial theoretical model of the mind. Of strong import in this model is the fact that the mind is endowed with innate mental structures and that new mental structures emerge through the normal maturational process and are constructed as development proceeds.

The view I express of the mental developmental process can be conceptualized as an object relations–structural view. Throughout the developmental process, children's object relationships lead to a complexity of stored internal representational structures that becomes their unique representation of their living experiences. These structures, together with the ongoing influences of the social environment, will forever affect the infant's and child's current and future object relationships. Simultaneously, as an infant's representational world begins to form, it forever influences how he or she perceives the current social world and the kind of thoughts, feelings, and memories that are generated in response to these perceptions.

Also integrated into the discussion of normal mental development are the following concepts:

- The mental constructs of the id, ego, superego, and self
- The conscious, preconscious, and unconscious mental domains
- Implicit versus explicit memories
- The development of the internal distress signal (or internal signaling function)
- Defense mechanisms
- Transference reactions
- Major principles by which mental development is organized

When these topics are not included or are given only superficial treatment in a book on normal mental development, there is a tendency to put these topics in the category "concepts to think about when evaluating troubled children, adolescents, and adults." When this occurs, these normal developmental concepts are not integrated into evaluatory and treatment work with mentally disturbed children, adolescents, and adults.

Organization of the Book

One reason for the difficulty many people have with conceptualizing that children progressively construct a complex representational world as they develop—a world that gives continuity to their ever-developing identity—has been the tendency in books on normal mental development to present information on each developmental phase through series of topics that address events occurring during each phase. The topics that are discussed for one developmental phase may not be repeated for succeeding developmental phases. This tends to make it difficult for students of child and adolescent mental development to follow in sequence the changes in one topic area (e.g., the maturation and development of emotions) from one developmental phase to the next. For this reason, I have chosen to follow the same basic organizational outline throughout this book, with only minimal deviations. The basic outline of each chapter is as follows:

- Major Developmental Tasks of [Particular Phase]
- Functions of the Social Environment
- Maturation and Development of Innate Needs
- Maturation and Development of Physical Capabilities
- Maturation and Development of Cognitive Capabilities
- Maturation and Development of Temperamental Characteristics
- Maturation and Development of Emotions
- Maturation and Development of Verbal Language Abilities
- Continuing Influence of the Preexisting Representational World
- Development of the Self and Object Relationships
- Development of the Superego
- Development of Adaptational Capabilities

It is my hope that this schematic organization will emphasize that children's mental development is continuous as well as discontinuous—continuous in the sense that their representational world provides the continuous "landscape" from which they progressively perceive the social world using their increasingly complex perceptual and cognitive capabilities, and discontinuous in the sense that children's maturational advances, coupled with new life events, will produce relatively unexpected developmental changes in them.

Acknowledgments

I am indebted to several faculty members of the Uniformed Services University of the Health Sciences who encouraged me to develop a course in normal development for medical students, a course that ultimately became the impetus for this book. They are John Duffy, M.D.; Harry Holloway, M.D.; Robert Ursano, M.D.; and Robert Hales, M.D. An added thanks goes to Richard Fragala, M.D., for his meticulous reading of the first draft of this book and his many insightful comments.

I am also grateful to Marilyn Benoit, M.D., and Jerry Wiener, M.D., faculty members of the George Washington University School of Medicine, for encouraging me to develop the concepts expressed in this book by supporting my teaching about normal development to medical students at George Washington University and to child psychiatric residents, psychology interns, and social work interns at the Children's National Medical Center in Washington, D.C.

I am indebted to the following faculty members of the Washington Psychoanalytic Institute: Judith Viorst, a professional writer, encouraged me to be forthright in expressing my views about normal development; Harvey Rich, M.D., and Judith F. Chused, M.D., read sections of the initial manuscript and were generous in supporting my bringing this book to fruition; and James L. Hatleberg, M.D.; Frances K. Millican, M.D.; and the late Dexter Bullard, Jr., M.D., taught me about the importance of using normal developmental concepts in helping children and adults with psychiatric problems. I am especially grateful to the late Helen Ross, who encouraged me to believe as she did, that children can teach adults much about what they need in order to develop normally. And finally, special thanks go to Jill S. Scharff, M.D., who read my entire manuscript and provided me with much empathic support at a time when my energies were depleted.

I want to express my appreciation to Sue Allison, a professional writer, for her meticulous reading of the final manuscript, her helping me to express my thoughts more clearly, and her helping me to understand the psychology of completing a major writing task.

My appreciation also goes to Marni Brooks and Vernita R. Hughes, who worked diligently in typing my original manuscript. Major accolades go to Cecilia Amtower who effortlessly worked to meet deadlines in retyping and organizing the many revisions of my manuscript. Amy Conrick did an outstanding job in the final editing of my manuscript and in carefully preparing my list of references.

I am also grateful for the special mentorship of J. Alfred LeBlanc, M.D., of the Washington Psychoanalytic Institute, whose insights about development helped me organize and integrate my overall view of the developmental process.

The challenges and triumphs of many children and adolescents and their parents are recorded in the pages of this book. I am indebted to all of them for what they have shared with me about their efforts to master developmental tasks. They have enhanced what I have learned about normal development by studying the many important contributions made to the child developmental, psychological, and psychoanalytic literature by the likes of Sigmund and Anna Freud, Jean Piaget, Erik Erikson, Robert Emde, Daniel Stern, Joseph Lichtenberg, Jerome Kagan, and the many others referenced throughout this book.

Chapter 1

Theoretical and Historical Perspectives on Children's Mental Development

The process through which a child's mind, or inner mental world, develops has become a serious interest for scientific thinkers only in the 20th century. As I document in this chapter, the content of children's minds was neglected throughout most of history. In addition, scientific methods for collecting data about the inner workings of children's minds were undeveloped, even into the early 20th century when Freud and others began to construct theories of normal child development. Further, as these theories were constructed, they were influenced—as they still are—by the biases of the researchers. Before turning to the biopsychosocial theory of children's development, I address this and other issues that continue to be encountered in constructing theories of normal development.

1

The Process of Developing Theories

A *theory* is one or more hypotheses with which one attempts to understand and integrate aspects of phenomena that are not directly observable. In contrast, an *empirical fact* is based on phenomena that are directly observable and are believed to be provable by investigative methods based on objective reality. For example, a human behavior such as walking can be directly and objectively observed; therefore it can be proven to have occurred as an empirical fact. However, the hidden mental structures—the perceptions, wishes, emotions, or memories—that precede and accompany a child's walking are phenomena that are not directly observable. They can be "observed" only indirectly through the child's internally perceiving his or her own mental phenomena and then expressing these perceptions, wishes, emotions, or memories in words.

Despite the difficulty in directly observing mental phenomena, theories guide researchers in better understanding mental development. Within the natural sciences, there is a growing *postempiricist philosophy of science* that supports the hypothesis that theories generate specific questions and focus the observer on what to perceive (Gardner 1994; Goldberg 1994). In other words, scientists first generate a hypothesis—based on other theories that are accepted as the best approximation of the truth—and then "see" what they assumed might have been there in the first place.

In studying the development of the human mind, theories guide not only the beginning student but also the experienced clinician and researcher in selectively perceiving and then focusing on the data that they believe or assume exist. Thus it follows that, when new theories generate new theoretical questions, new data are looked for and subsequently may be observed. *Knowledge-enhancing theories* are those that are retrospectively judged to have generated hypotheses and predictions that enabled new observational data to be gathered and new knowledge to emerge. *Knowledge-inhibiting theories,* on the other hand, are judged to be so when one realizes retrospectively that they have become an impediment in the acquisition of new knowledge. One example might be a theory that originally included only children of a certain age span when, based on later-formed theoretical concepts, it is determined that that theory should have included children of a wider age span.

■ Observational Methods for Collecting Data on the Development of the Mind

Various methods have emerged since approximately 1900 to collect data about children's thoughts, feelings, memories, and surface behaviors. In the early 1900s, Sigmund Freud gathered data by interviewing and psychoanalytically treating adult patients. This retrospective method was followed by other psychoanalysts and psychiatrists as they attempted to identify adult patients' childhood memories. In the 1930s, others (e.g., Anna Freud, Melanie Klein) began to gather direct data about children by directly interviewing children and their families. Since the 1970s, much progress has been made in understanding how to collect data about children, their parents, and important others to be used in evaluating children's preexisting representational world and their current mental and behavioral functioning. In the following sections, I delineate the different data-collecting approaches currently used to study the process of development, particularly in identifying 1) the variations in development between same-age children, 2) the occurrence of continuities and discontinuities in the developmental process, and 3) the pivot points that usher in new developmental phases.

Cross-cultural methods. Studies from different cultures show that wide variations exist in the physical contexts surrounding children. One child may live in an overly crowded boat in the harbor of a city enveloped in extreme air pollution, whereas another may live in an environment with clean air and abundant physical space. Wide variations also exist in child-rearing patterns. For example, in some cultures, children are weaned as early as age 6 months, whereas in other cultures they are not weaned until after age 2 years. Finally, wide variations exist in what behaviors parents developmentally task their children to learn as they become members of their particular society. Most parents intuitively know the major developmental tasks that their society expects of children, tasks that derive from long-standing cultural practices. For example, in one culture, female children may be taught that they must always wear a veil in public to conceal their faces; in another culture, pictures of both male and female children, from birth onward, may be put on open display within the home.

Retrospective methods. In these studies, data about earlier phases of mental development are drawn from the recollections of older child and adolescent patients about their pasts. In addition to past events, older children will remember aspects of their current and past relationships with important people in their lives. Another type of remembering is recalling past relationships through *transference reactions* which can lead to the genesis of *fantasies, verbalizations,* or *behavioral enactments* (R. Tyson and Tyson 1986). Transference reactions—which are, in fact, a ubiquitous aspect of human mental functioning—reveal 1) important elements of children's relationships with significant people in the past, and 2) later constructions and reconstructions (i.e., beliefs, symbols, and fantasies) of these relationships. Memories of these relationships are stored in children's representations; the transference reaction results from the externalization of these representations onto the present relationship with the interviewer. Through the transference, then, the reconstructed, past relationship is relived in the present.

Retrospective studies have produced a profound level of knowledge about how one's childhood can influence his or her feelings, thoughts, beliefs, and fantasies throughout adolescence and into adulthood. This knowledge has been used by mental health professionals to assist many children and adults in understanding the varying influences of their memories and present perceptions, thoughts, and emotions in the genesis of dysphoric emotional states (e.g., depression) and troublesome thinking (e.g., an obsession).

Retrospective research has also been used to generate theories of normal and abnormal development. Sigmund Freud (1920/1963) partially attributed the cause of the depression and psychogenic paralysis (e.g., hysterical illness) experienced by some of his adult patients to the persistence of infantile and childhood wishes stored in these patients' unconscious mental domain. He later challenged researchers to provide direct observational data to prove or disprove his retrospective theories. Anna Freud (1951, 1965) reaffirmed many of her father's theories, discarded others, and added some of her own theories based on her developmental research with both children and adolescents.

Melanie Klein (1935) developed a hypothesis, based on work with mostly verbal preschool children, that, before age 6 months, infants have the capacity for complex thinking in relation to their mother (e.g., that infants react to physical discomfort by thinking that the discomfort was caused by an angry mother). Although this hypothesis was refuted by later research, her attempt to understand the mental activity of the young infant stimulated much scientific activity in the 1940s and 1950s involving observation of young infants and children (Noshpitz and King 1991).

Heinz Kohut (1970), in his work with adult patients, hypothesized the importance of parental empathy for, and acceptance of, children's need to perform for their parents and experience a magical sense of power and omnipotence both in themselves and in their parents. Kohut emphasized the need for parents to help their children gradually relinquish these childhood wishes of omnipotence for themselves and their parents and to gradually accept their own and their parents' imperfections.

One important issue in evaluating the data that emerge from retrospective studies is to what degree the recalled memories of and the transferences related to the past are reasonably close replicas of past events. Children react to events in their lives by constructing individualized representations of those events—representations that are colored by their thoughts, wishes, emotions, and prior memories. These collected representations—which compose a child's inner world—will forever influence the child's perceptions, thoughts, and emotions as well as the child's future construction of representations of external events. The reality, therefore, that each child deals with in his or her life is both the external reality of the child's social world and the internal reality of the child's representational world, which includes memories of his or her past. Thus, any question asked of children about their past is a question about how they have constructed and undoubt-edly reconstructed (or reinterpreted) that past. A child's memory is not an exact photograph of a past event but, as Terr (1994) noted, is a "slightly flawed product from an active and developing mind" (p. 29). Abrams (1995) made a similar point when he stated,

> Minds are active synthesizers and organizers, not merely passive receptors. . . . Memory lies "between what happened and what is remembered." (p. 31)

For this reason, many retrospective theories are considered valid only when they are based on data that reveal similarities in child-hood experience among different adolescents or adults, rather than on data accumulated from the reported pasts of one or a few patients.

Longitudinal methods.   In longitudinal studies, the central re-search question is often whether a particular surface behavior or mental structure (e.g., a belief) will manifest continuity over time (i.e., have temporal stability). In these studies, a group of infants or children is selected and evaluated for certain sets of surface behaviors or mental phenomena, or both. Evaluations are then conducted periodically for several years. Andrews and Harris (1964), for example, investigated the incidence of stuttering in children by selecting 1,000 physically healthy, neurologically intact newborns and performing a standardized set of systematic, peri-odic evaluations on them for the next 18 years.

Longitudinal research is highly valued by child researchers but is quite costly and encounters many problems in follow-up (Ver-hulst and Koot 1991). For example, complications such as parents divorcing or losing their jobs or unexpected tragedies such as par-ents dying can cause children in the study to move to a new geo-graphic location. In the Andrews and Harris (1964) study (admittedly, a rather long study), there was a 24.8% attrition rate during the 18-year course of the study.

Another drawback to longitudinal research is the change in compliance by some children as they grow older. A child may show good motivation during one follow-up period and poor motivation during the next. This change is often attributable to changes in the child's beliefs about the usefulness of the study or about how further participation in the study will affect him or her.

The evaluators may also change over the course of the study, with a resultant potential change in what is actually studied in the follow-up evaluation sessions over the span of the entire study (Farrington 1991). When this occurs, the observations reported by different researchers decrease the reliability of the study's results.

Another potential problem in longitudinal research is the effect of an ever-changing social environment constant during a several-year evaluation period (Kovacs et al. 1993). For example, Appelbaum and McCall (1983) noted that, in any longitudinal study of a group of children, the changes attributable to age will have to be differentiated from changes attributable to environmental factors. For example, if a group of children born in 1985 were then studied in 1990 and 1995, the changes noted in those two follow-up sessions could be attributable to the children's being older as well as to changes in their environments over the 10 years since the original session.

One other difficulty in designing longitudinal research is the need to have a control group of children that is matched with the experimental group. This minimizes the number of potential variables that would be involved in explaining the changes in the behaviors and mental competencies that are studied. For example, if the goal of the longitudinal research is to study whether a temperamental trait from birth (e.g., distractibility) shows high temporal stability, the experimental group would consist of infants who manifested distractibility, and the control group would consist of infants who did not manifest this trait but who were matched to the experimental group in age, sex, cultural background, and socioeconomic status. At the completion of the study, if distractibility showed high or low stability, age (as a variable to explain the change in stability) could be much better assessed than if the other variables had not been controlled.

Despite these limitations, the longitudinal study is still the best method to 1) study the issue of phases in mental development, 2) investigate continuities and discontinuities in the mental developmental process, and 3) separate those maturational and developmental changes that would occur with the natural age progression of the child from those changes that would occur because of the historical eras in which the child was born and in which the evaluative measurements were carried out (Appelbaum and McCall 1983). Through such studies, developmentalists would hope to discover a body of data that establishes longitudinal links between a person's behaviors and mental activities in childhood and that person's behaviors and mental activities in adulthood. For example, what specific childhood standards and values for different socioeconomic groups of children show high temporal stability from childhood to adulthood? Not a great deal is known concerning this question, but well-designed and well-constituted longitudinal studies would help answer this and other questions about what aspects of a child's past moral standards persist as that child matures into an adult and how this occurs.

Cross-sectional methods. Cross-sectional studies are designed to measure developmental changes by evaluating different groups of children at different ages. In these studies, researchers use *cohorts*—that is, groups of children born at approximately the same time. For example, if researchers were attempting to answer the question, What are normally expected moral beliefs possessed by children (in a particular culture) at age 3 years? through a longitudinal design, they would select a group of 3-year-old children and evaluate them at yearly intervals for the succeeding 3 years. However, if they were using a cross-sectional design, they would evaluate a group of 3-year-old children and a different group of 6-year-old children concurrently.

In a longitudinal study, the family environment is more controlled, or assumed to remain relatively stable; hence, the child's specific changes in moral standards can be attributed to continuities or discontinuities in the child's developmental process. Using the cross-sectional design, the changes in moral standards between 3-year-old and 6-year-old children could be attributable to different parenting practices and different environmental beliefs about and attitudes toward morality.

The cross-sectional method is useful in developmental research in identifying, in a rather short period of time, differences in capabilities, abilities, and overall functioning between groups of children at different ages or between groups of children of the same age. In the latter situation, for example, researchers might investigate the differences in moral standards between Protestant, white, urban-dwelling children; Catholic, Italian-American, urban-dwelling children; and recently immigrated Vietnamese children.

To avoid the pitfalls of both longitudinal and cross-sectional study designs, researchers in many modern mental developmental studies have used a combination of these designs (Yussen and Santrock 1978).

Twin method. Twin studies incorporate a longitudinal design, cross-sectional design, or some combination of these two. They are often used to assess the influence of nature (biological stimuli) in the genesis of a normal or abnormal surface behavior, belief, fantasy, and so on.

There are two genetically different types of twins: *monozygotic twins* (i.e., those derived from one fertilized ovum) and *dizygotic twins* (i.e., those derived from two fertilized ova) (Rainer 1980). When a higher rate of concordance (i.e., occurrence of a given behavior or mental phenomenon in both members of a twin pair) is found in studies of monozygotic twins, it is more probable that the behavior or mental phenomenon being studied is more related to genetically controlled maturation (nature) than to the influences of the environment (nurture).

Twin studies are difficult because of the problem of identifying the type of twin pairs (monozygotic versus dizygotic) and the need to incorporate appropriate control subjects into the study. Also, in twin studies it is important that the disorder being studied not be more prevalent in twins than in singletons (Rainer 1980). For example, a familial incidence of stuttering has been found (Gemelli 1982a, 1982b; Van Riper 1973). If researchers wished to investigate how the presence of stuttering in the father affects the development of the same behavior in his son, the twin-family observational method could be used. Specifically, the question addressed in the study would be, Does stuttering in the father influence the development of stuttering in the son primarily through the effects of nurturant modeling, or primarily through the transmission of a genetically induced speech vulnerability? Subsequently, mono-zygotic twin pairs would be studied, and, if the concordance rate for stuttering was high, then a genetic transmission for stuttering would be considered as one of the etiologies for the disorder. How-ever, this conclusion can be considered only if the number of cases of child stuttering at any point in time is no higher in the general population of twins than it is in the general population of singletons.

Twin studies can also be difficult to do because of many of the same problems encountered in longitudinal studies (i.e., financial cost, availability of subjects, and controlling the social environment of each twin pair over time).

■ Effect of Observer's Beliefs on Interpretation of Data

In learning new information about human mental development, every developmental observer, whether an experienced researcher or a beginning student, will possess personal beliefs about the pro-cess of mental development and about which of the three types of stimuli—biological, social, and psychological—involved in chil-dren's mental development are of more significance in their se-quentially learning new information about themselves, their parents, and the external world. The observer's personal beliefs may not function as biased beliefs, in that they may not interfere with the observer's impartial judgment of the data being observed. But more often than not, the observer's personal beliefs function to some degree as hidden or unknown biases. This occurs when the observer rigidly holds to his or her personal beliefs and is not open to new data or information that challenges partially, if not totally, his or her personal beliefs.

A developmental observer's biased beliefs can arise from two sources: 1) what the observer learned about mental development during his or her own childhood and adulthood experiences, and 2) what the observer learned about mental development in his or her formal training experiences.

Biases formed from personal experience. In the follow-ing case example, I illustrate how a psychiatry resident approached his first formal interviews with a child unaware that he possessed a biased belief about child mental development that had been formed in his childhood.

A first-year psychiatry resident who was interviewing a 6-year-old boy told the boy that he was not allowed to mess up the interview playroom. The resident repeated this when the boy's crayon ran off the paper and left a mark on the table and when the boy scattered toy figures around a wide area of the playroom floor.

Later, in discussing the child's playroom behavior in a supervisory session with a staff psychiatrist, the resident stated this belief: "Little boys shouldn't be encouraged to mess up a room; otherwise, they'll never learn to behave socially." In a further discussion with his supervisor, the resident recalled how his own boyhood wishes to mess up a room were severely restricted by his parents. These restrictions were enforced by regular and excessive physical punishments. The resident believed these punishments had been necessary to teach him to be neat and organized. The supervisor suggested that, even though the resident seemed to have grown up believing it was wrong to mess up a room, the 6-year-old boy's messing behavior in the playroom would be considered a normal expression of this boy's assertiveness and playful aggression. The resident listened intently and the supervisory session ended.

When the resident left, the supervisor made a note to himself that this resident seemed unaware of his own biased interpretation of this child's behavior; the degree of this 6-year-old boy's messing behavior in the playroom was developmentally normal, but the resident interpreted it as being abnormal based on what his parents had taught him.

For the next several weeks, the resident returned for his regularly scheduled supervisory session. He had begun to see this 6-year-old boy for twice-weekly psychotherapy, and, in conducting this therapy, the resident maintained his same negative view of the boy's messing behavior. In a later supervisory session, however, the resident shared with the supervisor an intriguing dream he had had the night before. In the dream, he was yelling at his parents while he was throwing blocks around the family living room. Suddenly, in relating this dream to his supervisor, he became consciously aware of his past anger at his parents for their restriction of his childhood messing behaviors and strict rules of cleanliness. In expanding on this observation, he recalled how he had submitted to his parents' demand that he make his room "look like a girl's room, all neat and pretty." With the supervisor's help, the resident was able to recognize that, in identifying with his parents' demands and prohibitions, he had grown up believing that he always had to be extremely neat and organized. For example, he noted that in college, "I kept my room neat all the time. And when my friends complained that it looked like it was still being cleaned by my mother, I'd get angry at them and keep it even more spotless."

Prior to the resident's achieving the insight noted above, his interpretation of the boy's behavior as abnormal was a manifestation of the influence of what his parents had taught him. Now, having experienced the triggering social stimuli of interviewing this 6-year-old child and receiving the support of his supervisor, this resident was able to reconstruct his childhood biased belief. In a subsequent interview with the 6-year-old boy, the resident was able to tolerate and even enjoyed sharing in this boy's messy play. The resident's originally biased interpretation of what was normal behavior in this child had been replaced by some new unbiased beliefs about what constitutes normal play in young children.

Biases formed during formal training. As is discussed in the next section, the major developmental theories are all partial theories in that each emphasizes only a part of the developmental life cycle and only one, or possibly two, of the three stimuli (i.e., biological, psychological, and social) affecting children's development. Consequently, an observer often follows the developmental theory that emphasizes the stimulus or stimuli he or she has learned to believe is primarily implicated in the genesis of a particular mental phenomenon, social behavior, or both, and which he or she feels most competent in investigating. Thus an observer's selection of data—whether biological, psychological, or social—that he or she sees as the most important in investigating a child's psychological development may be anything but a purely objective selection (see Figure 1–1). The following clinical example illustrates this point.

One morning after a 5-year-old boy saw his father had left for work, he went to his room and drew a fake mustache on his face

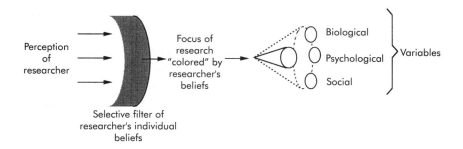

Figure 1–1. Researcher bias in developmental research.

with a marking pen. He then surprised his mother by walking up to her and showing her his new mustache. In believing that his new mustache looked just like his father's real one, he told his mother, "Mom, kiss me on the lips the way you kiss Dad. I have a mustache like him. Will you let me sleep next to you when Dad's away?" His mother, a bit nonplussed, nevertheless gave him a kind smile and said, "You're like your Dad in a lot of ways and I love you for it, but some things I do only with Dad because he's Dad, like kissing him on the lips and sleeping with him."

Suppose this mother-son scene is reported to three experienced, but differently trained (and most probably differently reared), developmental observers. They are asked to relate what each perceives (i.e., in his or her mind's "eye") in this scene and what each believes the scene reveals about this boy's normal or abnormal mental development, or both.

The first observer interprets this scene by stating,

This is a good example of a normal boy in his oedipal phase. In having already developed a masculine gender identity, he is motivated to identify with his father. Also, in already manifesting a heterosexual identity, his sexual object choice—the gender he pursues for sensual-sexual pleasure—is a female, his mother. Consequently, he wants to have what his father has and do what his father does in certain sexual interactions with his mother.

This researcher is specifically focusing on psychological stimuli: this boy's prior formation of a gender identity representation as a male (a preconscious memory) and his current wishes to gratify his sexual fantasies (as stimulated by his innate need for sensual-sexual pleasure) of what it means to him to be heterosexual in his family. The perceptual focus of this researcher, therefore, initially causes her to cast her mind's eye on the inner mental or representational world of the child—that is, on the child's innate need for sensual-sexual pleasure, the fantasies this need generates, and the influence this child's prior memories of his experiences in possessing a masculine gender have on him.

The second observer is one whose training has focused on the psychological maturation and development of children's cognitive abilities (i.e., their abilities to compare and comprehend new and old conceptions, emotions, and memories, and arrive at new conceptual understanding). Accordingly, he has studied how children attempt to assimilate current perceptions of the outside world into what they already know (as stored in their long-term memory structures), to sort similar perceptions into categories, and to accommodate to completely novel perceptions by either restructuring preexistent representations, constructing new representations, or both. These then become new psychological stimuli that are stored as long-term memories. This researcher notes the following:

> This mother-son interaction is interesting because it demonstrates the increasing development of a cognitive ability in this normal 5-year-old boy. This ability, with its beginnings in infancy, enables him to learn to collect objects of similar name or quality into categories. Consequently, he is showing us how he has the knowledge of being a member of the category made up of males and is demonstrating this knowledge to his mother.

This researcher's perceptual focus causes him to cast his mind's eye on psychological stimuli, as did the first researcher. However, unlike the first researcher's focus on the child's innate need for sensual-sexual pleasure and the influence of this need in stimulating the child's oedipal wishes toward his mother, this researcher has focused on the child's maturing cognitive abilities to understand the concept of categories in organizing, integrating, and comprehending his perceptions of himself and others.

The third observer is one who has chosen to become an expert in the study and clinical application of behavioral modification techniques in influencing the observable behaviors of the developing child. Accordingly, he attempts to bring about behavioral change by rewarding child behaviors that are desirable or normal, and by withholding rewards for child behaviors that he assesses as undesirable or abnormal. Consequently, this observer interprets the mother-son scene as follows:

> This is a good example of the effect of a normal mother's (social) shaping of her son's normal sex-typed behavior. In this shaping process, she probably has been using a set of rewards (e.g., providing verbal compliments) in her attempt to reinforce her son's imitation and identification with his same-gender parent, his father. The boy's behavior in this scene may also be attributable to the tendency in boys, more than in girls, to display more wishes for dominance and control in their social relationship with their mothers.

All the above developmental observers are "correct" in their individualized interpretations of the mother-son scene, even though each focused on and gave more weight to certain aspects of the scene and less weight to other aspects in accordance with their personal and professional beliefs. Given that each was correct in his or her individualized interpretation, the following question might be asked: In what way could a researcher's beliefs about normal mental development make that researcher biased in his or her selection of the stimuli chosen to study? The answer is that an observer's beliefs as generated by his or her training will become biased beliefs only if the observer cannot acknowledge that the stimuli he or she has omitted from an analysis of the data may have as much relevance as the one or two stimuli selected for study. In such a case, the observer will use his or her biased interpretation to reinforce a theory that he or she believes to be truthful or to formulate a new theory. In this type of biased selection of data, a climate can exist in which each researcher selects patients who produce data that corroborate his or her theory, or the researcher reconstructs his or her interpretation of the data in order to fit his or her theoretical bias (H. Holloway, personal communication, July 1982; Spence 1994).

An observer's biased beliefs, therefore, can lead him or her to generate new theories that are knowledge inhibiting. The observer may be either consciously aware or unaware of these biased beliefs. When the observer is consciously aware of the biases—assuming the observer is an ethical person—he or she is aware of how those beliefs influence the selection of the stimuli he or she chooses to study. This awareness enables him or her to perform a more unbiased or objective analysis of the data he or she "sees" and measures. In the current day pragmatics of doing research, it is often necessary to focus on one and possibly two stimuli rather than focusing on all three stimuli at the same time. However, the consciously aware, ethical, and open-minded researcher does not ignore his or her biases, but attempts to recognize when they have prevented him or her from studying one or more stimuli that may also have significance in generating the mental activity or surface behavior selected for study.

Developmental observers also possess differing capacities to learn new beliefs—that is, restructure their preexistent beliefs—based on their new experiences with children and others. Observers who maintain one or more of their biased beliefs about normal development will misperceive or fail to perceive new observations about a child that may run counter to those preexistent beliefs, but will selectively perceive the data that corroborate the truthfulness of their beliefs. In essence, these observers tend to project onto children their own biased beliefs and identify (i.e., misidentify) certain child behaviors as proof of their beliefs about normal mental development. This process—defined as *unconscious projection*—has throughout the ages been one of the major impediments that has prevented, and still prevents, certain adult developmental observers from truly observing the mental development of infants, children, and adolescents. Observers (whether medical students, psychiatric residents, or experienced child psychiatrists) who are able to remain open minded to perceiving new child observational data and interpreting it in a new way are the new theory makers of the present and the future.

Historical Beliefs on Children's Mental Development

For many centuries, infants and children were believed to be incapable of creating complicated thoughts and feelings in response to what they experienced in the world around them. Childhood was thought of as a time in life in which the mind was unorganized and unformed. This led to the general belief, persisting well into the early 20th century, that the events experienced in childhood had little, if any, effect on the mind of the future adult the child would someday become. It is not surprising, therefore, that recorded Western European history contains no significant theories about mental development that extend from infancy to adulthood. (For two excellent historical reviews of childhood through the ages, the reader is referred to Aires 1962 and Boswell 1988.)

There has always been a paucity of primary sources—that is, parent and child diaries, memoirs, letters, and documentation of direct adult observation—of developmental changes in a child's behavior and thinking (Boswell 1988; Fogel and Melson 1987). Instead, beliefs about children have been based largely on secondary sources of information about their internal experiences (i.e., their wishes, feelings, fantasies, and beliefs). These sources, according to Fogel and Melson (1987), included "medical advice books, religious sermons, . . . philosophical writings . . . and legislation." Information in these sources was based on adult hypotheses, fantasies, and conjectures about what children needed, wanted, and feared. It was not until 1787 that the first published record of an adult's observations of a child's sequential development appeared: a man named Tiedeman recorded his son's development from birth through age 2½ years (Boswell 1988).

In the last quarter of the 19th century, a new appreciation emerged for the importance of directly talking to and observing the behaviors of children in order to understand their mental development. A catalyst of this new appreciation was Charles Darwin and his seminal hypothesis that humans evolved from lower animal species. In 1877, Darwin published a diary in which he documented his close observations of his own son's early development. In describing these observations, he espoused his belief that adults could add to the understanding of their origins by directly observing and talking with their children.

During the 30 years following publication of Darwin's diary, other scientists began to recognize the scientific value of sequentially observing the language and behavior of children. Knopf (1984) has documented how the early 20th century American psychologist, G. Stanley Hall, used questionnaires he had developed for parents, teachers, and children along with interviews of parents and children to collate a description of children's fears, dreams, emotional expressions, and so on during different stages of childhood. His goal was to investigate the development of the uniquely complex inner mental world and observable (or surface) behaviors of each child.

Beginning after about 1875, researchers such as Freud, Erikson, and Piaget laid out theories about how the mind develops from infancy into adulthood. In 1885, Freud participated in a postgraduate training fellowship in Charcot's hysteria clinic. He eventually discovered that all of the hysterical patients he treated had experienced, in addition to the recent traumatic event, one or more similar traumatic events during their childhoods. Freud hypothesized, therefore, that there was a causal association between experiencing a traumatic event in childhood and the occurrence of hysterical symptoms in adulthood in response to an adult traumatic event. In 1900, Freud published *The Interpretation of Dreams,* in which he elaborated his theory that childhood events affected adults in ways they were not aware of (i.e., in producing hysterical symptoms).

In the United States, at about the time that Freud was publishing his theories about childhood associative links to adult hysteria, Adolf Meyer, a Swiss-born psychiatrist and a professor of psychiatry at Johns Hopkins University, was also emphasizing the association between the childhood memories of adult patients and the genesis of their mental illness. He strongly influenced American psychiatric training in sending a message to psychiatrists that was similar to Freud's: what happened during an adult's childhood was important in understanding his or her adult thinking and behavior. Meyer subsequently established the childhood developmental history as an integral part of the adult psychiatric patient's evaluation and treatment.

At about the same time, Alfred Binet and Theodore Simon developed a scale to test children's intellectual capabilities. The first Binet-Simon scale was published in 1905 (Binet and Simon 1905) and the revised scale in 1908 (Anastasi 1988). In the 1908 scale, the authors described intellectual norms of performance, known as the *mental age* for each *chronological age* of childhood. Thus a child's chronological age could now be matched to his or her mental age. When both ages matched, the child was considered to be of average intelligence. Likewise, when a child's mental age exceeded his or her chronological age, that child was considered to be of above-average intelligence, and when a child's chronological age exceeded his or her mental age, that child was considered to be of below-average intelligence, or in the retarded range. Binet and Simon's work expanded on Darwin's and Hall's messages to the adult world: not only were children worthy of scientific study, but also they were intellectually heterogeneous.

Developmentalists, as they now could all be called, such as Freud and Meyer, sparked the interests of many within the discipline of psychiatry. Consequently, in the era from 1900 to 1940, many psychiatrists began studying their adult patients' childhood memories. This eventually led to an interest in directly interviewing children. In the United States, Kanner, in remembering his experience as a psychiatric resident under Meyer in the 1930s, recalled how professionals working with mentally disturbed adults developed an interest in directly interviewing children to learn firsthand about their difficulties (Kanner 1957). Concurrently, disciples of Sigmund Freud, such as Anna Freud and Melanie Klein, began to interview emotionally disturbed children. They discovered that, by playing and talking with these children, they could learn much about what was contained within their inner mental worlds and thereby understand their unique view of their life experiences.

John B. Watson (1878–1958), working directly with infants and children, eventually established one of the first developmental laboratories to study infant behavior. B. F. Skinner, another psychologist, documented in 1938 how he could modify a child's behavior by granting rewards to the child if the child repeated a behavior. Watson and Skinner, in studying children's observable behaviors and how they were modified in response to rewards and punishments, developed the new discipline of behaviorism, with its focus on behavioral modification. *Learning principles* (i.e., principles that explain how a current experience will enable a child to modify his or her behavioral and mental responses to future experiences) were now discovered. For example, one learning principle is *operant conditioning,* which states that a child will tend to repeat behaviors that have brought positive responses from the child's environment and not repeat behaviors that have brought negative responses from that environment. Through this line of study, explanations were formulated of how children learn to behave through experiences with their parents. Based on these learning principles, for example, it would be hypothesized that children learn to eat with utensils because this behavior pleases their parents. However, learning principles did not explain why a particular child did not respond as expected (e.g., why a child did not obey his or her schoolteacher despite the child's being told that obeying would bring certain rewards). What learning principles failed to include were the individual child's thoughts, feelings, and memories that led to his or her manifestation of certain behaviors.

Children's internal mental responses became the focus of inquiry of people such as Anna Freud and Melanie Klein who, in ushering in the new discipline of child psychoanalysis, took the view that both children's memories and their thoughts, beliefs, feelings, fantasies, and fears became the motivational variables that ultimately determined their choice of surface behaviors. These early child psychoanalysts focused on the child's inner world; they placed less emphasis on the learning theorists' focus of how the behavioral response or lack of response by others influenced the child's choice of surface behaviors.

Both the disciplines of behaviorism and of child psychoanalysis made equally important and complementary discoveries about the development of children's surface behaviors: the behaviorist emphasized the environmental or social motivational variables affecting their behavior, and the child psychoanalyst emphasized the psychological or internal motivational variables.

In the 1950s and 1960s, two other developmentalists made important contributions to how children's minds develop. Jean Piaget (1950) began publishing his theories about the sequential development of intelligence in children from infancy into adolescence. Simultaneously, Erik Erikson (1963) published his theory of psychosocial tasks, which were a series of beliefs the normal child needed to construct to develop normally.

It has been only since the 1960s, when developmentalists began to observe children with a more open-minded and less projection-distorting attitude, that adults truly discovered the inner world of the child's developing mind. Since that time, there has been an explosion of new observational research concerning the developing infant and child (see Chapters 3 and 4). Adult beliefs about the child are certainly still evolving. It is now accepted that new beliefs about the child's mental development must come primarily from direct observational data, not from adult conjectures and assumptions, which have often been fueled by adult projections of their own needs, feelings, and beliefs onto children. The late 20th century child, therefore, has begun to teach the adult about the child's true self.

Developing an Integrated Model of Mental Development

A current quest of modern developmental researchers is to attempt to arrive at a more encompassing and integrated theoretical model of mental development. Spence (1987) has cautioned that such a model of the mind may forever prove limiting because it would be difficult for any model to explain the genesis of the myriad mental phenomena that are produced by the human mind. As he stated,

> General laws may be found which will account for some of the variance (in mental activity), but an explanation of the rich texture of any momentary state of mind may be beyond their reach.

. . . The randomness of everyday life may be a part of the natural order of things. (p. 95; parentheses in the original)

Sandler et al. (1973) made a related point:

The more one knows of specific features of the individual's behavior and his mental processes and experiences, the more certain one can be of the conclusions drawn. Generally speaking, no single cause is regarded as being a sufficient explanation (for an individual's behavior or his ideas and feelings), and the further assumption of multiple causes . . . is made. (p. 93)

Among current psychiatrists, psychologists, and other mental health professionals who ponder the development of the human mind, there is no general consensus about the existence of one integrated theoretical model of mental development. A theory of mental development should be an attempt to understand which mental structures and mental processes are present at birth, which ones emerge during maturational growth, and which ones undergo change during the developmental process from infancy through adulthood. A potential knowledge-enhancing, integrated theoretical model of the mind must be broad enough to represent each of the complexities of the developmental process. The model should also indicate the parts or aspects of the model for which knowledge is scanty and future theoretical additions are required.

Conceptualizing the Human Mind as a Biological System

A system, both in the physical and in the natural sciences, can be conceptualized as a complicated mechanism that uses energy in attempting to attain certain goals.

■ Components of a System

Energy. The type of energy needed by the system determines the system's structural design and the processes it performs. For example, a computer is a nonbiological system powered by electrical energy. Consequently, the specific characteristics of electrical energy (e.g., when and how electricity is delivered, the amount of electricity delivered) limit both the computer's structural design and the processes it can perform.

The human mind is a biological system whose energy is derived from physiological processes within the body and the brain. Sabelli and Carlson-Sabelli (1989) described this physiologically generated energy as follows:

> Biological [brain] and psychological [mental] energy are complex manifestations of simpler physical energy. Body and mind, matter and spirit, and physical, social, and psychological processes, no matter how apparently varied and heterogeneous, are all forms of energy. (p. 1543)

The recognition that mental energy and brain energy derive from physical energy, and that the mind uses mental energy to access its mental structures and run its mental processes, reemphasizes the following fact: there is no mind without underlying living and concretely visible brain and body tissue (Eisenberg 1986).

Structures. A system's structures vary in terms of the information they contain and the processes they perform (Arlow 1988). A mechanical computer contains structures (e.g., hard drives, microprocessors) that contain information called files. These structures also contain processes called word processing, formatting, and so on. Similarly, the human mind contains informational structures that contain information and cognitive structures that carry out mental processes (Boesky 1988).

Operating principles. In general, the operating principles possessed by any system, both nonbiological and biological, will bring a certain degree of either organization (i.e., regulation, order, stability, and predictability) or disorganization (i.e., disregulation, disorder, instability, and unpredictability) to that system's utilization of energy and how its informational and dynamic structures perform to carry out the system's goals (Meissner 1995).

For example, a nuclear-powered ship possesses a propulsion system that is designed in such a way that its chemical and physical propulsion processes follow organizing principles of science (e.g., heat transfer, thermodynamics, electricity). These principles are defined as organizing because they bring qualities of regulation, orderliness, stability, and predictability to the chemical and nuclear reaction processes performed by the propulsion system's structures. Organized processes of propulsion achieve stable and predictable goals, namely the attainment of certain speeds through the water while controlling the ship's maneuverability. In contrast, a nuclear fission reactor designed without an organizing neutron-capturing device becomes the nuclear bomb: a nonbiological system capable of bringing about maximal disorganization and chaos.

We view the mind as an organized biological system because, in its normal development and functioning, its structures and processes possess the qualities of regulation and order rather than the qualities of unregulation and chaos. This regulation and order enable the normally developing mind to effectively meet its goals (e.g., gratify its innate needs). For example, one organizing principle of the human mind is called the *representational principle*. Briefly, this principle states that each infant will mentally process sensory inputs and generate individualized perceptual, wishful, and emotional representations—and not exact replicas—of these sensory inputs. These unique representations become the substance of the developing infant's implicit memories and the older child's implicit and explicit memories (see Chapter 2). For example, two 7-year-old children will construct and store different explicit memories of the same second grade teacher. By the time they reach the third grade, one may remember the teacher, in both verbal and visual images, as being primarily kind, supportive, and accepting, whereas the second one may remember that same teacher as being primarily mean, demanding, and strict.

Disorganizing mental processes can emerge when the mind is malfunctioning. For example, in meningitis, a disease process that produces an inflammation of the outer layer, or meninges, of the brain, certain mental processes that emerge during the infection do not follow organizing principles. A child or adult with meningitis will often develop the pathological mental condition called an organic brain syndrome, one defining characteristic of which is the person's inability to mentally process incoming sensory stimulation in an organized manner. As a result, he or she is judged to be disoriented (i.e., is unable to generate a perception of the correct time of day, his or her physical location, and his or her identity).

Nature. Systems are either biological (i.e., living) or nonbiological (i.e., inanimate). The main characteristic of a biological system's aliveness is its ability to change its structures and processes through interaction with a nurturant environment (Rutter 1991). Every biological system is open to such changes; however, in the process, each system maintains its nature. A biological or non-biological system's *nature* is its "inherent character or basic constitution" (Merriam-Webster's Collegiate Dictionary 1993, p. 774); this nature is dictated by the system's genetic heritage.

Human beings' physical nature comprises the body's genetically controlled, innate structures and the structures that emerge during physical maturation. The innate physical structures are all of the defining characteristics that give a person an identity as a human being (e.g., major organs, such as the heart; structures within the brain, such as the optic nerve; structures that endow a person with a physiological need for nourishment). The maturationally emerging physical structures are the various new characteristics and abilities that emerge during the process of biological growth (e.g., the growth of teeth in the first 2 years of life; the emergence of axillary hair at puberty).

A person's mental nature is the genetically endowed informational and processing structures that either are innate or emerge during mental maturation. These innate informational and processing mental structures contribute mental characteristics that further define a person's identity as a human being. For example, the infant's innate need to engage in an emotionally pleasurable attachment relationship with at least one parent is in part fulfilled by the specific innate informational structures that enable the infant to selectively respond to the sound of his or her mother's voice. The other part of a person's mental domain—the maturationally emerging mental structures, both informational and processing—endow that person with various new mental abilities and characteristics. An example of a maturationally emerging mental structure is that which enables the infant, at about age 18 months, to recognize his or her own image in a mirror.

The Domain of the Mind
Understanding Mental Structures

The organizational constancy of the biological system known as a human being is even more remarkable than that of other biological systems when one considers how many biological subsystems (e.g., circulatory system, immune system, central nervous system) exist harmoniously within it. All of these subsystems can be divided into two broad domains: the body domain and the mental domain (Pardes 1986). *Domain* refers to the terrain where the structures reside and the actions or processes these structures perform (Reiser 1985). In this section, I give a brief description of the brain's domain, then focus in depth on the mind's domain.

The domain of the brain and central nervous system—both of which are within the domain of the body—can be conceptualized as neuroanatomic structures such as neurons and glial cells (Brodal 1969; Kandel et al. 1991). Neurons conduct nerve impulses, whereas glial cells serve in a supportive role in the overall organization of neurons in the brain. (See Kandel et al. 1991, pp. 15–16, for an introduction to brain morphology and histology.) Neurons also contain information, both innately present from birth (e.g., the brain's ability to regulate hormonal production in the body) and present as a result of living experiences (e.g., memories) (Gless 1988). In addition, they perform neurophysiological processes, which are series of actions that produce one or more products (e.g., the process of memory construction and memory storage produces the product called a memory).

The domain of the mind also consists of structures, called *mental structures* (Applegarth 1989; Hartman et al. 1946; Shapiro 1988;

Stolorow 1978). Mental structures vary from each other with regard to the following characteristics:

1. Genesis (i.e., whether they are innate, maturational, or experiential mental structures)
2. Type (i.e., whether they are processing or information structures)
3. Accessibility to the conscious and unconscious mental domains
4. Persistence over time
5. Ability to assist in the delay of action

■ Genesis

Innate mental structures. Innate mental structures are all those structures that are present at birth. They are a product of an infant's genetic endowment or genetic code.

Maturational mental structures. Maturational mental structures emerge as the mind undergoes the process of maturation. Their emergence is also controlled by the infant's genetic code. For example, the infant's capacity to understand more complex perceptions depends on the emergence of the specific mental structures necessary for that advanced understanding.

Experiential mental structures. Experiential mental structures are constructed by the mind as a result of life experiences. Examples of experiential structures are perceptions, wishes, and memories.

■ Type

Processing structures. Processing structures, also called *cognitive structures,* enable individuals to carry out the process of cognition. *Cognition* is any mental process that generates new or experiential information that is differentiated from the information contained within innate informational structures (see below). A *mental process* is defined as a simple or complicated mental action or a series of mental actions that are not directly observed but are inferred to be present in order to explain the products of their action[s] (e.g., dreaming would be the action and the dream, the product [Pulver 1988]). All mental processes occur outside of each person's conscious awareness.

The *innate processing structures* present in infants are perception formation, concept formation, memory formation, memory storage, and memory retrieval. These innate structures endow infants with the mental ability to respond to sensations emanating from their 1) body, 2) social world (e.g., parents, others), and 3) innate informational structures existing within their own mind (e.g., the ability to form a perception and eventually a conception of the innate informational structure that generates the emotion of anger). The result is that innate processing structures generate new experiential informational structures—perceptions, conceptions (wishes, ideas, fantasies, and beliefs), and memories. One or more of these mental structures will propel an infant to initiate observable surface behaviors. In short, the infant mind is preprogrammed to 1) generate perceptions and conceptions from sensory stimuli (e.g., the perception of his or her legs being lifted) and 2) store a memory of these perceptions and conceptions without having to first acquire these abilities through the process of learning.

Informational structures. *Informational structures* provide a person's mind with information or knowledge (Peterfreund 1971).

Innate informational structures. *Innate informational structures* include

- Innate need structures
- Innate emotional structures
- Innate temperamental structures

Traditionally, infants have been viewed as possessing a series of innate needs. (In this book I use the term *innate need* [Lichtenberg 1989] in place of Freud's term *innate drives*. Freud's innate drives were related to instinct. However, *instinct* is a term used to describe biological, and usually animal-like, propensities not usually influenced by the environment. Because the environment does affect human beings' innate propensities [i.e., they are able to learn and shape their innate needs accordingly], Freud arrived at the term *drive* to describe propensities in human beings that propel them to action but that can be shaped by learning.) The five innate needs are as follows:

1. Need for the gratification of physiological requirements that maintain bodily regulation and physical survival (e.g., temperature and stimulus regulation, nutrition, sleep, equilibrium)
2. Need to assertively explore the social environment in seeking novel stimulation in order to learn to differentiate these stimuli and generate adaptive responses to the same
3. Need to attach to at least one other person in a predominantly emotionally pleasurable interaction
4. Need for sensory and sexual emotionally pleasurable stimulation and gratification
5. Need to signal distress when experiencing an emotionally displeasurable experience and initiate fight-flight behavioral and mental responses

Each of these five innate needs generates specific sensations, based on which an infant's mind forms (through its innate processing structures) particular perceptions. These perceptions become internal motivators that propel infants to seek gratification of the particular need. For example, the need to attach to and engage in an emotionally pleasurable interaction with another person is stimulated both internally, through the state of being alive, and externally, through infants' sensory reception of stimuli emanating from their body and social world. When stimulated internally or externally, this need to engage in an attachment relationship becomes a mental perceptual impulse, an innate internal motivator that propels infants to activate behaviors in seeking interactions with their parents.

Infants' *innate emotional structures* are manifested in their capacity to generate several distinct emotions. The primary emotions are joy, fear, anger, sadness, disgust, and surprise (M. Lewis and Michalson 1983). By the time infants reach age 1 year, similar patterns of events will stimulate similar emotions, and these emotions will be manifested in similar facial expressions. For example, an infant is believed to experience anger when he or she is exposed to a highly displeasurable level of over- or understimulation and his or her distress signals (e.g., pushing away, visual gaze aversion, crying) do not result in the level of distressful stimulation being decreased. In addition, the infant's emotion, defined as anger, will be reflected in a unique facial expression.

Innate temperamental structures contain information about infants' innate unique behavioral style (Chess and Thomas 1986; McCall 1986; Weissberg-Benchell 1990), which refers to how infants behave as distinct from why they behave that way or what behaviors they generate (Chess and Thomas 1986). Various developmentalists include different dimensions of behavior in defining an infant's temperament. McCall (in Goldsmith et al. 1987) identified the following dimensions of behavior as defining an infant's innate behavioral style:

- *Activity*—how intense, vigorous, and fast-paced an infant's movements are
- *Reactivity*—how an infant approaches or withdraws from stimulation
- *Emotionality*—how an infant manifests feelings of anger, sadness, fear, joy, pleasure, disgust, surprise, and so on
- *Sociability*—how an infant expresses his or her preference for being with his or her parents and how much initiative he or she expresses in seeking social contact with, and in being socially responsive to, his or her parents

An infant's behavioral style becomes evident, for example, in his or her reaction to highly displeasurable stimulation (Izard et al. 1983). Whereas all infants will display the emotion of anger in such a situation, each infant will differ in the intensity of the anger he or she generates and the time it takes to ameliorate his or her angry feelings and soothe him or her.

Maturational informational structures.   Another group of informational structures emerge within the course of the mind's maturational growth. For example, as children grow older, they become more intellectually or cognitively adept because of the maturational emergence of new cognitive structures. These enhance their ability to compare new perceptions of their changing body and changing environment with prior perceptions and ultimately integrate both in comprehending the new perceptions.

Experiential informational structures.   This final group of informational structures consists of perceptions, conceptions, and memories that are constructed by a child's mind as a result of his or her living experiences.

One type of experiential informational structure is a *perception,* which is formed when the reception of a sensory stimulus activates the mind's generation of a perception. External sensory stimuli originate from the child's body and social environment; internal stimuli originate in the child's mind through its innate informational structures (i.e., innate needs, emotions, and temperamental characteristics).

A second type of experiential informational structure is a *conception,* defined as a mental structure that is formed when a perception becomes understood to some degree, or is given meaning, by an infant. Conceptions are ideas, wishes, fantasies, beliefs, and so on. The complexity of any infant's conceptions is a function of his or her cognitive capabilities, as contained within his or her innate cognitive structures, which are only beginning to undergo maturational growth. These structures enable infants to begin to compare and comprehend their day-to-day perceptions. This comparison of a present perception with something that was previously perceived and conceptualized involves infants' ability to form and retrieve memories (see below). As their cognitive processing structures mature, children can compare and comprehend new perceptions at increasingly more complex levels of intelligence (Flavell 1988). This increasing cognitive ability proceeds throughout their development. For example, a 4-year-old child's level of cognitive ability enables him or her to comprehend a puzzle or an emotion that he or she was unable to comprehend at age 2 years.

Various perceptions give rise to different conceptions within an infant's mind. For example, an infant's mind will first form a perception of his or her emotions and then secondly construct an emotional conception (i.e., attribute meaning to those emotions) (Lazarus 1984). Therefore, an infant will first form a perception of being sad before he or she will give meaning to this sadness (Sommers 1981).

A third type of experiential informational structure is a *memory,* defined as the mind's storage unit for information gained through living experiences. Through memories, infants progressively store a personal history of their living experiences. This personal history then becomes available to them through the process of remembering. The human mind encodes incoming stimuli into perceptions, and possibly conceptions, and temporarily stores this encoded information into short-term, working memory. Eventually this coded memory may be stored as a long-term memory structure. Long-term memories are later retrievable through the process of remembering.

In terms of how the human mind stores and retrieves information, there are two types of long-term memory structures: implicit ones and explicit ones (Clyman 1991; Schacter 1992; Squire 1986, 1992; Terr 1994). *Implicit memory* is defined as

> the way in which the brain encodes an experience and then influences later behavior without requiring conscious awareness, recognition, recall or an inner experience of a [consciously] "retrieved memory." Thus the skill of riding a bicycle can be demonstrated even if the youngster has no [conscious] recall of when s/he learned to ride. This is implicit memory without explicit recall. (Seigal 1993, p. 6)

An implicit memory is information received that cannot be described in words (Brenneis 1994). Hence, in the preverbal years (i.e., prior to about age 2–2½ years), infants have only implicit memories. Also, any life experiences that involve information about behavioral activities (e.g., tying shoes) and cognitive activities (e.g., solving a puzzle) that have become so well learned and automatic that conscious attention is not needed for their smooth execution can be stored as implicit memories (M. L. Lewis 1995).

Implicit memories are stored within an infant's unconscious mental domain (see below). When those memories are reactivated, the behaviors contained within them are repeated; however, the experiences that led to the formation of the implicit memory cannot be recalled. As a result, the presence of an implicit memory within a child's unconscious is known only through the child's automatic performance or enactment of one or more behaviors. For example, a 6-year-old boy will automatically know how to use eating utensils and feed himself without having to focus his conscious attention on those eating skills. However, he will not be able to recall when he learned these skills, regardless of whether they were learned before age 2 years or later. It is as if the human mind, even when it has stored memories of how behaviors were learned, no longer needs to engage in conscious recall and maintain attention to the task when the task has already been learned well. For example, a $4\frac{1}{2}$-year-old boy was demonstrating his knowledge of the different parts of an automobile by taking apart a toy automobile. When I asked him how he knew or had learned this, he stated, "I don't know! I just know it!"

According to the above definition of implicit memories as being based on experiences, the infant's mind is initially devoid of long-term memories. However, it should be noted that there has been early research indicating that the in utero fetus is capable of storing his or her experiences in long-term implicit memories. For example, if a bright light is placed on one side of the abdomen of a pregnant mother, the fetus can acquire the new behavioral skill of turning his or her head in the direction of this bright light (Noshpitz and King 1991). It is still unclear how this and other in utero experiences influence infants' behavioral and perceptual preferences when they begin life outside of the mother's uterus. (For a review of fetal learning research, see Graves 1989 and Noshpitz and King 1991.)

The second type of memory is *explicit memory,* which is the way in which the brain encodes an experience and then influences later behavior with conscious awareness of the inner experience of a retrieved memory (Seigal 1993). This conscious retrieval or remembering of facts or events can usually be stated in words. Consequently, explicit memories are storage units for information that is received after a child becomes verbal (i.e., about age $2-2\frac{1}{2}$ years). At this age, toddlers become capable of doing two things: first, they begin to become consciously aware of being a separate individual in a social world of other individuals, and, second, they begin to use verbal language. Consequently, perceptions or conceptions formed after this age can be stored as verbal information (e.g., the memory of a mother's words) and as visual, auditory, or olfactory perceptions or conceptions (e.g., the memory of the visual image of a mother's face and her words of anger when the child has disobeyed her). As Clyman (1991) stated,

> Declarative [explicit] knowledge stores memories for facts or events that have been experienced, and it is represented either in [verbal] language or in sensory images, such as mental pictures. (p. 351)

■ Accessibility to Conscious and Unconscious

Mental structures also vary with regard to their accessibility to the conscious and unconscious mental domains. In the human mind, three domains exist (Meissner 1986): conscious domain, preconscious domain, and unconscious domain (Ellenberger 1970; Gillet 1995).

Conscious domain. This domain is defined as the part of the mind in which perceptions, conceptions, and recalled memories—all having been formed from stimuli emanating from the developing child's mind or body or from the external world—are within the child's conscious awareness. The contents of this domain are available to a child's conscious introspection.

Preconscious domain. This domain is the part of the mind that stores those explicit memories that are retrievable or recallable. The preconscious domain does not come into existence until the child develops the ability to construct explicit memories (i.e., at about age 2–2½ years). The contents of this domain are also available to a child's conscious recall.

Unconscious domain. The mental contents within the unconscious domain come from 1) the biological components of a child's innate needs, 2) all of the implicit memories of experiences that take place before a child reaches age 2½ years, 3) all the implicit memories formed after age 2½ years of behaviors that have become so automatic that conscious attention is not needed for their smooth enactment, and 4) certain explicit memories of events that were highly emotionally displeasurable. The part of the unconscious that contains the contents from the first source is referred to as the systematic unconscious domain, whereas the part of the unconscious that contains the contents from the second through fourth sources is referred to as the dynamic unconscious domain.

The contents of the *systematic unconscious domain* are never accessible to a child's preconscious or conscious domains and thus are not available to a child's conscious introspection. No matter how much a child focuses his or her conscious awareness on one or more of the mental contents within his or her systematic unconscious mind, he or she will not be able to recall those contents. As noted above, within the systematic unconscious domain is the biological component of each child's five innate needs. The biological sensations created by each innate need, however, lead to the child's construction of perceptions about his or her innate needs; these perceptions are accessible to the conscious domain.

The *dynamic unconscious domain* refers to the part of the unconscious domain that is formed when implicit memories are constructed and when dynamic processes push an explicit memory from the conscious domain into the unconscious domain. In contrast to the systematic unconscious domain, which is present at birth, the dynamic unconscious domain does not come into existence until the child begins to construct explicit memories (i.e., at about age 2–2½ years).

Thus the human mind is endowed with the unique ability to segregate certain explicit memories of living experiences into either its preconscious domain or its dynamic unconscious domain. However, just how the brain determines which explicit memories are relegated to the preconscious (and hence consciously recallable) domain versus which are relegated to the unconscious (and hence consciously unrecallable) domain is not completely understood. One segregation rule, however, seems to be based on the overall emotional state that is associated with the memory.

As I noted earlier, infants are innately endowed with a group of emotions. The stimulation of each of these emotions is tied to the *stimulus seeking–stimulus avoiding principle,* or *stimulus principle* for short, which is another of the operating principles by which the human mind is organized. In essence, this principle states that infants will automatically seek quantities and qualities of stimulation that are within their optimal stimulation range. This stimulation range is unique for each infant. For example, a particular 1-month-old baby girl will seek and remain interested in a bright light of a particular level of intensity. In addition, she might be more interested in a bright light that flashes in a rhythmic fashion than one that does not flash. If she is interested, then the quality of the light's stimulation would be judged as being within her unique optimal stimulation range. Each infant's upper and lower thresholds of stimulation are defined by the infant's individual innate endowment and individual *stimulus barriers* (S. Freud 1900/1963). The possible maturation and development of such genetically controlled innate stimulus barriers are biological variables. Only recently have developmental researchers begun to understand the differences among infants in their vulnerability versus invulnerability to high levels of stimulation and in their ability versus inability to soothe themselves (Anthony 1985). These characteristics are now measured behaviorally with the Neonatal Behavioral Assessment Scale (Brazelton 1989).

When an experience generates pleasurable emotions (e.g., joy, excitement) because that experience provides stimulation within an infant's optimal stimulation range, the infant will assertively begin to attempt to repeat and prolong that experience. When a pleasurable experience is repeated several times, the infant inevitably constructs a representation of it and stores it as a memory. If this memory is stored before age 2–2½ years, it is by definition an implicit memory, and thus is stored within the infant's systematic unconscious. In the future, when this memory is activated by sensory stimulation, it will become an internal motivator that propel the infant to automatically enact the behavior(s) in an attempt to repeat this past emotionally pleasurable experience. However, the infant will never be able to consciously recall in words or visual images how the behaviors he or she is reenacting were originally learned.

If a memory is stored after age 2–2½ years—in which case it is an explicit memory—and is pleasurable, it is stored in the preconscious domain. In the future, when this memory is activated by sensory stimulation, it will be consciously recallable and will also serve as an internal motivator that propels the child to seek to repeat this past experience. In this case, the child older than age 2½ years will be able to describe the visual images or verbal content of the explicit memory of the original experience.

In the normal process of living, every infant will inevitably experience displeasurable feelings. It is then that the infant's mind will automatically activate behaviors that function as his or her distress signals. In order for the infant's mental development to be optimized, these episodes of signaling distress (e.g., crying) should not go too long without a response by one of the infant's parents or caretakers. When parents respond to their infants' distress signals, the infant gradually learns that episodes of emotional displeasure will eventually be relieved. Consequently, when an implicit or explicit memory of these displeasurable but consciously tolerable experiences is activated in the future by a sensory stimulus associated with the original memory, the memory will become an internal motivator that propels the infant to either unconsciously enact (if the memory was an implicit one) or consciously be aware of (if the memory was an explicit one) his or her signaling distress, with an expectation that the distress signal will be answered. If, however, an infant's distress signal is not appropriately responded to, and the infant's level of stimulation is not returned to an emotionally pleasurable range within a reasonable amount of time, then the infant will react by attempting to physically remove or deactivate or aggressively attack the source of the stimulation (Leigh and Reiser 1985). This reactive, aggressive response is termed the infant's innate *fight response.* When this fight response fails, the infant will attempt to physically withdraw from the source of stimulation. This is termed the infant's innate *flight response,* and may be manifested in the infant's crawling or running away or withdrawing into immobility.

When fight or flight responses are ineffective in alleviating highly displeasurable feelings in a child older than age 2½ years, these displeasurable feelings may become so intense and prolonged that they cause the child to experience a sense of helplessness and loss of control; that experience can then be defined as a *traumatic life experience.* Then, because of the highly displeasurable feelings and loss of control that are associated with the memory of that traumatic event, the memory is relegated to the dynamic unconscious domain; in this process, the mind is automatically activating its *defense mechanisms* (i.e., specific maturationally emerging mental processes that are automatically activated by the mind and that function to bar traumatic and other highly emotionally displeasurable memories from a person's conscious and preconscious mental domains). The barring activity of defense mechanisms spares a child from remembering and consciously reexperiencing the highly displeasurable emotions, the sense of helplessness, and the loss of control associated with traumatic memories.

The prototype of all defense mechanisms and the simplest memory blocking defense (Terr 1993, 1994) is repression. *Repression* is defined as an automatically activated (i.e., activated without conscious awareness) mental process in which a memory of a traumatic experience is relegated to, or repressed into, a person's dynamic unconscious. It is then stored there without the person's conscious knowledge of its presence. As long as it remains repressed, that memory cannot be retrieved.

Traumatic explicit memories formed after age 2–2½ years will be repressed into the child's dynamic unconscious domain. These memories are recallable only 1) after repression is relinquished by the child or 2) when repression fails (Laub and Auerhahn 1993). A child can relinquish repression only when he or she is able to tolerate the displeasurable feelings contained within the traumatic memory. One way this can occur is for the child to develop a high degree of trust in a certain person who enables the child to attain a sense of safety and support. The child then feels safe in exploring the traumatic memory within the support structure offered by the other person. Repression fails as a defense mechanism when the child is exposed to another highly traumatic event or is physically compromised in some way (e.g., the child experiences severe fatigue secondary to sleep deprivation). In the latter case, the breakdown in the defense mechanism occurs because, like all mental processes, a certain amount of mental energy is necessary in order for the mechanism to operate properly.

As noted earlier, traumatic experiences that take place during the infant's preverbal period produce implicit memories, which are then stored in the infant's dynamic unconscious domain. They are recallable throughout the child's life cycle only in their producing behavioral enactments.

Once a child possesses an unconscious traumatic memory, he or she not only will be unable to recall that memory, but also will not be consciously aware that certain of his or her current perceptions, conceptions, feelings, and behavioral enactments are being influenced by that traumatic memory. Use of a defense mechanism like repression effectively breaks the conscious connection between the child's unconscious traumatic memories and how these memories influence the child's current thoughts, feelings, and behavioral enactments. This break produces an advantage, but at a price. The advantage is that the traumatic memory does not enter the child's consciousness, and the child does not remember and reexperience the disturbing thoughts and highly displeasurable feelings associated with the sense of helplessness and loss of control experienced during the traumatic event. The price is that the child's current sensations, perceptions, thoughts, emotions, and behavioral enactments are influenced by the traumatic memory without the child's being aware of this influence.

For example, Terr (1988) demonstrated that the preverbal infant and toddler (from birth to about age 2½ years) uses primary repression to maintain traumatic implicit memories within his or her systematic unconscious domain. Terr described how these children, after age 4 years, automatically experience a vaguely sensed, trauma-specific fear and subsequently automatically enact behaviors to avoid situations that are not frightening to the normal child but that share common characteristics with these children's past traumatic situations. Their fear and automatic avoidant behaviors appear to be a partial behavioral reenactment of how they behaved during their original traumatic experience. They enact in their play certain events that are remarkably similar to traumatic events (e.g., they avoid certain people, animals, or situations) they experienced as young as age 6 months, but about which they now have no conscious recall or understanding. One example described by Terr is quite illustrative of this latter point:

> Sarah was ages 15–18 months old [when she was] in the day care home. She was 5 when she entered my office jauntily. First she drew a picture of a naked baby [a behavioral enactment]. She explained: "This is my doll. She is lying on the bed naked, [she hesitated], but covered up. I'm playing and yelling at my doll. She was bad! I yell at my doll [she hesitated again, looking up at me for some response]—not really yell—you get to bed, you!"
>
> I asked whether Sarah ever felt scared. "I'm afraid of some things but I don't know what they are [a trauma-specific fear]. I used to be scared of a cow. I never saw one. Moooooo! I thought that part [the udder] was real scary too. It looked like some kind of monster to me when I was little. I also remember [when] we went on a boat in Disneyland—an animal boat—some have stripes . . . there were some little Indians with spears pointed at us. I was scared of that." The child fingered her upper abdomen. I asked, "Did anybody ever scare you?" "Somebody scared me once," she said, "with a finger part."
>
> A few weeks later I saw the pornographic photos [taken when Sarah was 15–18 months of age]. Expecting to find a man's penis in or at the baby's genitals, I saw instead an erect penis [to this child with a 15- to 18-month-old vocabulary at the time of the experience, a "finger part"] on Sarah's upper abdomen—jabbing at the very spot she touched in my office. (Terr 1988, pp. 100–101)

In Terr's example, it should be noted how Sarah at age 5 years was not consciously aware of the connection between her current automatic trauma-specific fears and behavioral enactments and her repressed and unconsciously stored memories of traumatic events she experienced at ages 15–18 months. Also, although she had some vaguely recalled visual images of her infant traumatic experiences, she had neither verbal memories (e.g., of her own wishes and the wishes and demands of the perpetrator) nor emotional memories (e.g., highly emotionally displeasurable levels of rage and sadness) of these traumatic experiences.

Implicit memories have a timeless and fixed quality as they exist in the systematic unconscious domain. Those explicit memories, on the other hand, that are stored within the dynamic unconscious undergo a unique type of transformation. In a process that is still unclear, an explicit traumatic memory will be changed from the logical and rational form of thinking—called secondary process thinking—of the conscious and preconscious mental domains into the illogical and irrational form of thinking—called primary process thinking—of the systematic and dynamic unconscious domains.

Primary process thinking is so named because it is thought to be an evolutionarily older form of thinking than the more logical secondary process thinking that takes place within the conscious mental domain (Reiser 1984). *Primary process thinking* is defined as mental activity that does not maintain logical connections between thoughts; allows contradictions; does not maintain the logical progression of past to present to future time; and does not recognize negatives that contradict other facts (Meissner 1986). Reiser (1985) noted that primary process thinking is

> characterized by its lack of logic, . . . part representation for the whole, tolerance for mutually contradictory ideas to coexist or freely replace one another, . . . and predominance of the visual over the verbal mode in representing ideas. (pp. 83–84)

In general, primary process thinking exists within the unconscious domain, which would include both the systematic and the dynamic unconscious domains. An example is dreaming. Likewise, many aspects of every person's five innate needs that find expression within the content of a person's dream follow primary process rules. For example, an adult male consciously remembered the following dream from the night before:

> I was in a house that was my old house where I grew up as a child. At the same time it was the house I am living in now. [Contradictory thoughts and inconsistent time periods] Also, a woman was there who said she hated men who had blond hair like mine, but then she was passionately kissing me. [Another contradiction] The dream doesn't make logical sense, because time was not constant.

As evidenced by this man's conscious recall of his dream (which contained elements of primary process thinking), the conscious mind is capable of becoming aware of aspects of its primary process thinking. Indeed, it is normal throughout a person's life for the conscious mind to occasionally use primary process thinking in adapting to life experiences, (e.g., develop creative solutions to life's dilemmas, create new artistic interpretations of people, objects, and events [Zetzel and Meissner 1973]).

Conscious and preconscious mental activities for the most part follow the rules of *secondary process thinking,* defined as mental activity that follows laws of logic, identifies the causality of events with an appreciation of a sense of time, and uses a verbal and written language to express mental structures (Sandler et al. 1973). Secondary process thinking produces the goal-directed, sensible, logical, and rational thoughts and feelings that people verbally communicate in most of their interpersonal interactions. For example, secondary process thinking acknowledges that past is past, present is present, and death is irreversible.

Secondary process thinking is the principal mode of thinking that takes place within the conscious and preconscious mental domains. Primary process thinking can take place within the conscious domain, but to a far lesser extent than secondary process thinking.

■ Persistence Over Time

Some mental structures—such as visual, auditory, tactile, olfactory, and verbal perceptual images and transient emotional perceptions—do not have any significant degree of persistence over time. Memory is one mental structure that does persist over time. Although some memories—such as important autobiographical data and repressed memories—persist relatively unchanged, other memories—such as those of many insignificant daily life events—deteriorate over time (Terr 1994).

Both implicit memories and explicit memories involve how information is formed, stored, and retrieved. When addressing what a child forms into and retrieves as memories, human memory is separated into six types of memories (Terr 1994):

● *Immediate memory* (e.g., a child remembers why he or she put bread in the toaster)

- *Short-term memory* (e.g., a child remembers if he or she did homework the previous night)
- *Knowledge and skill memory* (e.g., a child remembers a fact about geography or how to hit a baseball)
- *Priming memory* (e.g., a child who knows about hiking will have fantasies about what it might be like to go mountain climbing)
- *Associative memory*—A memory in which a person automatically associates a perception with an action (e.g., a child sees another child drop an object and automatically picks it up and hands it to the child)
- *Episodic memory*—A memory of previously occurring autobiographical events

The modifiers immediate, short-term, knowledge and skill, priming, associative, and episodic describe the length of time a particular type of memory lasts within the mental domain, which will in turn dictate the duration of time in which the memory can be experientially recalled within the mind (Brodal 1969; Kandel 1981; Terr 1994). After this time period has passed, the particular type of memory can no longer be recalled because it is no longer present within the mind.

Immediate and short-term memories last from a few seconds to several minutes (e.g., the memory of a phone number, directions to a new store, the transient feeling of joy in seeing an eagle soar over a treetop) and from several hours to a few days (e.g., the memory of the previous night's dinner conversation). Immediate and short-term memories, which also are designated by Terr (1994) as forms of *working memory,* persist only for a short time because they are not stored within the mind. However, immediate and short-term memories are constantly used to transiently memorize various stimuli used in an individual's processing of information and communicating or interacting with others (e.g., memorizing a list of wines in order to impress another person at a restaurant several hours later). Knowledge, skill, associative, priming, and episodic memories, however, are long-term memories (e.g., they are placed in long-term storage).

During children's development, they are constantly selecting certain types of knowledge, skills, and episodes in their lives for long-term memory storage. As Terr (1994) stated, "Most of us shuck off tons of unnecessary information each day" (p. 10); this occurs as people select certain newly learned facts, skills, and autobiographical events for long-term memory retention. From the myriad perceptions children encode to form memories, they will select certain immediate and short-term memories for long-term storage. This selection process will then determine in great part how they subsequently perceive themselves, others, and the world for, once long-term memories are stored, they forever influence an individual's perceptions. Loewald (1980) expressed this idea in the following:

> Perception is shot through with memory. . . . The past would be irretrievably lost without memory; in fact there would not be any past, just as there would not be any present that has any meaning or any future to envisage. . . . Memory gives meaning to the present and helps to shape the future. . . . Memorial activity is linking activity. A before, now, and after are created in this linking and become mutually influential; continuity of our life as individuals comes into being. (p. 157)

Many of a child's preconscious long-term memories automatically undergo change as the child undergoes further development; for example, it is normal for a child to restructure preconscious long-term memories. Indeed, an aspect of new learning often involves adding something to or revising a prior long-term preconscious memory. Thus, a 2-year-old boy's long-term memory of his mother will obviously be restructured by the time he is age 18 years.

On the other hand, some of a child's long-term preconscious memories retain such a high degree of persistence over time that they do not undergo any significant developmental restructuring throughout the life cycle. For example, an elderly man expressed this lifelong belief: "Since I was a very young child, I believed in the existence of God, and at 90 years old I still have this same simple belief that God exists."

Traumatic memories that are present within the child's unconscious can undergo restructuring as the child develops, but they can also remain unaltered if that individual is never helped to consciously tolerate the highly displeasurable emotions contained within the traumatic memory. However, when the child is assisted in consciously tolerating these emotions, he or she is then open to new learning and the restructuring of the original traumatic memory (Osofsky et al. 1995; Pruett 1979; Terr 1993).

■ Effect on Delay of Action

The final way in which mental structures vary is their ability to assist in the delay of action.

For the developing infant to become better able to access and use his or her ever-expanding knowledge base of long-term memories, the infant's mind must begin to institute more of a delay between receiving sensory stimulation, forming perceptions and conceptions, and initiating or not initiating an action (including speech). This is because, during a delay, the developing infant has the chance to generate new perceptions and conceptions and to access memories of past perceptions and conceptions. During the delay of action, both new and old perceptions and conceptions are used by the child to comprehend past and present and to compare what is already known—that is, what he or she has previously learned—with what is new information—that is, what he or she has yet to learn. The infant can then achieve a more thought-motivated decision to act or not to act. As the infant's mind develops, it gradually becomes more able to retrieve long-term memories to understand and organize current perceptions.

Summary

In the following chapters, I begin to discuss the biopsychosocial model of mental development, based on the above understanding of mental processes. This model is then used in following the sequential mental development of the infant, child, and adolescent. It also aids in organizing and delineating some of the major questions that still remain unanswered about the infant's and child's mental development.

Chapter 2

Biopsychosocial Model of Mental Development

During the latter half of the 20th century, several researchers have contributed to the development of a biopsychosocial model of how the body develops disease (Alexander 1948; A. Meyer 1991; von Bertalanffy 1968). G. L. Engel (1977, 1980), who is usually credited with modifying and crystallizing this model, hypothesized that biological, social, and psychological variables or stimuli contribute to every defined disease in the human body (Eisendrath 1988). In recent years, this biopsychosocial model of disease has been extended as a model for understanding how the human mind undergoes normal maturation and developmental change (Reiser 1984). In this model, the process of normal mental development is viewed as emanating from the transactions among biological, social, and psychological stimuli. These stimuli are further defined in the biopsychosocial model as follows.

Biopsychosocial Stimuli

■ Biological Stimuli

Biological stimuli are defined as the sensory stimuli that emanate from the infant's physical nature, both in health and in disease. (Although I address normal development in this book, it should be noted that biological stimuli also emanate from disease or pathological conditions in the body.) As I note in Chapter 1, this physical nature is present at birth in the form of innate physical structures and undergoes chronological growth in the process of physical maturation. Biological stimuli can be categorized on the basis of the following:

- Biological stimuli emanating from inside the infant's body (including the brain):
  - Physiological stimuli (e.g., the sensation of thirst)
  - The body's position in space (e.g., the sensory stimuli emanating from the infant's legs when they are positioned above his or her head)
- Biological stimuli emanating from the surface of the infant's body:
  - Innate reflexive and central nervous system voluntary and involuntary motor abilities (e.g., the infant's voluntary motor ability to withdraw his or her hand from an external object whose temperature exceeds the infant's threshold for temperature tolerance)
  - The sequential emergence of all of the body's maturational advances in voluntary and involuntary central nervous system motor abilities, body growth, and hormonally induced physical body changes (e.g., the emergence of the 18-month-old toddler's ability to become visually aware of having a separate body from others and of possessing the characteristics of height, weight, and hair color; the emergence of the 2-year-old child's ability to begin to learn voluntary motor control over his or her urinary and anal sphincters)

■ Social Stimuli

Social stimuli are defined as all the sensory stimuli that emanate from sources external to the infant's body, brain, and mind. These would be stimuli emanating from people, things, and events that produce changes in one or more of the infant's sensory modalities (e.g., the tactile stimulation produced by the mother's finger placed on the infant's lips; the visual and auditory stimuli that the 2-year-old child learns are characteristic of the animal called a dog).

In the first few years of life, infants learn much about differentiating where their body ends and where the external or social world begins. Indeed, in a lifelong process of sensory differentiation, children will sequentially learn more about their own body (e.g., its different parts, what it can do, how it changes physically and functionally) and a social world of people, animals, and inanimate objects. Infants learn about these two worlds by being exposed to stimuli that vary in their frequency, intensity, and complexity. Furthermore, as infants continue to differentiate these stimuli, they slowly attain the knowledge that their social environment performs many functions, and that these functions are in the service of society's—as initially represented by the parents—goals of making them a socialized member of society.

The human *socialization process* can be defined as one in which a person learns the physical and social skills, moral and ethical values, and the overall knowledge that will equip him or her to function more or less satisfactorily so that he or she can fulfill the role of child, adolescent, and adult in their society (Maccoby and Martin 1983). Obviously, these habits, values, goals, and knowledge will differ from society to society, reflecting the cultural history of each specific societal group. For example, in addition to teaching children how to behave, one society might teach its children that a rigid social class system exists that does not permit movement from a lower to a higher class, whereas another society might teach that the social structure is flexible and not tied to one's status at birth.

Although societies differ in the particular goals they define for their children, certain universal social functions can be identified that are provided in the process of socializing children (see Chapter 3 for a fuller discussion of these functions). These five universal functions can be expressed as the social environment providing the following in a predictably reliable manner:

1. Truthful information about the child's body and the external world of people and things in which the child is being raised
2. Stimulus modulation and protection for the child from experiencing too many overstimulating or understimulating life events (See discussion of zone of proximal development below.)
3. Encouragement, support, and admiration for the child in response to the child's innate capabilities, maturational advances, and developmental accomplishments
4. Truthful information about how the child can begin to achieve gratification of his or her innate needs while concurrently adapting to the needs and developmental taskings of his or her parents and society
5. Adaptive solutions for children to cope with emotionally displeasurable life events, and special help, when needed, for children to deal with and eventually master traumatic life events

As infants and children learn about these social functions, they are encountering the social stimuli in the biopsychosocial model. How these functions are taught differs from one society to another; but, in most societies, infants first learn about each of these functions first through their parents' behaviors and verbal communications, and then further through the behaviors and verbal communications of others and through the social context or social circumstances in which these behaviors are manifested. Thus, although parents may attempt to provide their infant with the same social functions, each may differ greatly in the context in which these functions are provided. For example, one mother lives in a social environment in which she carries her infant in a cradle strapped to her back for several hours a day, whereas another mother lives in a social environment in which she leaves her infant with a caretaker for several hours a day. The social context in which each of these mothers attempts to provide her infant with (the social function of) encouragement, support, and admiration is different: different in terms of the total time each mother spends with her infant (which may or may not affect each mother's ability to provide her infant with the support and admiration needed) and each mother's societally based beliefs about how she should go about fulfilling this social function for her infant.

■ Psychological Stimuli

The psychological stimuli in the biopsychosocial model of normal mental development are defined as sensory stimuli emanating from 1) the infant's innate and ever-maturing mental nature and 2) the infant's ever-growing representational world of thoughts and feelings and long-term memories of developmental changes and associated learning experiences. By definition, psychological sensory stimuli emanate from within the mind—that is, they are generated from within the conscious, preconscious, and unconscious domains. This is in contrast to biological and social stimuli, which are generated from the infant's body, brain, and social environment.

Psychological stimuli emanate from the following:

- The innate informational structures within which an infant's five innate needs, a set of emotions, and temperamental characteristics are stored.
- New maturational informational structures that emerge in the process of mental development.
- Current and past experiential informational structures (i.e., perceptions, conceptions, emotions, and memories).
- Long-term memories of developmental changes and associated learning experiences stored within an infant's preconscious and unconscious mental domains. Stimuli from this source are either conscious stimuli, when preconsciously stored memories are recalled, or unconscious stimuli, when unconsciously stored memories are activated.

■ Differentiating the Various Types of Stimuli

Although the infant mind is innately prepared to receive and begin to form perceptions of biological, social, and psychological stimuli, infants must slowly learn where each type of stimulus comes from, what it means, and whether they are able to modify it. At birth, infants are not able to differentiate a biological stimulus from a social stimulus. For example, an infant boy may feel the same tactile sensation if his mother accidentally rubs a coarse towel on his lower abdomen (a social stimulus), if he rubs his own lower abdomen on the towel (a biological stimulus), or if he develops a skin rash on his lower abdomen that makes his normal diaper feel like a coarse towel (another biological stimulus). How, then, does this infant come to know that the first stimulation was caused by someone or something outside of his body; the second, by the actions of his own body; and the third, by a skin ailment? The answer is that, shortly after birth, he slowly begins to learn to organize, differentiate, and thereby distinguish which tactile stimuli emanate from his actions and which emanate from the actions of his environment.

Eventually, infants also learn to differentiate biological and social stimuli from psychological stimuli. For example, up until about age 18 months, infants are not able to

> differentiate a perceptual act (occurring now) from a memorial act (having occurred). Memory, as registration or recording, and perception are identical for the infant. (Loewald 1980, p. 155; parentheses in original)

In essence, in eventually discovering their own psychological stimuli, for example, a memory, infants discover that they possess a mind that generates sensations of need, emotional sensations, ideas, memories, and so on (Frye and Moore 1991). They also discover that their mind can produce memory sensations of past experiences. Mayes and Cohen (1994) emphasized this point in the following:

> For young children, appreciating that they and others have a mental life that guides talk and action requires the minimal understanding that there is a difference between the subjective mental world and the externally perceivable world, or more fundamentally, that things and people exist in memory and thought even when they are not directly perceivable. (p. 206)

Developmental Change

Developmental change can be defined as a process in which a biological system undergoes changes in its structures and the processes they perform. These changes can be triggered by maturation (i.e., the process in which new structures emerge through chronological, genetically controlled growth and differentiation of various parts of the biological system), events in the system's environment, or both. The maturation of an infant's mental nature, as well as his or her physical nature, takes place within an environment that provides nurturance. *Nurturance* within the human context is defined as those caretaking activities that are provided to an infant by one or more people in his or her environment that ensure the infant's 1) physical survival and 2) development as a socialized member of his or her society. One characteristic of the human infant is that, for any degree of physical and mental maturation to emerge, a life-sustaining amount of physical nurturance (e.g., nutrition, thermal regulation, physical activity, protection against bodily injury) must be provided by the infant's caretakers.

Developmental change, according to the biopsychosocial model, begins as the developing child's mind processes all input—that is, the transactions among biological, social, and psychological stimuli—and then generates one or more of the following as initial outputs: perceptions, conceptions (i.e., wishes, fantasies, or beliefs), feelings, and memories. Next the child's mind processes these internal responses to generate a new representation that integrates the transactions among the biopsychosocial stimuli. This new representation becomes a potential piece of developmental change. If the child stores the new representation as a long-term memory, developmental change has occurred, and the child will invariably begin to practice and consolidate this new knowledge by engaging in new learning experiences. Stated in the form of an equation,

Developmental change (as a potential for new learning) =
mental processing of transactions among biopsychosocial stimuli

The new responses generated by infants as a result of interactions among their nature, the actions of the people who make up their nurturing environment, and their prior use of developmental changes as contained within their long-term memories will lead to new learning experiences and new developmental changes. Therefore, the process of mental development is one of sequential developmental changes and associated new learning experiences—a process in which infants gradually acquire knowledge about their mind and body, their caretakers and others, and the animate and inanimate occupants of the world in which they live.

This mental development occurs at a higher level of complexity than the more simple processes that enable infants to construct their first perception of their mother. This more advanced type of mental processing involves the mind's abilities to form conceptions—that is, the cognitive ability to integrate and organize the transactions among biological, social, and psychological stimuli and arrive at an understanding of their relationships to each other. In contrast to perception-forming and emotion-generating processes, which are operative at birth, cognitive processes emerge at about age 18 months and then undergo progressive maturation and development. For example, whereas a 6-month-old baby girl is able to construct a simple perceptual representation of her mother's face and simple perceptual representations of her own hands as she puts her fingers in her mouth, she is not be able to construct a more complex conceptual representation of the transactions between her actions (as emanating from her biological, physical nature), the actions of her mother (as emanating from her social world), and her own first long-term, implicit memories of her mother (as emanating from her psychological world).

Applying the Biopsychosocial Mental Developmental Equation

In the process by which infants undergo sequential developmental changes and increasingly learn about themselves and the social world, all three types of input—the biological, social, and psychological stimuli—do not become activated simultaneously. At any point in time, usually one stimulus becomes activated and then it in turn activates varying degrees of responses in the other two realms. Also, although all three types of stimuli are equal in being able to activate prior responses in the other types of stimuli, they are not equal in their ability to generate a new response in each other. This is because the generation of biological and psychological advances—becoming new biological and psychological stimuli—are controlled by one's genetic code. Thus no amount of triggering stimulation from either social or psychological sources (e.g., wishes, memories) can trigger a new maturational biological or psychological advance. If it could, a child's wish (psychological stimulus) to grow physically (a biological response) or become intellectually smarter (a psychological response) could stimulate advances in the child's body growth or intellectual ability. Likewise, parents' social expectations and taskings of their child are not capable of generating new maturational changes in their child's physical or mental nature. (Later in this chapter I describe some new research that suggests that a child's social learning experiences may trigger "alterations in the regulation of gene expression" [Kandel 1981, 1983; Kandel and Schwartz 1982] and bring forth hidden biological and psychological maturational abilities; however, this research is still in its infancy.)

Although it is generally accepted that social and psychological stimuli are not able to trigger new biological or psychological maturational advances, the reverse, however, is possible: a maturational advance is able to act as a stimulus in generating new social or psychological responses or both. As illustrated in the following examples, an adolescent boy's perception of the external physical changes that occur in his body as a result of his biological maturation (e.g., axillary and genital hair growth, voice changes) will trigger social responses within the boy's environment (e.g., the responses by the boy's parents and others), which then become social stimuli for the boy, as well as psychological responses within the boy's mind (e.g., the boy's perceptions of his external physical changes, his parents' and others' responses to these changes, his recall of his prior memories regarding experiences involving his body) that become psychological stimuli for the boy. Both adolescent boys in these examples live in intact families and are the eldest of the children.

> Dan's perception of his newly emergent axillary and genital hair growth triggers his remembering how his parents quite often complimented him for his physical exploits as a boy. His positive memories generate positive expectations that his father will react to his new axillary and genital hair with admiration and pride because he sees his son beginning to have a masculine body image, similar to that of his own. These positive memories and expectant thoughts act as internally motivating psychological stimuli and propel Dan to display his new axillary and genital hair growth to his father (and other male peers and men). Hence, Dan's prior development of a representational world of predominantly positive memories of his interactions with his parents helps him to maintain and continue to create a social world of predominantly positive interactions with his parents and others.
>
> With these prior positive memories fresh in mind, Dan asks his father if he can accompany him on one of his visits to his athletic club. Dan's father is pleased by his son's interest, and they go to the club. While showering after exercising, the father notices his son's new axillary and genital hair growth, and proudly says to his son, while handing him a stick of underarm deodorant, "Guys need to use this when their bodies are starting to look like that of a man."

In this example, the internal stimulation provided by Dan's biological maturational advance (i.e., his development of secondary sexual characteristics) became a biological stimulus that activated the recall of psychological stimuli (i.e., emotionally positive memories); those memories then influenced the emergence of social stimuli (i.e., Dan's positive interactions in the athletic club with his father and similar experiences with others).

In time, Dan will undergo a developmental change as a result of these experiences. The first step in undergoing this change will be his integrating the transactions of the above biopsychosocial stimuli. This process will involve his generating initial outputs in the form of one or more perceptions, feelings, ideas, fantasies, and wishes and recalling other memories. Eventually he will combine all these mental elements into a final output in the form of a conceptual representation that captures what it means to him to develop these secondary sexual characteristics within his social world of family, peers, and others. In accordance with the developmental equation, this new conceptual representation will become a new developmental change. This will occur when he stores this representation as a long-term memory within his representational world—in this case, within the preconscious part of his representational world. Dan's new conception—which becomes a new piece of knowledge about what masculinity means to him—could be summarized as follows:

> I am beginning to look more like a man and my father likes it, which makes me feel happy and proud. If I grow up to look like a man, my family will support me. Further, I expect to become a successful man someday like my father.

Recalling this long-term memory in the future will be emotionally pleasurable for Dan. As such, its recall will act as an internal motivator that will cause Dan to generate positive expectations of his interactions with others (i.e., expectations of social responses that will generate pleasurable feelings). These future positive interactions will become new learning experiences that in turn will further Dan's continued development of his view of himself as possessing a masculine body appearance.

In contrast to Dan's experiences, Tim, in revealing the emergence of his secondary sexual characteristics to his father, receives a quite different response. This response contributes to Tim's constructing a completely different long-term conceptual memory of his experiences.

> Tim perceives his newly emergent axillary and genital hair growth as an indication of his beginning to have a masculine body image, similar to that of his father. This perception causes him to remember how often he had been angry at his father, not only for failing to compliment him for his physical exploits as a boy, but also for criticizing these same exploits. Tim's representational world has become an internal source of emotionally displeasurable psychological stimuli. These stimuli unfortu-

nately cause him to negatively color his expectations of his future experiences involving his own maturational advances and his social interactions with others.

Consequently, Tim's negative memories generate expectations that his father will react to his new axillary and genital hair growth with disinterest, criticism, or possibly both. Tim consequently struggles with a wish to avoid his father in order to protect himself from becoming angry at his father, an anger he expects to experience when his father does not show pride in his new secondary sexual characteristics. Tim decides to withdraw and does not ask to go with his father to his father's health club. However, when his father announces that he is going to a large department store to shop for clothes for himself, Tim asks to go with him. Tim tells himself that, if he admires how his father looks in his new clothes, then his father might admire him if he tried on new masculine-looking clothes.

When they arrive at the store, Tim asks his father if, after they go to the men's department, they could go to the teens' department to look for a suit for Tim's upcoming grammar school graduation. The father agrees. While in the men's department, Tim waits patiently as his father tries on several suits. His father asks for and receives both the salesperson's and Tim's opinions and encouragements about which suit looks best. When the father makes his final selection, Tim tells him, "You look great!" The father purchases the suit and they then go to the teens' department. Once there, however, the father quickly becomes impatient with Tim. The first suit jacket Tim tries on produces the following response from his father: "That looks fine. I'd get that one. So why don't you get it and let's go." Tim responds, "Look, Dad, you took a long time looking for a suit that looked good on you. I'd like to try on some other suits, like you did, before I decide." Tim's father suddenly becomes enraged at him and states quite loudly in front of the salesperson, "Don't you call me conceited! Like I make a big deal about my clothes!" Tim angrily answers back, "I don't know what you're talking about. I wasn't saying you were conceited."

Tim's father then physically grabs Tim's shirt sleeve and pulls him out of the store. On the way to their car, Tim tells his father, "I wasn't saying you were conceited, but I waited for you and told you what suits looked good on you. Why couldn't you let me try on some suits and tell me what looked good on me, instead of just saying the first jacket I tried on was okay?" The father then slaps Tim across the back of his head and says, "Don't answer me back. Shut up!" They arrive at their car and drive home in silence.

Tim feels rage toward his father, but dares not verbalize it. After arriving home, Tim goes into the family garage and paces while feeling furious. He notices one of his prized possessions— a basketball given to him by his grandparents. Suddenly he picks up a screwdriver and pierces his basketball several times. He then perceives that he feels much less angry inside, but also realizes he feels sad as he looks down at his destroyed basketball.

Over the ensuing days, Tim's father and Tim avoid each other. Three days later, the father finds the destroyed basketball hidden in the garage under some old rags, but he does not ask Tim why he has destroyed it. He only punishes him for destroying the basketball by removing his allowance for 2 months and by not permitting him to play any basketball for the same period.

Similarly to Dan, Tim will also undergo a developmental change in the form of a new conception about what growing up to look like a man means to him, and will then deposit this new conception within his inner world as a long-term explicit memory. Referring once again to the mental developmental equation, the "ingredients" that will go into his construction of his new conception are his perceptions, feelings, ideas, wishes, and fantasies in response to 1) his new axillary and genital hair growth; 2) his interactions with his father in the store, on their way home from the store, and during the next several days; and 3) his memories of past experiences involving his bodily changes and social interactions with his father.

Tim's new conception—which also becomes a new piece of knowledge about what masculinity means to him—could be summarized as follows:

My father doesn't want me to look like a man like him because he has to be number one. The rules he makes me obey aren't fair. So I won't tell him anything anymore. But I'll still grow up to look like a man. From now on, I don't need a father to help me grow up. I can take care of myself. It's stupid to ask a father for advice.

The maturational emergence of Tim's secondary sexual characteristics had initially propelled him to see if he could develop a closer relationship with his father, despite his negative expectations based on his past memories of his father's negative and disinterested responses to his bodily changes. However, his father's behavior in the department store and afterwards communicated his father's uneasiness and possibly unwillingness to support his son's wish to look more like him. Indeed, Tim's father seemed to possess more of a wish to sadistically dominate his son. Therefore, Tim's experiences related to the emergence of his secondary sexual characteristics reinforced his memories of his father's hostile responses to his emerging masculine body appearance. In addition, they triggered Tim's resurrection of his ideal self—his belief that he did not need either his father or other men to help him to grow up to be a man. The new conceptual memories he constructed of these experiences were emotionally displeasurable, but not so displeasurable that they were unconsciously repressed. In the future, Tim avoided activating and recalling these preconsciously stored memories by acting omnipotently around his father and other male authority figures that reminded him of his father. In essence, he was communicating to them, "I don't need you. I can take care of myself."

As a result of these negative experiences involving his pubertal bodily changes, Tim removed himself not only from interactions with his father but also from developmentally enhancing experiences with other men. In this regard, his memories of entering puberty will act as a developmentally inhibiting belief that will interfere with his future development in the sense that they will cause him to expect future experiences with his father and other men vis-à-vis exhibiting his masculine appearance and associated behaviors to be negative.

In summary, these two pubertal boys—who faced the emergence of the same secondary sexual characteristics (biological stimuli), lived in two different families (social stimuli), and possessed different perceptions, feelings, ideas, wishes, fantasies, and memories of their prior experiences with their fathers (psychological stimuli)—ultimately constructed different beliefs in reference to their pubertal physical bodily changes, beliefs that they then stored as new long-term memories. Each boy's mind was changed through his experiences involving his secondary sexual characteristics. Consequently, each boy's future social behaviors were then influenced by his individual beliefs related to those experiences. Thus Dan continued to readily approach his father and generate positive expectancies with regard to how other male authority figures would respond to him. In believing and then expecting them to support and admire him when he manifested his burgeoning masculine appearance, he would make his own active contributions to creating social responses that matched his positive memories. Tim, however, behaved quite differently around his father and other male authority figures. He exhibited a (pseudo)independence in situations in which he exhibited his masculine body appearance. In denying his need for interaction with other men, he also made his own active contributions to creating negative social responses, but these negative responses only served to reaffirm his remembered negative beliefs.

Biopsychosocial Triggers for Developmental Change

■ Biological Stimuli

A biological stimulus will trigger a developmental change when a new maturational physical advance occurs (e.g., as in the examples of Dan and Tim).

■ Psychological Stimuli

A psychological stimulus will trigger a developmental change when a maturational change occurs in one of the child's innate needs, emotions, language, temperamental characteristics, or cognitive abilities. With regard to cognitive abilities, three organizing principles help one to understand how the emergence of a new cognitive ability generates a developmental change: the transference-assimilation principle, the accommodation-transformation principle, and the hierarchical reorganizing principle.

Assimilation, accommodation, and learning.   New perceptions or conceptions can be integrated into a child's mind through one of two ways: assimilation or accommodation. *Assimilation* is the mental process in which a child "takes in" a current perception or conception into a preexisting representation. In trying to assimilate this perception or conception, the child attempts to achieve a sense of knowing or a sense of familiarity regarding the new perception or conception. If a child is not able to assimilate a new perception or conception, the process of accommodation may be activated. "Accommodation" occurs when the child perceives the new perception or conception as being novel, and, in integrating this perception or conception, either reconstructs an existing representation or constructs an entirely new one. Successful accommodation leads to new developmental changes because new representational mental structures are constructed.

Stillwell et al. (1991) explained the processes of accommodation and assimilation as follows:

> The [conceptual] meaning of events remains at a static level as long as new events can be assimilated into a particular framework of understanding [i.e., preexisting representations]. When cognitive disequilibrium develops in regards to events and the conceptual framework that explains them, either through new awareness brought about by neurological maturation or increasingly complexity in the environment, cognitive and emotional tension requires cognitive accommodation to a new conceptual framework. (p. 16)

Even though an infant may undergo a developmental change, it does not mean that he or she has also acquired new learning. For example, an infant may undergo a developmental change and become capable of cognitively understanding a more complex perception, but he or she may not use this new cognitive understanding to acquire new learning experiences through practicing and consolidating this developmental change (what J. Piaget [1972] referred to as *true learning*). The determining factor as to whether the developmental change is used to engage in a new learning experience is usually whether the infant's social environment provides adequate support for the infant to learn more about the developmental change (see the five functions of social environment, listed above). In summary, although many infants achieve similar developmental changes, not all are exposed to a social environment that allows them to learn and acquire the same amount or type of knowledge.

Transference-assimilation principle. The transference-assimilation principle states that infants, in formulating a perception or conception from current biological, social, or psychological stimuli, will unconsciously or automatically activate their database—stored within their long-term memories—of representations of people and things to generate predictive expectancies and transfer these expectancies onto the new perception or conception. This *transference* was defined by Lichtenberg and Kindler (1994) as "an expectancy of a human response or a situation involving humans and inanimate objects that may require very little cuing in actuality to seem confirmed" (p. 406). Thus, for example, an infant is propelled to automatically or unconsciously transfer one or more aspects of a previously stored representation of a person onto a new person that is currently being perceived. This transference becomes the initial inner referent for how the infant views the new person, a view initially colored by the wishes, feelings (including fears), conceptual beliefs, or fantasies that are contained within the representation that the infant has constructed of someone in his or her past. Following the transference of expectations, the infant then attempts to assimilate the new perception or conception into a prior representation.

Transference is mobilized by an infant's need to generate predictive expectancies about his or her perceptions and conceptions, and is enhanced when a majority of the infant's predictions are validated. The transference-assimilation principle also works in harmony with the stimulus principle I describe in Chapter 1. For example, when a current stimulus generates a perception, the infant's mind will transferentially expect—or at least, wish—this new perception to be within his or her optimal stimulation range. The infant automatically expects, therefore, that to pursue this perception will be emotionally pleasurable, and, consequently, assertively seeks to explore the stimulus. This transference of positive expectancies is called a *positive transference reaction.*

Successful assimilation automatically generates a pleasurable emotion within the infant when the new, assimilated perception or conception generates a level of stimulation that is within the infant's unique stimulation range. The memory of this pleasurable emotion is incorporated into the infant's long-term memory. Recollection of this memory then motivates the infant to repeat the behaviors or procedures in order to reexperience the pleasurable feeling associated with acting competently.

If the new perception is not within the infant's optimal stimulation range, the infant will experience displeasurable emotions and signal distress (e.g., begin to cry). When an infant begins to have more emotionally displeasurable than pleasurable experiences, he or she may gradually begin to transferentially view all new perceptions as outside of his or her optimal stimulation range and as something that will cause him or her to experience highly displeasurable feelings; consequently, the infant will automatically begin to avoid new perceptions. This transference of negative expectancies is called a *negative transference reaction* (Fosshage 1994; Roth 1990). As a defensive process, negative transferences lead the infant to avoid the new person or situation, signal his or her distress, and possibly generate a fight-flight response.

Psychologically aware parents attempt to raise their children so that they generate more positive than negative transferences. Children who have activated more developmentally enhancing positive transferences are more trusting and seeking of people, whereas children who have activated more negative transferences are more mistrusting and wary of people. (It should be noted that parents encourage development of a certain amount of developmentally enhancing negative transferences in the normal socialization process [e.g., when teaching their children about dangerous people and objects] so that they will avoid these people and objects in the future.)

Accommodation-transformation principle.   If an infant simply generates positive and negative transferences and uses them to assimilate new perceptions or conceptions into prior representations, then no developmental changes or associated new learning will occur. The continued growth of the infant's database of constructed representations—and their storage in long-term memory—depends on the construction of new representations and the reconstruction or modification of preexisting representations.

The *accommodation-transformation principle* becomes activated when new stimuli present an infant with new perceptions or conceptions that cannot be assimilated into prior representations. At this point, the infant's mind must accommodate the new perception or conception and either transform a prior representation or construct a new representation. This process is often activated when a new cognitive ability emerges through natural maturation, because such an ability enables the infant to comprehend a new perception or conception that was previously incomprehensible. These pivotal points are considered the triggers that usher in a transition from one phase in mental development into the next phase. The end result is the mind's achievement of a new level of comprehension—that is, a new sense of knowing about the stimuli that generated the new perception or conception. Thus the product of the accommodation-transformation process is developmental change.

Hierarchical reorganizing principle. The third principle that comes into play when a maturational cognitive advance occurs is the *hierarchical reorganizing principle*, which states that, as a child's cognitive abilities continue to mature and his or her mind continues to reconstruct prior representations to reflect a more advanced level of cognitive integration and comprehension, the child's mind will reorganize its representations in a hierarchy that reflects that child's unique preferences. Pine (1989) described this process as a slow and progressive reorganization of a child's inner (or representational) world in which the child prioritizes his or her innate needs (e.g., an attachment relationship with his or her parents and siblings may be ranked ahead of the child's assertively seeking new relationships outside his or her family), emotions (e.g., the expression of anger may be ranked ahead of the expression of loving feelings), personal interests (e.g., school may be ranked ahead of sports), and parents' developmental taskings (e.g., parents tasking their child to do well in school may be ranked ahead of their tasking him or her to be considerate to friends).

In attempting to explain how each child's priorities emerge and change in different phases of each child's life cycle, Pine (1989) noted that "the personal hierarchies evolve out of the accidents of personal endowment and personal history" (p. 59).

■ Social Stimuli

Social stimuli also act as potent pivot points in ushering in new developmental changes in a child's life. These stimuli include parental developmental tasks, child adaptation, and goodness of fit between the child and parent.

Parental developmental tasks. The five innate needs with which infants are endowed are psychological stimuli that internally motivate infants to seek the gratification of those needs. However, infants are not preprogrammed with the innate knowledge that permits them to know how they are expected to gratify those innate needs in their family and in society. Infants also do not know what societally defined tasks their parents (as society's representatives) will give them in terms of learning how to express their emotions, use their cognitive abilities, and temperamentally behave, tasks that are necessary for the infant to eventually become a productive member of society.

Parents' and others' developmental taskings of how a child is supposed to express his or her cognitive abilities, emotions, temperamental characteristics, and five innate needs help shape the normal development of each of these psychological stimuli. But these taskings are helpful only if the parents are knowledgeable about when their expectations reasonably match their child's maturational advances in innate needs, emotions, temperamental characteristics, and cognitive abilities.

Zone of proximal development. Although an infant may receive enough parental encouragement to convert developmental changes into new learning experiences, the infant's parents may or may not expose the infant to the type of social environment that will enable him or her to activate this developmental change in practice and consolidate this knowledge through the process of learning. For example, a 6-month-old boy might manifest the following maturational changes: he can sit up without his parent's support and at the same time grasp an object offered to him. These maturational changes then generate new transactions between the infant and his parents, and he eventually acquires a new developmental change: he constructs a representation of the pleasurable experiences generated by his sitting and grasping behaviors. For this infant to remain motivated to learn about his new developmental changes, his parents must provide objects for him that he is physically able to grasp. In other words, they must provide objects and interactional experiences that are within his *zone of proximal development* (Vygotsky 1978). Vygotsky defined this zone as the "distance" between an individual infant's "actual developmental level as determined by independent problem solving . . . [and a more cognitively advanced level of] potential development as determined through problem solving under adult guidance or in collaboration with more capable peers" (p. 95).

In this statement, Vygotsky emphasized that infants are stimulated to apply their already achieved developmental changes to new learning experiences—and eventually acquire completely new developmental changes—when their parents provide objects and experiences that are just proximal to (or slightly ahead of) their cognitive and physical capabilities. As Kagan (1984) noted, infants learn within a range or zone that has as its borders the completely learned and the completely bizarre (or too novel). Thus, in the example of the infant learning to sit and grasp objects, the parents must present the infant with objects that are not too boring and not too novel.

Societal tasks. Developmental tasks generally can be defined for each phase of the life cycle from infancy through adulthood. These tasks determine what knowledge and behaviors the infant will be more or less expected to acquire and master in order to become a productive member of society, and how each child must adapt his or her innate and maturationally emerging needs, emotions, temperamental characteristics, and cognitive capabilities to society's rules and guidelines concerning their proper verbal and behavioral expression.

Child adaptation. *Adaptation* involves children's attempts to behaviorally and verbally express and modify the expression of their innate needs, emotions, temperamental characteristics, and cognitive capabilities to fit the developmental taskings of their parents. One of infants' innate needs is to engage in emotionally pleasurable interactions, initially with their parents in the context of the *attachment relationship* (see Chapter 3) and later with others. This first relationship is crucial because it becomes the main vehicle through which parents progressively teach their infants how to adapt the expression of each of their innate needs, temperamental characteristics, emotions, and cognitive abilities to society's developmental tasks. The infant's need for this relationship is normally supported by the parents' wish to engage in a similar emotionally pleasurable relationship with their infant.

■ Goodness of Fit: The Parent-Child Context Within Which Developmental Change Occurs

In the beginning phase of a goodness-of-fit process (Chess and Thomas 1986), both the infant's innate needs and the parents' taskings achieve a reasonable degree of gratification in an emotionally pleasurable manner. This takes place when the parents' developmental taskings—which are usually in congruence with societal taskings—reasonably match their infant's current innate and maturing capabilities, and the parents guide the expression of their infant's innate needs in a certain manner.

If the parents either do not have knowledge of their infant's capacities or do not want to give their infant pleasure (e.g., they are more invested in gratifying their own needs at the expense of their infant's needs), then invariably they will ask their infant to adapt to developmental taskings that exceed their infant's capability. This would lead to a poorness of fit from the infant's point of view. In such a relationship, the infant becomes involved in a developmentally inhibiting adaptation in which he or she, in order to please the parents, begins to avoid attempting to gratify his or her own innate needs and instead attempts to adapt to the unreasonable developmental taskings of the parents. In such a difficult adaptational process, the infant invariably experiences displeasurable feelings because the parents' taskings are beyond the infant's capabilities and the infant repeatedly experiences levels of stimulation that are outside his or her optimal stimulation range. The following is an example of a poor fit:

A woman who had given birth to a girl was abandoned by the infant's father shortly following the birth. The mother avoided expressing her ongoing rage at her husband for this abandonment by repressing the rage within her unconscious. However, following the birth, the mother enacted an avoidance of any nurturant activities toward her daughter because they stimulated her unconscious memories of rage at her husband for leaving her alone to nurture their infant.

The mother decided she wanted to go back to her full-time job as an accountant as quickly as possible after her daughter's birth and find someone in the neighborhood to take care of her daughter, primarily to avoid nurturing her. During the 3 weeks of maternity leave she took from her job, she focused her thoughts on getting her infant on a regular eating schedule. The mother had avoided reading any books on how to feed her infant before and after the birth. She repeatedly tasked her infant daughter to drink from a bottle according to her adult eating schedule—that is, three times a day: at morning, noon, and evening. In keeping with this schedule, the mother attempted to get her infant to ingest much more infant formula than was physically possible for an infant of her age. This eating schedule was a developmental tasking that did not match her society's normal developmental tasking for an infant and that naturally exceeded her infant's capabilities.

At first the infant rebelled at this schedule, signaling her distress to her mother by crying during feedings, indicating that the feeding interactions were generating within her a highly displeasurable level of stimulation. The mother did not properly interpret her infant's continued crying during feedings as signaling her infant's distressful emotional state and the fact that she was being stimulated outside of her optimal stimulation range. On the contrary, the mother continued to feed her infant according to the thrice daily schedule.

Because the mother was too preoccupied with trying to repress and forget her own angry feelings at her husband, she did not tune in to her infant's distress as signaled by her crying behavior. Eventually, the act of eating generated such a high degree of emotional displeasure in her daughter that the infant began to reject most of her food. By age 2 months she was much below her normal weight and in danger of not physically surviving. So great was this infant's avoidance of ingesting food that, without intervention from her pediatrician and a child psychiatrist, this infant might not have survived physically.

Usually, a mother has access to a sufficient number of people (e.g., a husband, other family members, friends, professional colleagues) to enable her to reasonably gratify her own innate needs in an emotionally pleasurable manner. Thus, when her infant is born, she turns to her newborn with a desire to attune herself to her infant's behavioral and emotional signals and gratify her infant's innate needs in a manner that both satisfies society's developmental taskings and generates pleasure in her infant. To establish such a goodness of fit in her attachment relationship with her infant, she must know how to gratify her infant's innate needs in a manner that reasonably fits with the infant's capabilities (e.g., how much her infant is expected to eat, the proper manner of bottle feeding, how to prepare her breasts for breast-feeding). As a result, her feeding interactions with her infant will most likely lead to the emotionally pleasurable gratification of more than one of her infant's innate needs: the need for food, oral mucosal sensual stimulation, and behavioral stimulation and pleasurable interactions with other humans. Also, in perceiving her infant's emotional pleasure, the mother experiences pleasurable emotions within herself. Thus the mother and her infant engage in a transactional goodness-of-fit attachment process that is emotionally pleasurable to both and that actively changes the behaviors and feelings of both.

Interpersonal transactions between infants and their parents are viewed as a circular process in that the individualized perceptions and behaviors of one influence, and are influenced by, the individualized perceptions and behaviors of the other. Thus any transaction between infants and their parents changes, in varying degrees, both parties. Schaffer (1984) described this transactional relational model between infant and parents as follows:

> The relationship must be regarded as an ever-open system in which mother and child mutually and progressively modify each other's behaviors and remain malleable with respect to external influences. (p. 75)

(It must be noted, however, that, although infants are active in influencing their parents' behaviors toward them in the first 18 months of life, they do not have the capacity to be objective in being aware of both themselves and their parents as being separate others.)

Parents vary in the extent to which they believe they have the power to change their infant and the extent to which they attribute their infant with the power to influence them (Horner 1989). These beliefs can be either consciously perceived by a parent or unconsciously perceived and thereby exert a silent influence on how the parent perceives his or her exchanges with the infant.

For example, a mother who believed that she would fail to be a good mother perceived her infant son's first social selective smile when he reached age 6 weeks. The infant's smile invited his worried mother to engage in an emotionally pleasurable interpersonal transaction. Consequently, the infant's repeated smiling became a new and unexpected social stimulus for this mother. It eventually triggered the mother's reconstruction of her belief that she was destined to be a maternal failure. In her subsequently reconstructed belief, she began to believe that she was providing a good nurturant environment and that she was a good mother. A great part of this mother's now being able to attend to and utilize her infant's smile was the mother's attributing a powerful influence to her infant's smile (and other behaviors of her infant) in shaping her own feelings, beliefs, and behaviors as a mother. Also, her positive response to her infant's smile created a social context for the infant in which he received positive maternal mirroring smiles in response to his own smiles. Several months later, this same mother subsequently reacted to the emergence of her infant's normal 6-month anxiety in response to strangers with a new belief. She correctly believed that her infant feared strangers not because she had failed him as a mother, but because he now recognized his mother in comparison with a stranger and sought to be with her instead of with a stranger.

As the representational world of the infant grows, it continues to interact with the representational world of the parents. In the distinctly human tendency for each person to attempt continually to generate predictive expectancies about his or her new perceptions, the infant and the parents are each involved in an ongoing interpersonal transaction in which each attempts to have the other fit into his or her representational world of aspirations, fantasies, and beliefs about the other. This leads to the question, How does this potentially conflicting group of people survive and continue to mature and develop? For one thing, they are bonded through mutual needs for each other. In a developmentally enhancing goodness of fit, the capabilities of the infant are compatible with the demands and expectations of the parents, as is illustrated in the following example:

A husband and wife were faced with nurturing a profoundly, congenitally deaf newborn. In acknowledging their feelings of inadequacy, the parents sought professional parenting assistance. In time, they understood how much of their perception of the parenting demands made upon them was coming from their infant and how much was coming from their own representational worlds. In reference to the latter, they eventually became aware of feeling guilty about experiencing angry feelings in being given a deaf child. They had been attempting to assuage their guilt by tasking themselves with unrealistic caretaking goals and excessively perfectionistic parenting demands. However, in receiving parenting guidance, they realized that their reaction of anger was similar to that of other parents tasked with raising a seriously handicapped child. This realization helped them achieve the insight that their parenting expectations and feelings of guilt were irrational. In time, a developmentally enhancing goodness of fit began to evolve between these parents and their infant.

In the above-described family, as in all other families, the maintenance of a developmentally enhancing goodness of fit is not a static end point. Parents must continually assess their developmental taskings of their children as they mature. Parents are usually quite attuned to whether their developmental taskings have become pivot points that usher in normal developmental changes or pivot points for the development of a poorness of fit.

Each parent is assisted in his or her attempts to maintain a developmentally enhancing goodness of fit with his or her developing infant through several transactional phenomena. These are discussed below.

Raising a child stimulates parental aspirations and associated conflicts.

The infant, from the moment he or she is thought of, even before the pregnancy, stimulates conscious and unconscious parental aspirations of the type of child the parent hopes to raise, as well as the parent's conscious and unconscious conflicts associated with transactions he or she had with his or her parents regarding his or her own childhood aspirations and ambitions. The following case example illustrates this point:

> A mother wanted to be a lawyer when she was a girl, but never received the support of her parents to follow this career path. Her parents' aspirations for her were singularly focused: she should marry and have several children. Out of fear that her parents would criticize and reject her if she did not embrace their aspirations for her, she identified with those aspirations and married immediately after college. After having two sons, she had a daughter. Shortly after her daughter was born, she was surprised when her husband pointed out to her that she seemed to be preoccupied in mentioning, in an offhand and joking manner, to all their friends, that their daughter would probably be a lawyer. The mother, unaware of her strong unconscious aspirations that her daughter gratify her own frustrated childhood ambition to be a lawyer, laughed at her husband's observation, saying that her thoughts about their daughter becoming a lawyer were "some of my women's liberation stuff."
>
> The mother was not aware of possessing an unconscious abnormal belief that her daughter needed to become a lawyer in

order for the mother to feel that she was a successful mother. This abnormal belief caused the mother to unconsciously enact behaviors that subtly interfered with her daughter's developing autonomy.

During the ensuing first several years of her daughter's life, the mother maintained her unconscious aspiration that her child would be a lawyer. She was not consciously aware of how often she had made these "slips of the tongue" when she referred to her daughter's future. For example, when her daughter was age 5 years, she came home with a friend's doll and stated, "I'm going to be a mom and have lots of babies." The mother automatically, without any forethought, blurted out, "And a professional, too!" When her husband brought these comments to her attention, she angrily rebuffed him and, in an unconsciously generated negative transference reaction in "seeing" her husband as her father, she accused him of trying to hold their daughter back "the way my father held me back. Sometimes you are a jerk, just like he was!" In time, afraid of his wife's angry outbursts, the husband withdrew from her and began to distance himself from his relationship with his daughter.

As the daughter grew older, the mother continued to be unable to acknowledge her unconscious aspirations for her daughter. Any attempt by her husband or close friends to bring these unconsciously denied aspirations to her awareness would cause her to become angry. Her anger hid her inner guilt and shame, the shame she would consciously experience if she admitted to her husband and others that she wanted her daughter to become a lawyer. Her own conscience was telling her that this wish interfered with her ability to support her daughter's autonomy and aspirations. Instead of tolerating the guilt and shame and working on resolving her conflict, the mother reacted with anger and criticism toward her husband and her friends.

A developmentally inhibiting poorness of fit had developed in the relationship between this mother and daughter. Then, as the daughter matured and developed, a second transactional principle began operating that assisted the mother in acknowledging the presence of the inhibition she was unconsciously placing on her daughter's developing autonomy.

Raising a child can fuel or deplete a parent's self-esteem.

An infant is a production of the parents and, as such, becomes an expected source of pride. Most societies teach their adult members that one measure of self-worth is their offspring, and most future parents adopt the belief that, if they produce a thriving and active child, then they are competent and valued parents and respected members of their society. This belief, in addition to other individual, cultural, and religious beliefs, motivates parents to nurture their infants and assists them in assuming the greatest measure of responsibility for their infant's development.

A parent adopts a stance of authority or empowerment in believing he or she is a model with whom his or her children may identify (Kendler 1996). Maccoby (1980) noted that, in the process of good parenting, parents not only teach their children specific behaviors, but primarily offer their children models both of interacting with others and of learning ways of adapting to life's different challenges. Provided with these parental models, children subsequently behave and tend to think, at least initially, in ways similar to those of their parents. Through this process of modeling and imitation, it is as if children hold up a mirror to their parents when children behave or verbally express a thought, feeling, or a belief that is similar to their parents'. This mirror image can bring the parents closer to their children or cause them to distance themselves from their children. Recall, for example, Tim (see above) who, in using his father as a model, presented the father with an aspect of his own self that he, at the moment, could not tolerate, resulting in the father's becoming verbally and physically abusive toward his son. Consequently, the father's self-esteem was lowered to such a painful degree that he was unable to reassess his abusive behavior toward his son in light of his son's later reaction to that behavior (i.e., the son's destruction of his prized basketball).

In the more psychologically aware family, the child's behavior and verbalizations become a mirror image that generates a feeling of pride within the parents. Sensitively aware parents' eyes reflect their pride and self-esteem, which the child observes and eventually takes into his or her representational world. On the other hand, in all psychologically aware families, a child's behavior or verbalized thoughts, wishes, or beliefs can be an unpleasant mirror for the parents to gaze upon when the parents disapprove of those behaviors or verbalizations. When this occurs, parents may notice that their child is behaving or talking like one or both of the parents. The sensitively aware parent is able to use this somewhat painful image of himself or herself to reassess his or her relationship with the child. The parent will then use this reassessment to determine if the prior developmentally enhancing goodness of fit between himself or herself and the child needs some adjustment. A return to the story of the mother who had aspirations to be a lawyer illustrates this point.

> The girl, who was now age 7 years, and her family were gathered at her maternal grandparents' home for Christmas dinner. The mother's brother, a successful accountant, was there with his wife and two sons, ages 4 and 6 years. At one point, the grandparents asked their 7-year-old granddaughter and 6-year-old grandson what they were going to be when they grew up. The boy said he would be an astronaut and the 7-year-old girl stated that she would be a mother, "just like Mommy." Suddenly, the mother blurted out, "Oh no you're not. You're going to be a lawyer first, right?" Immediately noticing the emotional intensity with which she said this, the mother became acutely ashamed and remained silent. Her daughter looked at her intently. The family interaction eventually resumed and nothing more was said of the incident.
>
> Later that evening, the mother sat alone with her husband. She told him that she had been reflecting on what had happened that afternoon, and she acknowledged that he had been right in periodically telling her that she had been denying her (unconscious) wish to live out her frustrated ambition to be a legal professional through their daughter.
>
> The image of herself as a mother—an image her daughter had always focused on—had been held up to her that afternoon at her parents' home. At that moment, she had automatically rejected it. However, with her husband's support, the mother became aware of a conflict within her own representational world between two opposing wishes: one wish was that her daughter would become a lawyer in order for the mother to feel competent, and the other

was to support and nurture her daughter's autonomy and initiative in developing her own aspirations for the future.

The mother's abnormal belief that, to be a competent and proud mother her daughter had to be a lawyer, derived from her frustrated childhood ambition. The mother finally began to accept that she had failed to achieve her childhood ambition and realized that, in pushing her daughter to be a lawyer, she was repeating what had happened to her as a child: not getting support from her mother and father for her own independent adult aspirations. Once the mother began to acknowledge that her old frustrated ambition could not be gratified through her daughter, she became more able to use her good maternal empathy in sensing the negative effect she was having on her daughter.

This leads to the next transactional process that assists a parent in assessing and maintaining the degree of goodness of fit between himself or herself and a child.

Raising a child stimulates parental empathy. *Empathy* is an advanced perceptual ability in which an observer is able to intuit, to some degree, the feelings and thoughts of another. It is a uniquely human ability which becomes activated when a person temporarily suspends concentration on his or her representational world and comes close to experiencing what another person is feeling or thinking.

For children's innate empathic ability to emerge and develop, they must receive ministrations of empathy from their parents. Parental empathy becomes one of the ways in which parents intuitively monitor the effects of their behaviors, aspirations, and beliefs on their children. The children then play back to their parents what they have been receiving. However, they do not play back an exact replica of what their parents send. Instead, they form their own representations of what they sense and play back their own impressions of their parents' actions. Parents, in using empathy, can become attuned to their children's emotional and behavioral reactions to their behaviors, beliefs, aspirations, and demands. When parents use empathy, they become more aware of their own representational world and more aware of conscious and unconscious motivations and personal beliefs in reference to their children.

I return once again to the example of the mother who unconsciously wished that her daughter would become a lawyer.

> A few days after the incident at the grandparents' home, the mother was alone with her daughter. The mother asked her daughter if she remembered what the mother had said to her at her grandmother's house, when her grandmother had asked her what she would like to be when she grew up. The girl now hesitantly answered her mother, "No, I just remember Grandma asked us what we would be when we all grew up." The daughter then sat quietly. Using her maternal empathy, the mother sensed a degree of tension and confusion in the quietly sitting child.
>
> The mother then was able to put herself in her child's shoes, and, in essence, spoke for her child in a way in which the mother believed her child was fearful of speaking herself. The mother told her, "I know it wasn't easy for you at your grandmother's house to hear me say that I wanted you grow up and be something other than a mommy. I don't want you to think that I wouldn't be happy if you wanted to be a mommy. Sometimes moms make mistakes in telling their children that they have to grow up to be just one thing, like I tell you a lot to be a lawyer. But it's better and makes children happier if they feel that their mom and dad want them to grow up and be whatever they want to be. Maybe you'll decide someday to be a mommy, or a lawyer and a mommy, but I want you to decide that for yourself as you grow up." The little girl looked pensively at her mother, and then said, "Well, you know, if I decide to be a mommy, you have to show me how to do it!" She then spontaneously leaned over and hugged her mother.

Whether this little girl understood all that her mother was telling her is less important than the following transactional message the mother was sending to her child: I will always listen to you and to myself, and I will always try to talk to you about things that happen between us that may be making you feel uncomfortable.

On another level, what the mother had actually told her daughter was something the mother, during her childhood, had wished she had received from her own mother or father. In giving her daughter a degree of empathy that she had not received as a child, the mother was tolerating her inevitable feelings of sadness for herself as a child who did not have a mother and father who supported the development of her autonomous identity. This mother was now able to use her transactions with her child as a catalyst to rework—through activating the assimilation-transference, accommodation-transformation, and hierarchical restructuring processes—and eventually reconstruct her previous belief that her daughter had to be a lawyer into a new belief that her daughter would arrive at her own future decisions. In so doing, the mother once again established a developmentally enhancing goodness of fit between herself and her daughter. She was able to achieve true generational progress—that is, she was not transferring faulty parenting transactions from one generation to the next and not repeating the same mistakes her parents had made with her (Hiatt 1971). Subsequently, the mother was able to construct new representations of herself as a competent mother and recognize that, in some respects, she had become a better parent to her child than her own parents had been to her.

In summary, the goodness-of-fit process is one of transaction and mutual change. Only recently have developmental researchers begun to realize the infant's earliest active contribution to this process. Now the infant's and child's own biological and psychological maturational advances and the organizing principles used in processing these advances to engage in social transactions with his or her parents are accepted as the ingredients for defining pivot points in the sequential progression of developmental phases.

Developmental Phases and Major Developmental Tasks

Given the manner in which representations are transformed, newly constructed, and hierarchically prioritized by the mind in response to developmental change, it is clear that personal development is "not a series of linear additions, but a gradual reorganization of the past and the present. Once reorganized the past or old elements or structures are transformed" (Sroufe and Rutter 1984, p. 20). Schaffer (1984) noted the sequential nature of these reorganizations and further noted that they periodically enable a new level of integration to occur in the child's mental life. These points of reorganization represent transition or pivot points that usher in a new phase in the child's mental development. Determining when these transition points will occur in each child is not easy, particularly because the developmental changes that ultimately lead to them evolve from the transactions between biological, social, and psychological variables.

One way of conceptualizing the normal life cycle of mental development is to postulate a series of developmental phases; the transition points between phases would then be those points in time when a child has mastered a cluster of major developmental tasks. Major developmental tasks, in essence, are what each particular society believes the child must first acquire as new knowledge and then apply in new learning experiences. The acquired new knowledge involves a child's learning how to gratify his or her innate needs, express his or her emotions, and demonstrate his or her cognitive capabilities while concurrently adapting to the needs of his or her societal group (e.g., family, peers). In other words, once children master their major developmental tasks, they are prepared to engage within relationships characterized by a developmentally enhancing goodness of fit, in both the familial and societal context.

It must be noted, however, that the remarkable complexity of the human mind—particularly its ability to process different combinations of biological, psychological, and social stimuli—makes it difficult to define the normal age at which each major developmental task should be achieved. The choice of the age span defined for each developmental phase depends on how a certain developmental researcher arbitrarily clusters major developmental tasks, and even this clustering will be influenced by the biases of the researcher (see discussion of the observer's bias in Chapter 1). It should come as no surprise, therefore, that different textbooks on normal development divide up the life cycle differently. For example, the developmental phase of childhood can be defined as the period between ages 2 and 12 years, or childhood can be divided, as in this book, into infancy (birth to age 18 months), toddlerhood (ages 18 months to 3 years), early childhood (ages 3–6 years), late childhood (ages 6–11 years), and adolescence (ages 12–19 years).

It is now recognized that the overall process of development is a flexible, fluid, and variable one. Developmentalists such as Emde (1983) have cautioned that the adverse effects of early life should not be viewed as irreversible and that there needs to be more faith in the power of later life experiences. Thus it is not necessarily required that a person attain a major developmental task during a particular phase for that person to be assured of making further developmental progress. On the contrary, the major tasks defined for each phase represent more of a beginning than an ending. Each child begins to attain each major task during the developmental phase in which it emerges and continues to develop it during succeeding developmental phases. Each task, therefore, involves the maturation and development of psychological stimuli (i.e., representations stored as long-term memories) that show high continuity throughout all developmental phases of the life cycle. The mental representations that are constructed by children when they attain these major developmental tasks become psychological building blocks that influence and either enhance or inhibit the child's attainment of later developmental tasks.

In the following chapters, one possible set of major developmental tasks is defined for each phase in the life cycle; however, again, it is important to remember that each developmental phase is not rigorously tied to a specific duration of time (Pine 1985).

■ Continuity Versus Discontinuity in Mental Development

The hypothesis that a child's life cycle can be organized into developmental phases is difficult to define operationally because the mental developmental process is both continuous and discontinuous (Emde and Harmon 1984; Kagan 1971a; Rutter 1984).

In stating that the mental development process is continuous, one accepts that the premise that a transition into the next developmental phase depends on having completed—at least to a certain degree—the developmental tasks of the preceding phase. Major theories of development have tended to be unilinear (Meissner 1980) in that each stage is built upon by the next.

R. Tyson (1986) described this approach as the *Lego view,* after the toy building blocks that interconnect. According to this view, when one block is damaged or faulty, then all further growth of the structure is destined to be potentially shaky or faulty. Many aspects of maturation and development can be viewed as manifesting the type of continuous growth that follows this model. For example, toddlers must become competent in walking before they can run.

Researchers espousing the Lego point of view have postulated that early experience is the crucial determining factor in shaping all later development. Consequently, they strongly support the position that, when early experience is faulty, all later development will be more or less faulty. Erikson (1959) espoused a congruent theory, known as the *epigenetic principle,* in which it was postulated that everything that grows has a plan or blueprint; Lego-like parts are stacked according to that growth plan, with each part having its own special time for growing and all parts being crucial building blocks for a functioning individual.

However, for many children, new, unexpected, developmentally enhancing life experiences often enable them to master developmental tasks that had not been mastered in earlier phases. It is these non-phase-related experiences that are emphasized in the discontinuous or nonlinear view of mental development. According to this view, there can and often do exist specific times in the life cycle in which unexpected physical or cognitive abilities emerge or unexpected social events occur, none of which appear to be the direct result of prior competencies or social transactions (R. Tyson 1986). These discontinuities represent significant times of transition in a particular child's mental and behavioral abilities and his or her social environment.

Kagan (1984), a proponent of the existence of discontinuities during the life cycle, has noted the following:

> Many observers want the past to seriously constrain the present through material links that join the universal milestones of growth into a forged chain. Each child must step on every link—no skipping permitted—as he or she journeys into maturity. . . . [However], one cannot explain a 10-year-old's phobia of horses or Proust's aestheticism by listing their respective experiences as

infants. Each person can be understood only as a coherence of many, many past events. . . . Each developmental journey contains many points where one can move in any one of several directions. (pp. 110–111)

R. Tyson (1986) referred to the *Playdough view* of mental development as one in which new, discontinuous abilities add to the overall developmental structure and thereby transform and remold a child's emerging maturation and development. According to this model, a "new piece of clay" can patch up defects present from earlier stages of development. This contrasts with the Lego view in which it is argued that a defect or deficiency from an earlier developmental stage remains an ongoing impediment.

■ Critical Periods Versus Sensitive Periods for Mastering Developmental Tasks

Closely related to the discussion of whether mental development is continuous or discontinuous is whether certain developmental tasks must be attained during certain periods to be fully mastered. The crucial aspect of Erikson's (1959) epigenetic principle is that, for proper mental developmental progress to occur, the person must engage and learn critical developmental tasks at the proper time and in the proper sequence. Implicit in this principle is the recognition that there are critical periods in which a certain task can be optimally learned; also implied is that, if a task is not learned during the critical period, it can never be attained to its full potential. R. Tyson (1986) also noted that, according to this view, a child's failure during one phase to attain a major developmental task, learn a new concept, or learn new information is believed to result in discernible vulnerabilities and incompetencies in all subsequent phases.

The variability of the developmental process as manifested by many children has led researchers to reassess whether these critical periods actually exist. Studies have revealed that adherence to a strict stepwise attainment of major developmental tasks at specific ages invariably causes developmental researchers to 1) overvalue the on-time achievement of major developmental tasks and 2) undervalue the positive effects of later life (e.g., unexpected achievements in a child who had failed to master one or more developmental tasks at the expected age). Some children appear to be able to learn developmental tasks usually conquered earlier in the life cycle at a later time in their lives. Thus many developmentalists have replaced the critical period concept with a *sensitive period concept.* This latter concept holds that a child will learn in the manner that is optimal for him or her, based on his or her own potential, and thereby attain certain developmental tasks better, and often with less training, at certain task-specific sensitive times in the life cycle than at other times.

It is my view that defined major developmental tasks can be only the most general road map to assess a child's progress along the developmental ladder, and that progress through defined developmental stages is highly variable. This view acknowledges that 1) sensitive periods, more than critical periods, exist in which developmental tasks can be eventually learned, and 2) it is difficult to predict what, if any, discontinuities will occur in each child's life and how the discontinuities will affect his or her mental development. A discontinuity can lead to the reconstruction of preexisting faulty representations and the formation of entirely new representations, aspects of the child's representational world can be repaired into a healthier overall structure.

Changes in the Child's Genotypic Expression as Influencing the Phasic Phenotypic Progression of Mental Development

Only since the 1970s have geneticists begun giving attention to theories about the continuities and discontinuities in the human developmental life cycle (Goldsmith 1986). Instead of just focusing on cross-sectional studies of specific temperamental traits and their genetic and environmental underpinnings (Goldsmith 1986), geneticists have become interested in conducting longitudinal studies that address temporal change in genotypic expression over time (Plomin 1986; Scarr and McCartney 1983).

The unfolding of infants' maturational advances in their biological and psychological nature points to the existence of a control mechanism that seems to physically regulate which genes are active during the child's overall maturational growth (Kendler 1995).

An infant's *genotype* consists of all the infant's preprogrammed innate and emerging maturational abilities. An infant's *phenotype* refers to the actual surface behaviors and mental activities manifested as the infant constructs a representational world through interaction with the environment. In processes yet to be understood, the infant's sociocultural environment has a shaping influence on the infant's genotype so that similar genotypes can give rise to different phenotypes (Plomin 1990; Reiss et al. 1991).

Earlier in this chapter, I emphasize that infants mature by demonstrating the emergence of biological and psychological competencies and abilities. These, in turn, influence and are influenced by parents and other caretakers and eventually by infants' prior memories (i.e., the psychological stimuli that make up their representational world). In the process of repeating behaviors, interacting with others, and using memories of prior learning, these maturational competencies develop. In addition, the goodness of fit between infants, with their genetically controlled emerging maturational capabilities, and their parents, with their caretaking behaviors and their reactions toward their infant's overall behaviors, will either primarily enhance or inhibit the infant's developmental process.

Kendler and Eaves (1986) have presented three models for the joint effect of genes and environment on influencing a child's vulnerability to develop psychiatric illness. These models can also provide a means for understanding the complicated processes that transpire in the transactional goodness of fit between most psychologically aware parents and their children.

Additive effects of genotype and environment. According to this model, an infant can possess a genetically controlled innate temperamental trait (e.g., distractibility). This aspect of the infant's genotype would encounter a parenting environment that may or may not be predisposed to provide a developmentally enhancing goodness of fit versus a developmentally inhibiting poorness of fit. However, in this model, the degree of the infant's distractibility is not a factor in creating the type of environmental response the infant encounters. Thus an infant with a genetic endowment that produces a high degree of distractibility would have no higher probability of being exposed to a developmentally enhancing or developmentally inhibiting parental response to his or her distractibility than an infant born with a low degree of distractibility.

Therefore, in this model, transactional changes are not viewed as significantly affecting the infant's phenotypic development. The effects of the infant's genotype and the parenting behaviors and attitudes the infant encounters are simply additive. One does not influence what the other brings to their goodness-of-fit interaction, and one does not change the other through a transactional process.

This model explains the poor fit between, for example, a blind infant and parents who have no tolerance for blind people; however, it was not helpful to a developmental researcher who was trying to understand how an infant boy born with high distractibility and his depressed mother were able to engage within a developmentally enhancing goodness of fit when the infant was age 1 year. That mother told the researcher that her infant boy's distractibility (his genotype) changed her in that his distractibility became a demand on her that distracted her from dwelling on her own depression. She stated,

> His fussiness pulled me over to him and out of myself. He made me realize that my being a mother was as important as being a wife. When he was born, my husband abandoned me, and I withdrew into myself. But my friends noticed how easily distracted and upset my infant was, right from the beginning. I gradually realized that he needed me to pay attention to what he was doing so that he wouldn't get too stimulated. (R. Solomon, personal communication, December 1992)

As Solnit and Neubauer (1986) stated,

> In many of these instances, the child's [genotypic] vulnerabilities activate potential resources within the parents. (p. 24)

Genetic control of the infant's sensitivity to the environment. In this model, the infant's genotype is viewed as dictating whether the infant is sensitive to a more nurturant versus a relatively nonnurturant environment (Kendler and Eaves 1986). Thus an infant can be born with a certain degree of sensitivity to his or her parents' distractibility. When such an infant's sensitivity is high, the emerging goodness of fit will be quite poor or developmentally inhibiting in this distractible parenting environment (e.g., when the parents are unpredictable in their soothing, when they do not protect their infant from excessive stimulation, when they are easily distracted themselves from following through on initiated caregiving activities). However, when the infant's sensitivity to his or her parents' distractibility is low, the emerging goodness of fit will not be as developmentally inhibiting despite the parents' providing a quite distractible environment. In this model, the parenting environment dictates whether an infant with a high degree of sensitivity to parental distraction will become engaged in a developing inhibiting goodness-of-fit interaction. This model tends to place the infant in the passive and reactive position, with the parents being the sole activators of the goodness-of-fit relationship.

Genetic control of exposure to the environment. In this model, the infant's genotype is viewed as having an influence on the type of parenting the infant will receive. Thus an infant can be born with a high or low degree of distractibility. The infant's genetically induced distractibility (his or her genotype) will then influence what kind of environmental response the infant receives from his or her parents. Thus the degree of distractibility present in the infant does not directly cause a developmentally enhancing or inhibiting goodness of fit to emerge. Rather, the goodness of fit between the infant and his or her parents depends on the parents' response to the distractibility in their infant. If the distractibility alienates them, the goodness of fit will become developmentally inhibiting. If the infant's distractibility does not affect them negatively, it will not adversely affect the emergence of a developing enhancing goodness of fit. In this model, the infant is attributed with an active position, and the parents are attributed with a relatively passive and reactive position.

A new model of developmental genetics. What is absent in these three models is an appreciation of the postulate that infants and their parents are mutually influenced by each other's behaviors. With such appreciation, a new model would emerge that combines aspects of each of these three models and adds to them. Definitely, the additive aspects of the first model have validity. In addition, the second model's highlighting of the presence of genetically induced infant sensitivities to the environment is also useful in understanding the process of goodness of fit. Finally, the third model highlights that genetically induced infant characteristics at birth can alienate or attract the parents.

What needs to emerge from further research within the new field of developmental genetics (Goldsmith 1986) is a new model that addresses how the ongoing transactions between infants and their parents affect the dynamic shifting on and off of the pool of structural genes that reside within each infant and parent. Consequently, it is presently not known if and how an infant's temperament can be the catalyst for the switching on within a parent of a group of structural genes that catalyzes the emergence of new parenting behaviors and abilities. It is theorized that new parenting behaviors may have been locked away as maturational potentials within the parent that required the triggering influence of having to parent a child with a particular temperament and during a specific phase of the child's development. Perhaps this is the genetically controlled maturational process that is captured in the observation given by one parent who was interviewed by me when the mother took part in a study of child development:

> I changed a great deal when I became a parent, and in particular, with one of my children I changed the most. I have feelings and do things now that I never thought I would have done. It's as if I've changed in a special way through each of my children.

Of course, the genesis of new infant behaviors and new parenting behaviors does not necessarily mean that their emergence is controlled at the level of genetic coding, and in particular, within the domain of a switching on and off of structural genes. The relevance of these recently enunciated genetic hypotheses to understanding the phenomena of developmental continuities and discontinuities can be assessed only through further research. For example, Kendler (1996) noted that a particular adult's parenting is

> influenced by attitudes derived from the parent's family of origin
> as well as genetically influenced by parental temperamental characteristics. The elicitation of parenting by children is influenced
> by temperamental traits of the offspring that are, in turn, under
> partial genetic control. (p. 11)

In this report, although Kendler postulated that both parents' and children's genotypes influence how they interact, further research needs to address how parents' and children's temperamental characteristics are modified through that interaction (i.e., which temperamental characteristics show continuity and which show discontinuity over time).

In summary, genetic influences play an ongoing part in the process of maturation and development. Two questions to add to the list of current unanswered questions and disagreements about the process of normal human development are, 1) How do regulating genes turn on and off structural genes? and 2) How are these switching events influenced both by social experiences and by the representational world that is constructed by the child?

Chapter 3

Infant Phase of Mental Development

Birth to Age 18 Months

Major Developmental Tasks of Infancy

During the infancy phase, which I define as extending from birth through age 18 months, the major developmental tasks are as follows:

1. *Infants begin to develop the awareness that they are separate from and valued and loved by their parents.* This awareness is achieved by their acquiring new knowledge through developmental changes, storing that knowledge within their long-term implicit memories, and then consolidating that knowledge through learning experiences in which their parents view and treat them as separate individuals with their own needs, feelings, and actions. It should be noted that this beginning self-awareness is only a subjective self-awareness, meaning that infants do not have the capacity to be self-reflective

and become aware of having a separate mind and body in a world of other separate minds and bodies. Instead, they experience their actions, sensations, and perceptions only subjectively. The sense of an objective self is not developed until about age 18 months.

2. *Infants begin to become aware that their parents can be trusted to feed, shelter, protect, and stimulate them in more emotionally pleasurable than emotionally displeasurable ways.* This awareness is achieved by their gradually learning that their parents are reliable and predictable in fulfilling their needs and exposing them to people and situations that similarly respect their needs.

3. *Infants begin to become aware that they are engaged in transactional relationships with their parents and begin to actively attend and reactively respond to what is going on in those relationships* (J. B. Miller 1991). This awareness develops in large part as infants sense and learn to act in response to their parents' emotions and parents sense and learn to act in response to their infant's emotions.

Functions of the Social Environment

Infants must learn that there exists a social world of people, animals, and inanimate objects that emit stimuli that vary in their frequency, intensity, and complexity. As infants begin to differentiate these social stimuli, they slowly learn that the social environment performs many functions; these functions are in the service of society's goals of nurturing, protecting, educating, and making them socialized members of society. As noted in Chapter 2, five distinct functions can be listed. Throughout all phases of the life cycle, these five functions support parents' provision of a dynamically changing, developmentally enhancing, transactional goodness of fit with their children. In this section, I describe how these functions pertain to the infancy phase of the life cycle.

■ Providing Truthful Information About the Infant's Body and Surrounding World

One major developmental task of infancy is for infants to become aware that they can trust their parents (Erikson 1959). Parents instill such a sense of trust in their infants by becoming consistently reliable conveyors of truthful information about the world the infant has entered (Magnusson and Allen 1983). For example, when a mother consistently provides her infant daughter with the appropriate type of food when she is hungry, and feeds her in a way that allows her to digest it, her daughter begins to perceive that this set of social stimuli is being provided by a reliable source of truthful information—namely, her mother. The infant eventually learns that, when she experiences a specific type of internal stimulation, her mother provides her with substances that cause this internal stimulation to be pleasurably abated. The infant then uses this knowledge to continue to learn about the world.

When infants learn to trust their parents, they can then begin to perceive that other human beings can be trusted to protect, nourish, and pleasurably interact with them. Only once they learn to trust others can children become adults who believe that cooperative relationships with others are necessary to ensure not only their own physical survival but also the survival of their society. Societies that teach their children to not trust others produce adults with a "dog-eat-dog" mentality. This mentality usually is anathema to a society's overall developmental progress.

By being a reliable source of accurate information, parents also teach their infants an important truth about how people remain in relationship to each other—namely, that the occurrence of certain behaviors and events in life are contingent on the prior occurrence of one or more behaviors or events. In other words, they teach their infant to trust that predictable cause-and-effect relationships exist between people and between events. For example, infants slowly learn that the provision of food is contingent on the actions of one or both parents. Later they learn that the provision of food is also contingent on their own actions (e.g., crying or reaching for the mother's breast or a bottle) and that their parents consistently and reliably respond to those actions.

Sensitively aware parents expose their infants to only those truthful aspects of life that they are able to understand and learn about and that will not expose them to harm. When these aspects of life generate more pleasurable than displeasurable feelings, infants learn that their world can be trusted as one that provides caretaking activities and reacts to their own behaviors in a consistently reliable and predictable manner. Infants then recall the reliability and predictability of these experiences and the pleasurable emotions they engendered so that, when they are presented with new stimuli, they are motivated to seek new pleasurable interactions with their parents or others.

■ Providing Stimulus Modulation and Protection

Infants are innately endowed with the ability to stimulate their own innate needs—that is, to generate biological stimuli—which in turn cause them to actively seek social stimuli. At the same time, infants are similarly endowed with the ability to perceive and react to social stimuli. Infants are not innately endowed, however, with mental structures that provide them with the knowledge that their self-initiated activities can also expose them to emotionally displeasurable and even life-threatening situations. Also, they are not endowed with the innate knowledge that they need parents or other caretakers to 1) protect them from danger, 2) signal them when danger is near, and 3) respond to their distress signals when they are being over- or understimulated. Consequently, when infants actively seek stimulation (e.g., reach out to touch an object), parents must be vigilant in protecting them from their own actions that might expose them to physically dangerous types of stimulation. For example, the visual stimulus of a bright light will cause an alert, satiated, and temperature-regulated 5-month-old infant boy to turn his head toward it, whether the light emanates from a flashlight or an exposed flame. If the light comes from an exposed flame, the infant obviously can be seriously burned.

When parents observe their infant approaching a dangerous situation, they communicate the impending danger by sending their own behavioral and emotional signals to the infant before the infant sends out any distress signals of his or her own. For example, if a father observes his infant daughter approaching the stairs, he may give her a behavioral signal (e.g., hold up his hands in a stopping gesture) to warn her of the potential danger. If this does not work, he will pick her up to prevent her from falling. Alternatively, he may send his daughter an emotional signal, manifested in his facial expression of fear and apprehension.

Infants are preprogrammed to sense and comprehend their parents' behavioral and emotional signals. Within days after birth, they display the ability to "read" their parents' looks of apprehension, an ability called *social referencing* by Emde and Buchsbaum (1989) but which I label *emotional referencing*; Emde and Buchsbaum defined social referencing as a form of "active emotional communication which occurs when a child encounters a situation of uncertainty and looks to a significant other for an emotional signal to resolve it" (p. 120). In using this innate perceptual ability, infants eventually learn that their parents are a point of reference to be used in guiding their future behaviors. This ability can be demonstrated in the following example (Walk and Gibson 1961; see also Figure 3–1):

> A normally developing 6-month-old boy is placed on a special table, the edge of which has been extended with a clear piece of firm plastic (a "visual cliff"). Then, in a demonstration of the innate visual depth perceptual ability that infants seem to possess, he crawls to the natural edge of the table, looks over it, appears to perceive the apparent drop off, and stops before attempting to crawl further. Once he stops, he automatically turns and looks for his mother. On seeing her, he specifically focuses on her face. Then (as documented by Klinnert et al. [1983]), if his mother shows a facial expression of fear, he will invariably maintain his hesitation and not go forward. However, if the mother smiles when he looks at her, he will invariably crawl over the natural edge of the table.

Thus infants learn to either trust their mother's emotional communications as reliably protective, as in this example, or mistrust them because they cause them to repeatedly experience emotional or physical displeasure.

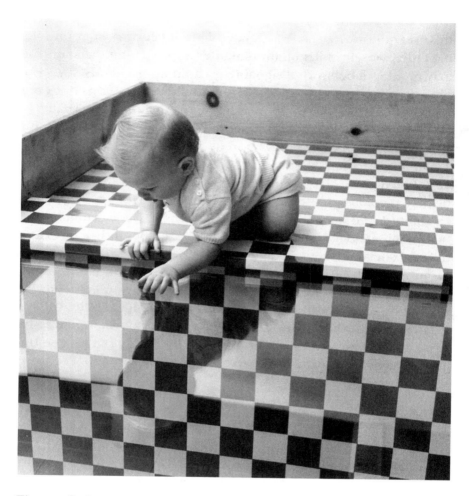

Figure 3–1. A 6-month-old boy crawls across a table and hesitates in reaching the edge, which has been extended with a piece of firm, clear plastic in a test of emotional referencing.
Source.   Photograph by William Vandivert; reprinted with permission from *Scientific American,* April 1960.

Parents must also provide the social functions of modulating the quality of the stimulation their infant is exposed to so that they can keep the overall stimulation within their optimal range. For example, they must protect their infant from the following:

1. *Receiving too much stimulation*—For example, whereas an infant girl will take pleasure in being rocked by her mother (when that stimulation is within her optimal stimulation range), she will begin to cry if she is rocked excessively.

2. *Receiving not enough stimulation*—For example, when parents repeatedly place their infant in a crib with no toys, or allow him or her to go for prolonged periods without interacting with either one of them or anyone else, the infant may show his or her displeasure by crying.

3. *Receiving overly repetitive and potentially monotonous stimulation*—For example, if a flashlight focused directly on an infant's face is left on for several hours, it becomes monotonous because the infant has already attained knowledge of this particular object, thus rendering the object no longer novel; however, if left on for only 1 minute, the light can be pleasurably stimulating.

4. *Receiving stimulation in a sensory modality that their infant will process into perceptions that are overstimulating*—For example, if parents present stimuli to their infant boy through a specific sensory modality that is difficult for him to process, and continue to communicate through that modality, their infant will become overwhelmed because the perceptions he constructs in response to those sensory messages will stimulate him above his upper stimulation threshold. The infant will then express his distress by crying. Greenspan (1989) illustrated this point in stating the following:

> In some families where the infant seemed to have difficulty organizing auditory experience, caregivers responded with anxiety and talked to the infant very rapidly, overwhelming the system that was having the most difficulty. Their infants often withdrew from the human environment. On the other hand, there were rare caregivers who intuitively slowed down their vocalizations and experimented with pitch and rhythm. They talked, for example, in low-pitched voices and repeated themselves, offering less novelty to the infant who was slow to process auditory information. They also appealed to the infants' visual, tactile, and other senses as a way to communicate information. (p. 607)

All of the above examples of inappropriate levels of stimulation will generate displeasurable feelings in infants and result in their displaying distressful behaviors, such as crying or visual gaze aversion and head turning.

Psychologically aware parents seem to be preprogrammed to interpret their infants' behavioral distress signals as meaning that they are experiencing displeasurable feelings. Even first-time parents who have little prior experience in caring for infants will intuitively know that their infant's cry is a signal of distress. They will then modulate or modify their infant's stimulation level. However, parents do not innately know which sensory modalities are innately preferred by their infant and which, if any, sensory modalities innately predispose their infant to experience emotional displeasure. In those cases, if parents use empathy to sense and understand what their infant is experiencing, they will often be able to sense that their infant is receiving a level of stimulation that generates displeasurable feelings. Parents then intuitively act to modulate the level of the infant's stimulation before the infant has to distressfully signal his or her approaching displeasure.

Once infants begin to acquire knowledge about whether or not their parents are to be trusted, they will recall this stored knowledge when faced with future overstimulating, understimulating, or ambiguous situations. Depending on whether these implicit memories contain an awareness that their parents can or cannot be trusted to protect them from highly emotionally displeasurable experiences, infants will evoke either a positive expectation that their parents will intervene with protective emotional signals and behaviors or a negative expectation that their parents will not intervene.

■ Providing Encouragement, Support, and Admiration

Just as infants turn to their parents for behavioral and emotional signals when they are embarking on novel or ambiguous behaviors, they will also turn to their parents for such signals when they are in the midst of or have recently completed a behavior stimulated by one of their innate needs (e.g., sucking on the mother's breast nipple), new maturational advances (e.g., initiating crawling), or new developmental achievements (e.g., eating with a spoon). Parents must respond to these infant behaviors with support, encouragement, and admiration. These become the crucial ingredients of infants' construction of internal perceptions of themselves as admirable and valuable. When these perceptions are stored as long-term memories, they become the forerunners of infants' future positive self-esteem. When infants recall pleasurable memories of their parents' encouragement and admiration of their previous behaviors, they will then evoke a positive expectation that their parents will respond to each new maturationally emerging behavior with continued admiration and support. Thus these memories become a source of internal stimulation that motivates infants to continue to seek actively their parents' admiration and support.

■ Providing Truthful Information About Achieving Gratification of Innate Needs

Although infants are preprogrammed to stimulate their own innate needs, they do not have the innate knowledge that permits them to know how to have those needs gratified. Specifically, they do not know what knowledge they must acquire and what behaviors they must master in order to become a productive member of society, nor do they know how they must adapt the expression of their innate needs and maturationally emerging capabilities to society's rules and guidelines. These behaviors are taught to infants and children by their parents (e.g., how to use the eating utensils preferred by their society, how to use speech to properly express anger) prior to sending their child to formal grade school. Once their children are in grade school, parents' work continues as they support other developmental tasks that society defines for the grade school child.

■ Providing Adaptive Solutions to Emotionally Displeasurable Life Events

In learning the above four functions of society, infants also learn that emotionally displeasurable events occur during their life, despite the best efforts of their parents and others to protect them from such events.

Parens (1979) described two types of displeasurable experiences for the developing infant: those that generate benign displeasure and those that generate excessive displeasure. *Benignly displeasurable experiences* are those in which the intensity of an infant's displeasurable feelings is not so severe as to prevent the infant from habituating, assimilating, or accommodating to the stimuli and ultimately adapting his or her needs to the situation at hand. At times, parents may directly assist their infant in dealing with benignly displeasurable stimuli, whereas at other times they may not intercede but instead will allow their infant to arrive at his or her own manner of achieving self-regulation. In the latter situation, the parents begin to allow their infant to engage in and attempt to regulate for himself or herself those experiences that are emotionally displeasurable. Parens's *excessively displeasurable experiences* are what I note in Chapter 1 to be traumatic experiences (i.e., those that cause an excessive and sustained degree of displeasurable feelings and from which an infant, child, or adult cannot withdraw or which the person cannot terminate).

Parents try to protect their children from experiencing severe physical hurts as well as other traumatic experiences. However, children gradually discover that moderately emotionally displeasurable and moderately physically painful experiences are a part of life, and that their parents are not omnipotent in being able to spare them from these experiences. Parents can only attempt to keep their child's number of displeasurable experiences within the benignly displeasurable category and try to protect their child from experiences in the excessively displeasurable or traumatic category.

As children grow older, their parents usually continue to monitor how much displeasure they can tolerate. In addition, parents begin to allow their children to gradually experience more displeasurable feelings without attempting to immediately alleviate the cause of those feelings. This eventually allows children to construct a belief in their ability to tolerate and eventually ameliorate their own displeasurable feelings, which in turn leads to their developing a belief that they have the ability to self-regulate their emotions. Children who are allowed to go through this process grow up prepared for life's inevitable minor hardships that occur as they asser-tively explore the world.

It is unfortunate that traumatic experiences do occur in many children's lives. In the most tragic cases, the perpetrator of the trauma can be one or both of a child's parents (e.g., in cases of physical or sexual abuse). More often, however, the perpetrator is either a criminal (e.g., a child rapist [Terr 1993]) or an unexpected calamity (e.g., an automobile accident). When children experience such traumatic events, they are led to question whether their par-ents can protect them from a future experience that is terrifying and potentially physically harmful. When such events occur, par-ents must fulfill the social function of assisting their child in learn-ing to tolerate and potentially master the displeasurable feelings associated with the trauma. Only then will their child begin to re-construct new representations of the traumatic event, which will prevent the original traumatic memory from becoming a develop-mentally inhibiting force in the child's life.

The Organizational Mental Structures of the Id, Ego, Superego, and Self

S. Freud (1923/1963) conceptualized the mind as developing into three major structures: the id, ego and superego. Although the self was also described by Freud, its more complete definition is attrib-uted to post-Freudian developmentalists such as Kohut (1971), Kernberg (1982), and Havens (1986). The id, ego, superego, and self are conceptualized as complex organizational structures, each containing a group of mental structures that carries out a set of mental functions. (A *mental function* is defined as the mind's ap-plication of one or more mental structures, mental processes, or both for the purpose of attaining one of the mind's goals.) As col-lections of mental structures, the id, ego, superego, and self are more complex than elemental informational and processing struc-tures, such as the representational structures labeled as perceptions, conceptions, emotions, and memories. The phenomena of the id, ego, superego, and self are merely theoretical constructs that segregate groups of mental functions under a particular overall goal.

Id. The *id* is the container of the infant's innate needs. As such, the id's goal is to generate psychological stimuli (i.e., sensory stimuli) of innate needs. Be definition, the id occupies the systematic unconscious domain and can never enter into the preconscious or conscious domain. However, innate needs present within the id become sources of internal sensory stimuli.

The id seeks the gratification of all its innate needs; the infant's self (see below) must learn how to gratify those needs in a way that is acceptable to the infant's parents and society. This is not an easy task because the innate needs "press" for unfettered gratification. As Sandler et al. (1973) noted,

> The instinctual wishes in the unconscious have a peremptory quality. . . . [They] can be considered as thrusting forward "blindly" toward overt expression in consciousness and behavior. (p. 32)

Because one of these innate needs is the infant's need to attach to another in an emotionally pleasurable relationship, the id is no longer thought of as some "wild horse" that must be eventually tamed by the developing child's ego, superego, and self and the child's parents and society.

Ego. Whereas the id is an internal stimulus generator of innate needs, the *ego* is a collection of informational and programming "files" of emotions, temperamental characteristics, and cognitive, verbal language, and physical capabilities. The ego receives stimuli from biological sources (the body), psychological sources (the id), and social sources (the actions of other individuals). After receiving these biopsychosocial stimuli, the ego integrates them into the mind's prior representations and conceptions in accordance with the mind's organizing principles (e.g., the stimulus principle, the representation principle, the accommodation-transformation principle, the hierarchical restructuring principle) and then generates mental and behavioral "products" or information (i.e., perceptions, conceptions, emotions, verbal language, surface behaviors, and memories) for the self.

To accomplish its goal, the ego performs a variety of mental functions and activates all of the infant's behaviors (Greenspan 1989; Hartman 1939; Kernberg 1987; Rapaport 1959); these mental functions and behaviors are grouped together as *ego functions*. These ego functions are usually listed as follows:

- Reception of sensory input
- Integration of biopsychosocial sensory stimuli
- Generation of emotions
- Formation of perceptions and conceptions
- Production of verbal language
- Formation, storage, and recall of memories
- Utilization of defense mechanisms
- Generation of transference reactions
- Activation of all surface behaviors

Thus ego functions cover all innate and maturationally emerging mental processing abilities and all surface behaviors, including language, that are either innately available or learned in adapting innate needs to the developmental taskings of parents and society.

Inherent in the process of conception formation is the ego's ability to comprehend new perceptual representations, compare them with preexisting representations, and engage in assimilation and accommodation integration processes. In this way, the ego's functions are organized under the goal of being the mind's overall integrating and comprehending structure and also allows the mind to differentiate more and more complex perceptions.

The ego operates silently and hence unconsciously. Infants and children will never directly experience their egos; they will experience them only indirectly through observing their own mental and behavioral abilities and surface and verbal behaviors.

Some developmentalists, such as M. L. Lewis and Volkmar (1990), view the abstract concepts of the ego and ego functions as unnecessary. In my view, however, the theoretical abstraction defined as the ego is a useful way of summarizing a great many of the mind's conscious and unconscious mental capabilities and behavioral responses to biopsychosocial stimuli.

Superego. The third complex organizational structure is the superego (S. Freud 1923/1963). The *superego,* or its synonym, the conscience, is another "container" of specific mental functions. The superego's functions, however, are organized under the goal of providing the developing child with an inner source of familial and societal rules and standards.

The term *superego* connotes an aspect of mental activity that is "super" or over the id and the ego. The id generates stimuli that propel children to attempt to gratify their innate needs. The ego receives not only id-generated stimuli but also other biopsychosocial stimuli and "looks up" at the superego to check if a particular generated thought, feeling, memory, or contemplated behavior is permitted. The superego forever monitors stimuli emanating from the id and responds by sending encouraging or prohibiting signals to the ego and the self (see below). Thus the superego is not only an inner guide but also a source of internal approval when the child behaves according to its rules.

Unlike the id and ego, which are viewed as existing from birth, the superego does not begin to fully function as an effective internal authority over the id and ego until about age 5 years. Even then it must undergo many more years of development before it functions most effectively. By midadolescence (i.e., ages 15–16 years), the two main goals that the superego effectively begins to accomplish are 1) control of the adolescent's behavior relatively independent of external constraints and 2) maintenance of the adolescent's self-esteem relatively independent of the external feedback the adolescent receives about his or her self-value and the quality of his or her performances.

Self. Viewed as present from birth, the fourth complex organizational structure is the self. The *self* is defined as the supraordinate organizational structure of the mind; according to this view, it exerts overriding control of the id, ego, and superego. The self not only occupies the conscious mental domain but also occupies, or has ongoing access to, the preconscious and unconscious mental domains. As such, the self makes both conscious and unconscious decisions about whether to act, activate a defense mechanism to repress a thought or feeling, or relinquish an operative defense mechanism to allow a repressed long-term memory to enter consciousness. This view of the self, however, is not a unanimous one. For example, whereas Kohut (1971), Stern (1985), and Emde (1988) viewed the self as the supraordinate structure of the mind, Greenspan (1989) viewed the ego, not the self, as the supraordinate—or "control room"—structure of the mind.

The self as used here must be differentiated from each person's self-representation. Earlier I noted how, during the first 18 months of life, infants have only subjective self-awareness; in essence, they are not aware of being a separate self in a world of separate others. At age 18 months, toddlers achieve objective self-awareness through their construction of a self-representation. This *self-representation* is not the self but is the experiential part of the self; it enables the toddler to become aware of having a mind that perceives and a body that acts. The self, however, of post-Freudian developmentalists is never experienced. It is a composite mental structure—or intrapsychic entity—that, like the ego, is a theoretical construct to give meaning to phenomena that occur but are not easily explained—in this case, the mind's ability to organize all of its component structures (i.e., the id, ego, superego, and all other structures) and process and use them to achieve certain goals. In this view of the self, I am in agreement with Meissner (1986), who stated,

> The self is thus seen as an intrapsychic entity which serves as a frame of reference or as an organizing principle for integration of the interactions of other psychic structures. (p. 384)

As the mind's main agent of organized activity, the self does not require conscious forethought and is never experienced mentally. The self is like a hidden person within one's mind who is using a computer in which all of the contents of the mind are contained within its various programs and databases. Included within its programs and databases are the id, ego, and superego. The self is the main "scanner" and ultimate selector of all of the mental activities and behavioral capacities that are produced by the id, ego, and superego.

Maturation and Development of Innate Needs
The Oral Phase

■ Innate Physiological Needs

Infants' innate need to gratify their physiological requirements (i.e., hunger, thirst, elimination, tactile stimulation, equilibrium, thermal control, and sleep) and their ability to generate feelings and activate distress signals both indicate that infants "greet" their parents with active, preprogrammed behavioral abilities that are then developed through a "goodness of fit" process with their parents.

Satisfying innate needs.   From birth to age 18 months, infants seek oral sensual pleasurable stimulation and gratification (Brenner 1965). The sensual pleasure achieved through oral stimulation motivates infants to use their mouth to acquire new knowledge about biological stimuli (e.g., their oral mucosa and tongue) and social stimuli (e.g., their mother's breast nipple). S. Freud (1923/1963) called this period of development the *oral phase* and labeled infants' sensual pleasure as *oral eroticism.* He viewed infants as possessing a sexual drive that propelled them to seek sensual pleasures and, following maturation of their sexual drive, sexual pleasures. (Lichtenberg [1989] used the term *innate need for bodily sensory-sexual emotionally pleasurable stimulation and gratification* in place of sexual drive; I use his term in this book.)

As noted earlier, infants possess an innate sucking reflex that is activated when any object touches their lips. In time, they learn to discriminate between stimuli and will sustain their sucking only when the object being sucked on produces pleasurable sensual oral mucosal feelings and gastrointestinal satiation. This pleasurable experience is enhanced by their mother's responding pleasurably to feeding them. Eventually infants mentally process the transactions among these biological stimuli (e.g., their sucking reflex), psychological stimuli (e.g., their innate need to seek nourishment), and social stimuli (e.g., their mother's feeding activities) into a composite representation of their feeding experiences. When they have stored this representation as a long-term implicit memory, they have acquired new knowledge about their innate need to seek nourishment.

In interactions between all their innate needs (i.e., their nature) and their parents' responses to them (i.e., the nurturing element), infants eventually construct representations in which each innate need is internally linked in their representational worlds to how their parents responded to that need and what emotions both the parents and infant experienced in expressing and meeting those needs. This is a good example of how infants' socialization experiences trigger developmental changes in their mind: parents teach their infants the social rules and the accepted manner of expressing or inhibiting each of their innate needs. In undergoing developmental change, therefore, infants acquire knowledge about their innate needs that is social in its orientation; they learn that, to become civilized, they must experience their innate needs in a socializing environment.

Signaling when innate needs are not met. Infant crying—an innate behavior that triggers socializing transactions between infants and their parents or caretakers—is found in all cultural environments. Crying has been proposed by several developmentalists (Ainsworth et al. 1978; Bowlby 1969; Lamb 1976, 1981a, 1981b) to be an innate capability that generates an innate or preprogrammed response in other humans—both children and adults. And when adult caretakers respond appropriately and consistently to infants' crying signals, infants learn to perceive their caretakers as predictable and reliable soothers.

In addition to signaling hunger, temperature-related discomfort, and the need for stimulating interactions with the parents, crying is also used as an active means by which infants attempt to shut out their reception of 1) sensory stimuli that have reached either their unique upper or lower stimulation thresholds or 2) sensory stimuli being received through a specific sensory modality (e.g., auditory stimuli) that generates a level of stimulation that is above their upper stimulation threshold.

Crying helps infants adapt to their social world in that it gives them a means of controlling their level of stimulation. As Brazelton (1989) expressed it,

> There is a kind of fussy crying which occurs periodically through-
> out the day—usually in a cyclic fashion—which seems to act as a
> discharge of energy. . . . After a period of such fussy crying, the
> neonate may be more alert and he may sleep more deeply.
> (p. 414)

The Neonatal Behavioral Assessment Scale (Brazelton 1989) is used to measure infants' ability to withstand high levels of stimulation and to soothe themselves. The scale includes two behavioral items related to crying: "rapidity of build up to crying state" and "attempt to console self and control state behavior."

Infants also have the innate ability to signal distress when their physiological needs are not gratified by engaging in rhythmic behaviors. These self-soothing actions help infants remain within their optimal stimulation range. Some rhythms seem to be common to all infants (e.g., infants will suck on a pacifier at an almost identical rate [Wolff 1968]). Other rhythms are unique to each infant and help attune his or her rhythms to those of his or her parents (Schaffer 1984). A transactional process takes place between mothers and their infants as they gradually adjust to each other's rhythms (e.g., infants appear to have the innate ability to adjust their sleep-wake rhythms to those of their mother). This adjustment occurs when the mother is attuned to her infant's innate and maturationally changing rhythms and responds to them positively so that the infant's rhythms develop into more synchronous patterns that fit into her patterns. Mothers can developmentally shape their infants as long as they are flexible enough to perceive their infants' rhythms and adjust their activities accordingly.

Sleep.   In adults, sleep is separated into two different types. *Active sleep* or *rapid eye movement (REM) sleep* is so named because of the presence of synchronous and rapid eye movements during it. During this phase, there is an increase in heart rate, respiration, and blood pressure, but, at the same time, there is a profound decrease in motor movement, with virtual paralysis of the large muscles of the extremities. The bulk of human dreaming takes place during this sleep. The function of this REM dreaming state has, therefore, been postulated as allowing the person to dream quite active, creatively vivid, and uninhibited dreams while concurrently preventing the person from behaviorally acting on this dream stimulation (S. Freud 1900/1963). *Quiet sleep*, *deep sleep*, or *non-REM sleep* is broken down into four stages, ranging from Stage 1 (mild drowsiness) to Stage 4 (profound somnolence). During non-REM sleep, adults' respirations and heart rate are slower than during REM sleep and they engage in virtually no muscular activity (Roffwarg et al. 1973). Dreaming also occurs during adult non-REM sleep, but it is more mundane and associated with a replay of thoughts related to the past day's activities.

Infants' sleep is not fully understood. In the first days of life, an infant's sleep-awake cycle is very disorganized (Sander 1989). However, by the second week of life, as Schaffer (1984) noted, the infant and his or her primary caretaker begin to become more coordinated in that the infant's sleeping periods begin to take place more at night and the infant's periods of alertness and crying take place more during the daytime. Most infants gradually settle into a diurnal rhythm of sleep and wakefulness and will sleep through the night somewhere between ages 3 months and 4 months.

By the second week of life, infants' sleep-awake cycle is further differentiated into six qualitatively different states that occur in a cyclical fashion (Wolff 1966). Parents can almost predict these states and can gradually shape their infants into experiencing cycles of sleep and nonsleep, alertness and relaxation. Brazelton (1989) delineated these six states as follows:

- *State 1: Deep sleep*—Regular breathing, eyes closed, spontaneous activity confined to startles and jerky movements at quite regular intervals. Responses to external stimuli are partially inhibited and any response is likely to be delayed. No external eye movements and state changes are likely after stimuli or startles than in other states.

- *State 2: Active REM sleep*—Irregular breathing, sucking movements, eyes closed but rapid eye movements can be detected underneath the closed lids, low activity level, irregular smooth organized movements of extremities and trunk. Startles or startle equivalents occur in response to external stimuli, often with a change of state.
- *State 3: Drowsy*—Semi-dozing, eyes may be open or closed, eyelids often fluttering, activity level variable, with interspersed mild startles and slow smoothly monitored movements of extremities at periodic intervals; reactive to sensory stimuli but with some delay, state change frequently after stimulation.
- *State 4: Wide awake*—Alert, bright look; focuses attention on sources of auditory or visual stimuli; motor activity suppressed in order to attend to stimuli. Impinging stimuli break through with a delayed response.
- *State 5: Active awake*—Eyes open, considerable motor activity, thrusting movements of extremities, occasional startles set off by activity. Reactive to external stimulation with an increase in startles or motor activity; discrete reactions difficult to distinguish because of high activity level.
- *State 6: Crying*—Intense crying, jerky motor movements, difficult to break through with stimulation.

It is presently unknown what function REM sleep serves in children during the first 18 months of life. Although REM sleep and dreaming are identical in children and adults, the presence of dreaming during the REM sleep of the nonverbal infant (i.e., prior to age 18 months) is unknown. Dunn (1981) observed the following regarding phases within infant sleep:

> [In the full-term infant] it is not possible to classify the physiologic phases [of sleep] simply: besides phases of sleep that resemble active REM sleep and quiet sleep there are phases of intermediate sleep. . . . The proportion of this "intermediate" sleep phase decreases over time and by 3 months it has usually disappeared. . . . The newborn baby at term spends 45%–50% of sleep time in active REM sleep, and 35%–45% in quiet sleep. . . .

With increasing age these proportions change, with quiet sleep increasing and REM sleep decreasing, so that by 8 months there is twice as much quiet sleep as REM sleep, and by 10 years the normal adult proportions of 20% REM and 80% quiet sleep are reached. (p. 121)

Various hypotheses have been generated concerning the functional significance of such a high quantity of REM sleep (45%–50%) from birth to about age 10 years. Roffwarg et al. (1973) hypothesized as follows:

In infancy, when the proportion of time awake is smaller than in any other period of life, there is a large amount of REM activity. . . . We are now aware that during REM sleep brain activity is vigorous . . . [and we] hypothesize that REM sleep affords intense stimulation to the central nervous system, stimulation turned on periodically from within by a mechanism capable of stimulating the rest of the central nervous system. . . . The REM mechanism serves as an endogenous [or biological] source of stimulation, furnishing great quantities of functional excitation to higher [brain] centers. Such stimulation would be particularly crucial during the period in utero and shortly after birth, before appreciable exogenous [or social] stimulation is available to the central nervous system. (p. 135)

It would appear, therefore, that even in the passive-appearing activity of sleep, infants may possess innate central nervous system competencies that are "silently" activated during periods of sleep.

■ Need to Assertively Explore the Social Environment

Infants' need to act assertively. Infants are equipped with an innate assertiveness, or "assertiveness system" (Stechler and Halton 1987), that internally motivates them to explore their social environment. Assertiveness involves activity that is directed, focused, and not easily prohibited or deflected from its goal. Infants' innate need to assert themselves propels them to seek stimulation, perceive novelty in their environment, and attempt to assimilate and accommodate themselves to new stimulating experiences. As described by Stechler and Halton (1987),

> Assertion derives from the universal tendency to be active, to seek stimuli, to generate plans, and to carry them out. It is a self-activating system and is generally associated with the positive affects [emotions] of joy, interest, or excitement. (p. 821)

Through the stimulation of their need to assertively explore the environment, infants begin to use their innate perceptual ability to perceive contingent events in the environment (Lichtenberg and Kindler 1994). Through this ability, infants can perceive that there exists a contingency between two external events (Greenspan 1989; Greenspan and Lieberman 1989). For example, say an infant girl is placed in her crib with a mobile overhead and that, every time she kicks her legs, she activates a shining light in the mobile. Each time her kicking produces this result, she produces a joyful smile. She then tries to repeat the event to regenerate her enjoyment.

What would be occurring in the above example is the following: An infant becomes interested in a novel stimulus. If the infant then perceives that he or she is assertively doing something to bring about the novel stimulus, then the infant becomes more thrilled with producing the stimulus than with the stimulus itself (i.e., in the above example, the flashing light becomes less interesting than the kicking actions performed by the infant to make the light flash). The infant now feels *competency pleasure*—a pleasure in acquiring new knowledge in mastering a novel stimulus—that takes precedence over the initial novel pleasure in recognizing the novel stimulus of the flashing light. As a corollary, when a novel stimulus is repeatedly presented to an infant, the infant will become bored. He or she will already have acquired new knowledge, practiced it, and mastered the object or event, and subsequently will become distressfully understimulated (see habituation below). In social interactions with parents the same principles apply: the infant will become bored if parents always have the same look on their face, or if they never allow their infant's activity to influence them, especially if their infant's activity does not generate pleasurable emotional facial expressions in them (Stern 1985).

Parents' interpretation of their infant's assertiveness. In order for infants to experience the joy of causing things to happen in their environment, parents must want their infant to learn about their assertive abilities. While allowing their infant a certain amount of flexibility in initiating his or her assertiveness, parents must also behave as consistently reliable sources of stimulus modulation and protection to prevent their infant's assertiveness from leading to displeasurable feelings or physical pain. Winnicott (1965) described this function as parents providing a *holding environment*. As infants develop, their parents increasingly allow them to explore assertively and experience a sense of doing things competently, including fostering certain behaviors in them. As Lichtenberg (1989) noted,

> Parents intuitively allow themselves to be manipulated so that their infants can express individualistic rhythms of activity and learn that their parents attune to their rhythms and regulate back—a mutual experience of defining and developing competence. (p. 141)

The pleasurable emotions that infants begin to experience in activating certain transactions with their parents and being allowed by their parents to assert themselves appear to become a major, if not the major, motivator in infants' continued assertiveness in seeking new stimuli. Being assertively active and reactive within a transactional relationship with each parent whom an infant is learning to trust is one of the major developmental tasks of infancy. In slowly achieving this task, infants begin to organize their representations of their experiences in which they were assertive into those that generated pleasurable feelings and those that generated displeasurable feelings. These representations are then stored as long-term implicit memories and become future motivators of other actions (Schacter 1992; Terr 1994).

Parents can respond to their infant's assertive behaviors with varying degrees of acceptance and support as well as prohibition (e.g., gaze aversion, verbal disapproval). They perceive their infant's assertive behaviors through the selective filters of their representational worlds, and they develop both a subjective and objective response to those behaviors based on their past experiences. For example, one mother viewed her 2-week-old infant boy's assertively extending his hand toward her face after he appeared satiated after feeding at her breast by saying,

> See, I have an infant that is just like me. I was always hungry when I was an infant and my mother told me that the only thing that made me happy was a bottle in my mouth. I was overweight as an infant and as a child. So I'm not going to spoil my infant and feed him when he keeps asking for more milk.

This mother was having difficulty in perceiving her infant's normal assertiveness in wanting to explore her face. She was projecting what she was told by her mother—and still believed—about her own voracious infant hunger onto her own infant. In this transferentially influenced and, hence, distorted perception of her infant, she "saw" his assertion as a demand for more food.

S. Freud (1926/1963) postulated that infants were born with an innate destructive aggressiveness that he conceptualized as the *death instinct,* defined as the innate need to strive toward the elimination of all inner tension and seek the nonliving or nonstimulated inorganic state. He saw this instinct as being opposed to all the life instincts (e.g., Freud's sexual instinct would be a life instinct) and as being directed outward, particularly toward the infant's primary caretaker in the form of aggressive attacks on him or her. Freud believed that this instinct propelled infants and children to destroy their parents, others, and even themselves. For example, Freud pointed to an infant's tendency to bite his or her mother's breast while nursing as behavioral proof of the existence of the destructive and cannibalistic aspects of the death instinct. He interpreted this behavior as the infant trying to devour his or her mother's breast, especially when the infant was uncomfortable while sucking from the breast.

Thus, early in the 20th century, infants' assertiveness in exploring their world was virtually unrecognized by both society in general and developmentalists in particular. Even today, many parents attribute malevolent aggressive motives to their infant's normal assertive behaviors or their infant's reactive aggressive responses to displeasurable levels of stimulation (e.g., sources of physical threat, physical pain). This parental projection can prevail when parents believe, based on their physically abusive childhood experiences with their own parents, that, as one mother described it to me,

> [Infants] are greedy and just want to be fed, held and changed and then go back to sleep. When they don't get fed, changed and rocked right away, they get mean and angry and need to get a good whack on their bottoms.

Stechler and Halton (1987) explained how some parents confuse their infant's normal assertive need to 1) initiate social transactions with their parents, 2) take control of an interchange with their parents, and 3) explore their inanimate world as an expression of the infant's hostile destructiveness:

> [The surface behaviors of assertive exploration] include reaching, grabbing, pulling, throwing, smearing, banging, kicking, scratching and even biting. Taken as isolated acts, there is a high degree of overlap with the motor acts that may be involved in aggression. Thus, it easy to confuse the two. What is needed . . . [is] an appreciation [by the parents] of the context of the acts and the accompanying affective expressions [by the infant], as well as the drawing of inferences [by the parents] about the infant's intent, all combined into an empathic connection with the infant. (pp. 826–827)

A determining factor in whether or not parents misidentify their infant's normal assertive activity as hostile aggression is how well they learned as children to differentiate their own active behaviors. Most adults learned to differentiate between when they were being assertive and when they were being angrily, or even destructively, driven to ward off what they perceived as a threat or dangerous situation. However, some adults may not have been taught to make this distinction, and thus may view any assertion in themselves as destructively aggressive and therefore view their infant's assertion accordingly. Other adults may have learned as a child not to acknowledge their own episodes of reactively driven destructive aggression and so they view all activity in their infant as assertive. For example, one father I interviewed after his 3-year-old daughter had almost seriously injured her 1-year-old brother by roughly pushing him into a sandbox stated, "My daughter never would hurt her infant brother; she was just being a bit too rambunctious." In asking the father to explain his use of the word "rambunctious," he described his daughter as an "assertive normal little girl." Obviously, parents' own interpretation of their infant's innate behaviors will affect how they socialize their infant and how the infant eventually learns to view his or her own assertiveness.

When infants begin to learn that their assertive needs will be eventually gratified, they begin to be able to delay their acting assertively. During this delay, they have time to perceive their innate needs. As I note earlier, prior to age 18 months, infants have only a subjective or self-absorbed awareness of their needs. They do not possess the ability to be aware that they are separate from others and possess their own assertiveness in a world of other assertive people. One aspect of their gradually becoming aware of their innate needs is the existence of what Pine (1985) designated as *periods of ease-continuity,* during which the infant is neither hungry nor sleepy nor exposed to external stimuli, and the infant, in being enveloped in his or her mother's calm ministrations, experiences a sense of ease and continuity. This concept of ease-continuity is a derivative of Winnicott's (1958, 1965) belief that it is important to infants' mental development that they have periods of being quietly alone with their mother or father. It is during these relatively unstimulated and quiet periods that an infant will suddenly experience a sensation and a resultant spontaneous perception of one of his or her innate needs.

Maturation and Development of Physical Capabilities
Reflexive and Perceptual Abilities

Traditionally, infants were considered to be passive with respect to their parents in that they did not stimulate interactions with their parents. They were also thought to be equipped with a limited number of genetically endowed or innate reflexes. If adults attributed any purpose to these reflexes, it was that a few—such as sucking and rooting—were present to assist infants in their physiological, innate need to eat. However, since the 1940s, the virtual explosion of researchers' interest in systematically observing infants (Dowling and Rothstein 1989; Lichtenberg and Kindler 1994; Stern 1985) has provided a large body of evidence that infants are also equipped with a sophisticated, genetically endowed perceptual apparatus that selectively orients them to attend to other human beings (Schaffer 1984). In addition, infants are also biologically prepared with a number of innate and progressively maturing behavioral abilities that are oriented toward attracting and interacting with other human beings.

■ Reflexive Abilities

Infants' preprogrammed or innate reflexes are automatic, involuntary responses that appear to orient them toward reacting to, as well as stimulating transactions with, their parents. Two tactile reflexes are especially important in early infant-parent transactions: 1) the *sucking reflex,* stimulated by stroking the infant's lips, which causes the infant to produce a sucking movement of the lips and mouth; and 2) the *rooting reflex,* produced by stroking the infant's cheek or lips, which causes the infant to turn his or her head toward the stimulus and initiate a snapping movement with the mouth. Both reflexes are nurturant and socializing signals to the mother and father who interpret them correctly. For example, an infant's sucking behavior in response to having his or her lips stroked could mean that he or she is hungry, causing the mother to respond by feeding him or her, or could mean that the infant needs nonnutritive sucking, causing the mother to insert a pacifier or her finger to gratify this need.

■ Perceptual Abilities

An infant's innate perceptual apparatus is highly developed at birth. In this section, I address four specific innate perceptual abilities—visual, auditory, olfactory, and intermodal perceptual matching behaviors—in which infants display selective biases (see Table 3–1).

Visual. Shortly after birth, infants show a preference for disks with facial patterns painted on them over disks with nonfacial patterns (Fantz 1963; Kagan 1984). In addition, by age 1 month,

> when scanning live faces, infants act differently than when scanning inanimate patterns. They move their arms and legs and open and close their hands and feet in smoother, more regulated, less jerky circles of movements. (Stern 1985, p. 63)

Also by this age, infants are more attracted to a moving rather than a stationary face (Girton 1979). Schaffer (1984) noted that faces easily attract the infant's attention because the infant is perceptually preprogrammed to respond selectively to the human face.

Auditory. Fantz (1961) and Hutt et al. (1968) showed that, within the first days of life, infants preferentially respond to sounds that demonstrate auditory patterns similar to human speech over other types of sounds. Mills and Melhuish (1974) demonstrated that 3-week-old infants choose to suck on a nipple when the sucking is associated with their mother's voice. Two other researchers, DeCasper and Fifer (1980), discovered an even earlier selective attention to the mother's voice. They demonstrated maternal voice recognition in 3-day-old babies who had had no more that 12 hours of contact with their mothers. Another remarkable discovery was made by Condon and Sander (1974), who

Table 3–1. Infants' innate preferential perceptual responses to the environment (birth to age 2 months)

Visual	Facial patterns (bias toward moving face)
Auditory	Human speech patterns; synchrony with mother's voice
Olfactory	Mother's breast milk
Intermodal perceptual matching	Visual and auditory recognition of mother

showed that, at birth, infants move in unique interactional rhythmic synchrony with their individual mother's speech patterning.

Olfactory. Infants' innate abilities to form olfactory perceptions also show an early preferential bias for, and a discrimination of, human tastes. Stern (1985) reported on the following study carried out by MacFarlane (1975):

> [He placed] 3-day-old infants on their backs and then placed breast pads, which contained breast milk taken from their nursing mothers, on one side of the infants' heads. On the other side, he placed breast pads taken from other nursing women. Each infant reliably turned his or her head toward his or her own mother's breast milk pads, regardless of which side the pads were placed on. The head turning answered MacFarlane's question in the affirmative: infants are innately endowed with the ability to perceptually discriminate the smell of their own mother's milk. (p. 39)

Intermodal perceptual matching. It has been proposed that infants, in the first month of life, possess *intermodal perceptual matching,* which has been defined as "the capacity to know or comprehend that two identical objects are similar even when they are perceived through different sensory modalities, such as touch and vision" (Dowling 1981, p. 293). This perceptual ability has not traditionally been attributed to the early infant but has been viewed as being acquired later in life. In possessing intermodal matching, infants are able to match, for example, a voice (which is heard) with a mouth (which is seen). Stern (1985) identified another innate infant capacity called *amodal perception,* which he noted to be the "innate general capacity . . . to take information received in one sensory modality (e.g., a sucked breast) and somehow translate it into another sensory modality (e.g., a seen breast)" (p. 51). The result is that the infant experiences the mother's breast as a whole rather than as two unrelated breasts, one on which to suck and another at which to look.

Seigal (1993) referred to another related cognitive capacity present in the infant: the capacity for *stimulus generalization.* He wrote,

Infants can note both similarities across stimuli and differences. . . . In infancy and onward, the human mind is able to establish a "summation" of prior stimuli and experiences. This process can be thought of as the creation of a "mental model" for a category of objects, persons or interactions. (p. 5)

Stimulus generalization enables infants, for example, to begin to recognize characteristics in their father that were previously learned to be present in their mother, as long as the characteristics in the father were similar to those in the mother (Gleitman 1987). A great deal of the developing infant's ability to group similar perceptions and conceptions into categories depends on the infant's ability to use stimulus generalization. In a classic study by Watson and Rayner (1920), Albert, a 9-month-old infant, was shown a white rat (the researchers were reasonably sure that he had never seen a rat before). Albert expressed a joyful excitement in seeing the rat and reached for this novel stimulus (Wesley and Sullivan 1980). Independently, the researchers discovered that the stimulus of a loud noise made Albert cry. The authors then went on to do the following experiment:

[Whenever] Albert was playing or reaching for the rat at different occasions, a loud noise was made that made Albert withdraw from the rat and cry. . . . After about seven pairings of rat and noise, the presentation of the rat alone would make Albert cry and move away from the rat. . . . [Watson and Rayner also] showed Albert a [white] rabbit, a white piece of fur, and a Santa Claus mask with a [white] beard. Albert cried and withdrew from all of these objects. This additional testing showed clearly that cues (or different stimuli) can transfer to similar cues with which the child had no previous experience. (Wesley and Sullivan 1980, p. 132)

Thus infants have the cognitive capacity to begin to sort their representations of perceived events, objects, and so on into categories in which each category is defined by some common feature or quality. In using stimulus generalization, it appears that infants' cognitive processing abilities automatically begin to associate stimuli that share some commonality without having to directly experience each of the members of the category. For example, an infant boy who has learned that the family dog will bite when threatened may automatically become vigilantly hesitant when he is approached by a neighbor's cat. This shows that he has recognized certain salient features in the cat that have already been learned about the dog; recognition of these similarities causes him to hesitate in threatening the cat. In time, this infant will learn to discriminate a dog from a cat. For the time being, however, his assigning both dogs and cats into the "animals that bite" category has obvious survival and emotional regulatory value in maintaining his experiences within his pleasurable stimulation range.

Maturation and Development of Cognitive Capabilities

Cognition, as an innate and maturing mental capability, generates both primary process and secondary process forms of thinking. In Chapter 1, I describe how cognitive processes within the unconscious mental domain mostly follow primary process rules of thinking. This form of thinking is characterized by the absence of logic, the existence of contradictions, the absence of time, and the inability to recognize negatives. It is irrational and magical thinking. Conversely, cognitive processes within the preconscious and conscious domains primarily follow secondary process rules of thinking. This form of thinking is characterized by laws of logic, identification of causal factors, and the permanence of elapsed time. (See Table 3–2 for a comparison of these two types of thinking.)

S. Freud (1911/1963) postulated that primary process thinking was an archaic form of thinking that was contained only within the systematic unconscious. This idea has been discarded by modern developmentalists (Weiss 1993). Now it is recognized that, throughout the life cycle, both primary and secondary process thinking take place in the unconscious, preconscious, and conscious mental domains. In addition, both types of thinking undergo maturation and developmental change. As P. Tyson and Tyson (1991) noted,

Cognitive processes can be looked at as operating along a spectrum with the primary process and the secondary process occupying opposite ends. Most mental functioning, then, would represent a balance between the two. . . . The primary and secondary processes provide lenses through which to view the maturation of an underlying cognitive system. (p. 169)

■ Sensorimotor Phase

In the acquisition of all knowledge, infants' cognitive processes slowly begin to differentiate into primary and secondary forms of thinking. This happens more clearly after age 18 months. Before this age, infants' thinking processes are still mysterious, given that infants cannot speak to describe their thoughts and, even if they could, are not objectively aware of themselves or their thoughts. Nevertheless, subjectively self-aware infants do construct perceptual representations of their innate needs, emotions, temperamental characteristics, and transactional experiences with parents and other caretakers. Some of these representations are stored as long-term memories within their dynamic unconscious domain. In Chapter 1, I describe long-term memories constructed within the

Table 3–2.   Modes of mental activity: primary process thinking versus secondary process thinking

Primary process thinking (unconscious domain)	Secondary process thinking (conscious domain)
Instinctual, wish directed	Goal directed
Irrational thinking	Rational thinking
Illogical	Logical; recognizes causality of events
Tolerance of mutually contradictory events and conceptions	Recognition when events and conceptions are mutually contradictory
Timeless	Sense of time
Communication primarily through visual imagery	Verbal and written communication

first 18–24 months of life as implicit memories. According to P. Tyson and Tyson (1991), implicit memories are formed from thinking activities in the infant that are "related to his actions—that is, he enacts in relation to objects that are perceptually present, and he shows a wholly practical, perceiving-and-doing, action-bound kind of intellectual functioning" (p. 175).

During this period, infants' cognitive processes are organized around their seeking novel stimuli, forming perceptions of biopsychosocial stimuli, acting on these perceptions, and eventually forming implicit memories of these experiences. This is why Piaget (1952) labeled this phase of cognitive maturation and development the *sensorimotor phase;* infants sense, perceive, and act through their motor central nervous system.

Through recent research, it has become increasingly apparent that infants are endowed with innate cognitive abilities that direct them to assertively seek and selectively form specific perceptions, such as the sight of their mother's face, the sound of her voice, the feel of her skin, and so on. These perception-forming abilities attest to the fact that a segment of early infant knowledge is greatly influenced by cognitive structures that are preadapted to selectively focus on certain perceptions. These cognitive competencies enable infants to acquire knowledge quickly when the appropriate social stimuli are encountered, stimuli usually automatically provided by parents in the socializing environment they provide for their infant. For example, an infant's preprogrammed perceptual preference for visual configurations that are similar to the human face (Fantz 1961; see discussion above under perceptual abilities) enable the parent's face to attract the infant's attention much more easily than if this attraction had to be completely learned by the infant.

In addition to cognitive perceptual preferences, other forms of cognitive information are also present in infants. Existing as innate informational structures, they await the appropriate environmental stimuli to develop. This theory of preexisting innate informational structures differs from Piaget's postulate that all infant knowledge is acquired through infants' actions on their environment. For example, Piaget posited that children's language evolves through their imitating their parents' language and then experimenting with speaking according to what they have heard. However, according to the theory that informational structures are innate, it is assumed that infants are innately preprogrammed to begin to understand a verbal language when maturationally ready and when exposed to the verbalizations of others (Kagan 1984). For example, by age 6 months, infants are able to distinguish the approximately 150 sounds that make up human speech (Ferguson and Farwell 1975). By age 1 year, they show the cognitive capacity to understand certain words (e.g., no, mom, milk) a full 8–12 months before they can verbalize them.

Thus it is now believed that certain forms of knowledge—such as that necessary to acquire language—are more easily acquired by infants because of their genetically preprogrammed informational structures. Parents do not teach their infants every word they eventually learn. Once an infant's innate, language-related mental structures are actuated near age 1 year as a result of normal maturation processes, the infant seems to become highly attuned to words he or she hears in the environment. Later, a specific cognitive competency for learning language, initially mediated by preprogrammed mental structures, enables children to go from knowing about 20 words at age 2 years to knowing about 2,000 words at age 5 years! Kagan (1984) summarized this as follows:

> The basic cognitive competencies are best viewed as processes that are prepared to be actualized given proper experience. (p. 312)

I now turn to two basic types of cognitive activity that fuel infants' acquisition of knowledge about their animate and inanimate social world: those involving Piagetian types of learning processes and those involving classical and nonclassical learning processes. It should be noted that, despite the fact that different cognitive processes lead to infants' development of their knowledge base, their total fund of knowledge is not compartmentalized within their representational world. An infant's mind uses all existing knowledge in its never-ending attempts to integrate and comprehend its present perceptions. Knowledge gained through interaction with inanimate objects will fuel the acquisition of knowledge of the animate world and vice versa.

■ Piagetian Learning Processes

A great portion of infants' waking hours is spent in using their innate need to be assertive in seeking novel stimulations. In essence, they conduct daily "experiments" on their parents, siblings, and a variety of inanimate things, thereby coming to know the external world. Piaget devoted much energy to studying this form of knowledge acquisition.

Before Piaget's work, traditional views of infants held that they were passive in seeking knowledge and were primarily interested in the gratification of their innate instinctual wishes (seen primarily as wishes to gratify their physiological needs). According to this view, all of an infant's motivation to acquire knowledge was extrinsic. Thus parents had to create a motivation within their infants to acquire the knowledge they wanted them to possess.

Piaget had a different conception of children. He viewed infants as innately active seekers of knowledge, as innately motivated learners who used their innate reflexes and innate abilities to form perceptions to act on their social world. In the process, they acquired knowledge. Beginning with his studies in the 1930s—from which he produced his seminal work, *The Origins of Intelligence in Children,* in 1952— Piaget postulated that children become more intelligent as their cognitive maturational competencies evolve with increasing age.

According to Piaget, there are four major phases of cognitive maturation and development, each of which is qualitatively and quantitatively different from the other:

1. The *sensorimotor phase* (birth to age 2 years)
2. The *preoperational phase* (ages 2–7 years)
3. The *concrete operational phase* (ages 7–12 years)
4. The *formal operational phase* (age 12 years and onward)

The age spans listed for the phases are only approximations of when most children can be expected to show the specific cognitive developmental achievements that characterize that particular phase. Piaget believed that every child must pass through the phases of cognitive development in the same sequence, but not necessarily at exactly the same age span. The maturation of new cognitive structures dictates that the cognitive functioning of children at different phases of their life cycle is quantitatively and qualitatively different. Not only are children capable of an increased amount of thinking at a later phase, but they can think at a more advanced level of integration and comprehension. This phasic theory has been labeled as *epigenetic.* In expanding on many of the concepts first expounded by J. Baldwin (1894), Piaget fostered a theory of *genetic epistemology,* which was the "study of the manner in which a subject comes to attain objective knowledge of the world" (Case 1992, p. 164). (*Genetic* here refers to the progressive unfolding of new cognitive dynamic mental structures in accordance with a set plan, and *epistemology* refers to the study of the limits of children's acquisition of knowledge at each phase in their life cycle.) In essence, Piaget's cognitive genetic epistemological theory was an epigenetic one, as were Freud's and Erickson's theories.

Piaget was a pragmatist, believing that infants and children seek to master stimuli they encounter while acting on the environment through intelligent adaptation. (In Chapter 2, I refer to this process as infants attempting to fit their need to seek stimuli [an innate need] into what the social environment tasks them to learn.) Sternberg (1985) noted that Piaget's theory of cognitive development primarily focused on the notion that "survival depends on adaptation to the environment, and hence, intelligent survival requires intelligent adaptation" (p. 1116).

Acquiring knowledge in the sensorimotor phase.　During this preverbal phase, the knowledge that infants acquire in response to what they sense and perceive is manifested in their actions. According to Piaget, infants' innately endowed reflexes—defined as biological stimuli in the biopsychosocial model—become activated at birth and mediate the acquisition of their earliest knowledge of the world. Piaget put forth the following postulates for understanding how infants use their innate reflexes to acquire knowledge about their body and environment (see also Table 3–3):

1. *Infants' innately endowed reflexive apparatuses are not only exquisitely reactive to any available sensory stimulation, but*

also active in seeking out more and more complex stimuli with which to interact. Thus infants possess an intrinsic motivation to acquire knowledge. Bidell and Fischer (1992) noted that, according to Piaget's theory,

> Action, not perceptual abstraction, is the primary source of information about the world. According to Piaget, perceptual information [e.g., the newborn's innate perceptual ability to selectively focus upon a human face] may be indispensable, but it is limited to relatively static knowledge of configurations in the world. Knowledge of action—what we can do with the world—is much more powerful because . . . one gains fundamental knowledge about relations with and between people and objects. (p. 105)

2. *Newborns' and growing infants' perceptions trigger innate reflexive surface behaviors.* For example, any object that touches the lips of a 1-day-old infant will stimulate the infant's innate sucking reflex, and sustained sucking will occur.

3. *Once an inborn reflex has been activated, an infant's maturing mind seeks to repeat the reflex.* Different stimuli initiate innate reflexes as infants continually use these reflexes to acquire new knowledge and become "intelligent." For example, at birth, when an infant is hungry, any object that touches the infant's mouth will activate his or her sucking reflex (providing it does not overly stimulate or harm the infant). By age 3 days, however, only a nipple on a bottle with palatable fluid within

---

Table 3–3. Piaget's major postulates

- Infant's mental apparatus seeks sensory stimulation.
- Infant's brain is genetically programmed to repeat activated reflexes.
- Sensory stimuli trigger inborn reflexive patterns of behavior.
- Infant acquires intelligence by action on the environment.
- Schemata are the basic cognitive structural unit.
- New intelligence arises when existing schemata cannot deal with a new object: through assimilation, new schemata are constructed; through accommodation, old schemata are reconstructed.

---

it or a breast nipple that produces milk will continue to be sucked on for any length of time. The infant has already begun to learn to differentiate stimuli that touch his or her mouth.

4. *Infants continue to acquire knowledge and learn by acting on and reacting to their environment; in this way, motor actions become the initial basic triggers for acquiring new knowledge.* Through repeated sucking actions, the infant learns that a nipple that is sucked on produces fluid that, when swallowed, relieves a displeasurable feeling (hunger) and produces a pleasurable feeling (satiation). In actively seeking to repeat the sucking reflex, the infant learns that sucking on certain types of nipples gives satisfaction. The repetition of these behaviors makes up a set of experiences that eventually become an internal representation called a *nipple schema*. This schema then becomes a new unit of knowledge for the infant. (*Schema* was originally defined by J. M. Baldwin [1894] and then extensively used by Piaget [1954a]. Kagan [1984] defined it as "an individual's way to represent an event," a description similar to that of a representation. The difference is that the word "schema" is most often used to describe knowledge about the inanimate world acquired in a nonsocial context, whereas representation is most often used to describe knowledge about the social world acquired in a social context. As I note throughout this book, both schemata and representations are constructions of the mind and never exact replicas of outside phenomena.)

5. *Infants are motivated to initiate action when existing schemata cannot be used to integrate and comprehend new perceptions.* In essence, this is the process described by the transference-assimilation principle (see Chapter 2). According to this principle, an infant will attempt to transfer a prior schema onto a new perception and then try to assimilate the new perception into the prior schema. This process of acquiring new knowledge by changing a preexisting schema into a new schema involves the following mental processes:

   a. *Habituation*—According to the *habituation principle,* when infants become selectively focused on a stimulus that appears novel in some way, their response to that stimulus will decrease over time as the stimulus is repeated and has no noxious effects. Hence the novel stimulus that was once capable of producing a response of excited interest becomes ineffective in maintaining the infant's interests. The infant now reacts to this stimulus with a sense of boredom. Habituation is not discussed by Piaget in his description of his sensorimotor phase of cognitive development. However, it needs to be included here because habituation is even more basic than Piaget's processes of assimilation and accommodation.

Habituation does not require any preexistent schema to be present within the infant's mind; instead, the novel stimulus generates a response in the infant until the infant has formed a new schema or representation of his or her perception of the stimulus. Whether that stimulus continues to generate interest or excitement depends on what gratification the infant expects to achieve through interacting with the stimulus (e.g., if an infant's play with a favorite toy becomes repetitive and monotonous or the infant's play does not bring a positive response from the parents [which would encourage the infant's play with the toy], then the infant's interest in the toy will abate).

b. *Assimilation*—This is the process of initially taking in or incorporating a new perception into an existing schema. In assimilating the new perception, the infant attempts to make the new perception fit into a familiar schema (or representation) of a prior experience. In effect, assimilation helps the infant achieve a sense of pleasure in knowing and mastering an external experience by making it equal to an existent inner experience. (See Chapter 2 for a more detailed discussion of assimilation and the transference-assimilation principle.)

c. *Accommodation*—In this process, infants who are confronted with new stimuli that do not fit into an old schema must then restructure the old schema to accept those new stimuli (Sternberg 1985), thus constructing a new schema. An infant's or child's accommodations are always limited by the cognitive phase he or she has reached developmentally (e.g., 6-year-old children are not asked to accommodate to arithmetic principles usually comprehended only by 8-year-old children). (See Chapter 2 for a more detailed discussion of accommodation and the accommodation-transformation principle.)

d. *The circular reaction*—This is the mental process, which can sometimes be observed behaviorally, in which an infant continues trying to assimilate a new object into an old schema, and then eventually accommodates the new perception into a new schema. For example, a 1-month-old infant literally can stumble on a new experience as a consequence of activity (Flavell 1963) and thereafter will try to repeat the same activity.

The following is an illustration of Piaget's postulates on how infants and children gain knowledge through acquiring new and more complex schemata:

A 14-month-old boy has played before with a box and has already constructed and stored within his representational world the schema that boxes open and close. Now, for the first time, he drops a toy into a box purely by chance. When he closes the box he cannot see the toy; when he opens the box, there is the toy! He is pleasurably excited and yet uncertain. He repeats the process of dropping the toy in the box, closing the box, then opening the box and finding the toy (the circular reaction). He experiments and experiences competency pleasure by causing the toy to appear and disappear within the box.

The boy then tries to assimilate his actions involving the toy into his old schema: boxes open and close. A state of mental disequilibrium now emerges, created by his possessing an old schema that cannot be used as a piece of knowledge to integrate and comprehend this new experience. He is now helped, without being consciously aware of this internal process, by his mind's ever-maturing cognitive ability to reconstruct a preexisting schema into a new one through the mental processes of accommodation and transformation. Consequently, he is once again able to achieve mental equilibrium by accommodating to the new experiences of toy and box through reconstructing and transforming the old box schema. This new schema—his new piece of knowledge—is: Boxes are objects that open and close and can hold and hide things, like toys.

This 14-month-old boy has performed an experiment and acquired new knowledge about his inanimate world. In the future, maturationally emerging new cognitive competencies will enable him to perform new and more complex experiments on the world, and continue to construct new schemata or reconstruct preexisting schemata. In Piaget's view, once schemata are constructed and stored as long-term memories, they become internal sources of motivation (psychological stimuli in the biopsychosocial model) that propel the infant to seek new stimuli and assimilate or accommodate them, thereby acquiring more complex schemata.

Piaget also emphasized that all schemata constructed by infants and children are based on direct environmental experience. For example, when a 10-month-old girl wants to reach an object that is far from her on a blanket, she pulls the blanket toward her to get to the object. She then plays with the object. Suddenly and excitedly she throws the object away from her but still on the blanket. She thereupon experiences competency pleasure in pulling the blanket toward her in order to once again retrieve the object. For Piaget, this repetitive action was an act of intelligence, indicating that the infant has acquired knowledge through constructing a schema, one that can be characterized as: Things can be used to make other things come to me.

Discrepant events.   The processes of assimilation and accommodation are optimized when new experiences are initially perceived as both similar and dissimilar to preexistent schemata. These types of new experiences are called *discrepant events,* defined as "events that are a partial transformation of existing schemata" (Kagan 1984, p. 37). Discrepant events attract and sustain a child's attention and concentration more than nondiscrepant events. Furthermore, discrepant events clearly produce a pleasurable emotional response in infants and children. Although Piaget did not address children's emotions in his study of how they acquire knowledge, if a learning experience is pleasurable, an infant will be more motivated to acquire new knowledge. For example, if sucking on a certain nipple is pleasurable, in the future the infant will seek that nipple to suck on. However, if an infant's assimilation processes begin to fail, a state of disequilibrium will ensue as the infant experiences a certain degree of pleasurable uncertainty.

Understanding object permanence. During most of the sensorimotor phase, infants continually acquire knowledge through the process of assimilation and accommodation. But they remain objectively unaware of possessing this knowledge until they achieve the capacity for objective self-awareness (at about age 18 months).

One of the most significant cognitive developments during the sensorimotor stage begins to emerge at about age 6 months. At this time, infants become able to construct the schema of *object permanence,* a principle that can be verbalized as: All objects are permanent and continue to exist even when not seen. Like many schemata, an infant's schema of object permanence undergoes reconstruction through the dual influence of the maturation of new cognitive competencies and new environmental experiences. The process of constructing the schema of object permanence develops as follows:

- *Before 5 months*—Infants will cease to look at a spot from which a familiar person or an object they had been gazing at was suddenly removed. This behavior indicates that the person or object is no longer present within the infant's mind as a perceptual representation. At this age, infants are capable of using their long-term implicit memories only in a recognition process: they remember only familiar people and objects that are currently generating stimuli. Thus, in using only recognition memory, the infant's mind functions along the lines of out of sight, smell, hearing, or touch equals out of mind.
- *By 5 months*—Infants watch while a familiar object or person is hidden from their view. Now they use their hands to reach for the place from which the object or person disappeared in order to try to retrieve it. These behaviors reveal their development of retrieval memory (Kagan 1984). Now, recently out of sight, smell, hearing, or touch does not equal out of mind.

● *By 6 months*—When infants see a familiar object or person, are then distracted from looking at it, and eventually look back at it and find it is gone, they can still recall the object or person and initiate actions to find it. This seeking-and-finding behavior is interpreted as indicating that they can now recall an image of an object or person in its absence.

The cognitive processing ability to evoke a memory of an object or person when the subject of the memory is not within the infant's immediate sensory field is called *evocative memory*. Along with evocative memory comes the cognitive ability to compare past (i.e., the memory) with present perceptions and eventually come to know what is novel from what is familiar or already known. Stern (1985), however, has questioned whether evocative memory really exists, postulating that all memories are triggered by some sensory stimulus or cue and that therefore all memories are forms of recognition memory.

■ A Critique of Piaget's Theories

Piaget's cognitive phase theory was a monumental contribution to the knowledge of how infants and children acquire knowledge about their world and become socialized in the process. Gelman and Baillargeon (1983) highlighted three important ways in which Piaget's epigenetic cognitive phase theory has contributed to the fund of knowledge about human development:

1. Piaget emphasized infants are endowed with reflexes and later behaviors that enable them to be innately motivated to actively acquire knowledge as a result of the interactions with their environment. This view was a departure from the more traditional one that portrayed the child as passive in terms of what and how much knowledge infants and children acquired.
2. Piaget was one of the first developmentalists who underscored the view that infants' and children's innate and maturationally emerging cognitive competencies determine for them "their perception and understanding of the world and delimit the nature and range of knowledge they acquire at each point in their development" (Gelman and Baillargeon 1983, p. 185).

3. Piaget provided a plethora of facts concerning cognitive development (e.g., assimilation, accommodation).

Piaget's cognitive phase theory has thus become another valuable piece of the complex developmental "patchwork quilt" (Erikson 1980), a metaphorical quilt made up of various and partial theories of normal mental development. However, as typically occurs when a new developmental theory is proposed, as it is further explored it is inevitably critiqued and revised. Some of these criticisms with regard to Piaget's cognitive phase theory follow.

Piaget offered no definitive principles to explain what stimulates the transition from one developmental phase to the next (Kagan 1984). In defense of Piaget, it is my view that he did accept that psychological stimuli—both innate and maturationally emerging cognitive structures—activated at birth and at certain transition or pivot points in a child's life become the age transition points that separate one cognitive phase from another. However, Piaget was not concerned with attempting to describe the makeup of these cognitive structures. He was a pragmatist who observed the effects of these processes taking place within mental structures on children's acquisition of new knowledge as well as their acquisition of ways to transform knowledge (Kagan 1984). Kagan has suggested the analogy that, if Piaget were to study the development of human breathing, he would focus on the physiological processes involved in breathing and not the structure of lung tissue. Thus Piaget offered descriptions, not explanations, of phases of cognitive maturation and development. If he had proposed explanations, he would have had to describe antecedent mental developments necessary for a transition to occur from one phase to another (Brainerd 1978).

Piaget also did not address how children's social experiences with their parents affected their acquisition of knowledge either in one phase or during their transition into a new cognitive phase. Instead, Piaget focused on innately motivated infants—those who were not bothered by displeasurable levels of stimulation or threatened in any way, and those who acted on and reacted to their environment, acquiring knowledge and new learning experiences in the process. If parents rewarded this knowledge-acquiring activity, so be it. If they did not, Piaget viewed this as an individual issue—an issue he did not address in his cognitive theory of knowledge acquisition in the normally developing infant and child. For Piaget, emotions supplied only the energy for thinking (Lane and Schwartz 1987), whereas cognition (i.e., using thoughts to integrate and comprehend biopsychosocial stimuli) supplied the structure for thinking. As Tenzer (1984) wrote,

> Piaget made the point that affect and cognition are inseparable—affect being the energetic or motivational component of [mental] structures. His focus was on the development of knowledge in general rather than on the intraindividual or interpersonal differences. (p. 25)

It is not surprising that Piaget also did not address infants' and children's temperament. More recent researchers (Goldsmith and Campos 1982) have shown that infants' temperament, operating as another innate psychological stimulus, can affect their capacity to both acquire new knowledge and engage in new learning experiences. Campos et al. (1983) observed that

> temperamental dispositions predict subsequent cognitive performance. . . . There is plenty of evidence that temperamental traits related to the emotion of interest—namely, persistence or its variants, such as attention span, goal orientation, and distractibility—predict individual differences in cognitive functioning . . . and infants who tend to explore the environment, orient to interesting features in it, and respond in a well-modulated fashion to stimulation are likely to develop superior cognitive skills. (p. 139)

Thus social and emotional and associated temperamental influences on infants' and children's acquisition of knowledge are not part of Piaget's theories. He considered infants and children as being in a state of calm alertness, ready to experiment on their social world, and as having parents who were supportive and admiring of their efforts in acquiring knowledge. Because infants' current representational world was quiet, and children's outer world of objects, parents, and others was similarly quiet, they were both free to activate their innate motivation to acquire new knowledge and thereby add to their inner, representational world. Many years after he first offered his cognitive phase theory, Piaget stated, "Generally speaking—and I am ashamed to say it—I'm really not interested in the individual. I'm interested in what is general in the development of intelligence and knowledge" (Bringuier 1977/1980, p. 53).

Piaget studied only universals in the maturation and development of infants' and children's cognitive abilities (Feldman 1980) and neglected developmental variability in their cognitive development (Bidell and Fischer 1992). Universals are cognitive developments that occur in all infants and children, as long as they are free of brain deficits (as a form of biological stimuli) and major environmental deprivations (as a form of social stimuli). According to Piaget, for each child to acquire universal knowledge, he or she must pass through each phase to acquire the same universal cognitive achievements, although the rate of each child's progress might vary.

Piaget did not study non–spontaneously occurring cognitive processes, also called *nonuniversals* (i.e., cognitive developments not achieved by all children regardless of their passing through each of Piaget's cognitive phases) (Feldman 1980). Nonuniversal cognitive processes appear to require unique cognitive maturational competencies (as psychological stimuli), certain types of transactions between children and their parents (as social stimuli), or both. An example of a nonuniversal cognitive achievement is the emergence of a creative idea. Cognitive competencies, as well as the types of environmental transactions that produce the creatively fertile mind, remain a mystery.

Piaget's system of phases also neglects variability in cognitive development. Bidell and Fischer (1992) noted that "Piaget's stages mark off the course of cognitive development in the crudest fashion, dividing the reorganization into units that can cover 3 to 5 years per stage" (p. 124). They describe how passage from one cognitive phase to the next cognitive phase is related to the following:

1. *Variability in age at acquisition of specific cognitive skills* (Bidell and Fischer 1992)—Post-Piagetian research has demonstrated that children can attain certain cognitive achievements both later than Piaget predicted (Elkind 1964; Fischer and Canfield 1986) and earlier than Piaget predicted (Halford 1989).

2. *Variability in the social environment's assistance as a child acquires specific cognitive skills*—Bidell and Fischer (1992) summarized the effect of environmental conditions on a child's acquisition of knowledge:

   > An individual's cognitive level varies widely depending on the degree of contextual support immediately available. . . . A given child's cognitive level will vary from high to low over a period of a few minutes depending on the degree of support. (p. 120)

3. *Variability in the sequence of acquiring specific cognitive skills*—This aspect of variability is less absolute than the first two. In two studies of large groups of children (Case 1992; Fischer 1980), there was little variability in Piagetian phases of cognitive acquisitions. But other researchers have shown that some children vary in the sequence of their cognitive phase development depending on variations in their cultural background, academic history, and performance and style (Gelman and Baillargeon 1983; Kofsky 1966) or variations in their temperamental characteristics (Bidell and Fischer 1992). These children appeared to progress through all of Piaget's cognitive phases earlier than suggested by Piaget's age predictions (Gelman and Baillargeon 1983).

Piaget postulated that all schemata are constructed, and not inherited, by infants and children. Piaget did not believe that infants' innate perceptual competencies significantly contributed to their early acquisition of knowledge. Others have maintained that certain innate cognitive structures contribute significantly to the process of habituation, assimilation, and accommodation (Chomsky 1957; Piatelli-Palmarini 1980). Hence all knowledge is not constructed only from direct experience; instead, as Gelman and Baillargeon (1983) observed, the complexity of the final structures that are constructed is to some extent limited by the complexity of the originating innate structures.

For example, in reference to speech, Chomsky (1957) postulated that inborn cognitive structures are present from the moment of conception as inborn schemata that need only the stimulating exposure of a human speech environment to become manifest. Piaget, however, postulated that the acquisition of speech knowledge depends on the action of talking in the context of a trial-and-error modeling of the speech children have heard. Kagan (1984), supporting Chomsky's position, observed that many words (e.g., you, is, why) that are acquired by children have no relation to covert actions performed in acquiring them.

In summary, despite some of the above limitations of Piaget's theories, his phases of cognitive development are still quite valid and continue to stimulate further research and new discoveries about the child's cognitive development.

■ Knowledge Acquired Through Classical and Operant Learning Processes

A child's learning ability is always limited by whatever cognitive competencies the child possesses. This is usually defined according to Piagetian cognitive phases. In such a definition, it is assumed that a child's cognitive capabilities are up to the task of a particular phase. This learning theory, however, does not address a child's representational world, conscious and unconscious beliefs, feelings, fantasies, and memories. The data focused on in generating learning theories are how stimuli influence the child's behavioral responses and how these stimulus-response associations are learned and remembered (Bandura 1974; Yussen and Santrock 1978).

Other learning principles focus more on the way in which infants and children become motivated and practice in modifying their surface behaviors based on the response or lack of response they receive from the environment. A learning theorist would focus on these principles and not on the private thoughts and emotions of child subjects.

Learning theorists divide learning into 1) classical or Pavlovian conditioning, and 2) instrumental or operant conditioning. According to either, infants experience a contingent relationship between a stimulus (which can be an infant behavior, a parental behavior, or some event in the environment) and a behavioral response. They then construct a representation of an association between a stimulus and a behavioral response.

Classical conditioning learning processes.   In classical conditioning, a specific stimulus produces a specific response. Classically conditioned learning experiences involve not only infants' discovery of this specific stimulus-response association, but also their learning of new stimuli that will produce the same response as the original stimulus. The stimuli used to initiate the learning experiences are "natural" stimuli that produce innate behavioral responses, not learned responses. For example, most infants' innate response to a sudden very loud noise is one of crying and agitation. Thus a very loud noise could then be used as the initial specific stimulus to produce the initial specific response of crying.

Pavlov conducted pioneering research in identifying early principles of learning (Pavlov 1927). Pavlov's classic experiments involved a hungry dog who was first presented with food (the specific, unconditional stimulus), following which the dog began salivating (the specific, unconditional response). The term *unconditional* is used to describe the food stimulus and the salivation response because the association between them did not depend on prior learning, but instead was innately or unconditionally present. In Pavlov's experiments, a new stimulus was then introduced: the ringing of a bell while the dog was in a hungry state. Pavlov found that after the unconditional stimulus was presented concurrently with the new stimulus (the bell), the dog eventually would salivate in response to the bell alone. In this case, the bell would be labeled a conditional stimulus and salivation the conditional response, signifying that this stimulus-response pattern was developed under a specific set of unnatural conditions. Pavlov also found that if he repeatedly presented the bell stimulus to the conditioned dog without providing food after the dog salivated, the conditioned salivation response to the bell would eventually become extinct.

Another discovery Pavlov made was that he could teach a dog to establish links or mental associations between unrelated stimuli. For example, if a dog who was conditioned to salivate when a bell was rung was shown a light during the ringing of the bell, in time the light itself would produce salivation. (This is an example of stimulus generalization, described above.)

Instrumental (or operant) conditioning learning processes. In operant conditioning, the stimulus initiating the learning experience would be, for example, a parent's response to a particular behavior an infant has been taught. For this type of teaching to be successful, however, the behavior being taught must be one that the infant can produce based on his or her mental and behavioral capabilities (e.g., no type of behavior by the parents will be able to elicit talking in an 8-month-old infant).

Through operant conditioning, infants are assisted in maintaining self-regulation through their feelings. New surface behaviors can be gradually produced in infants when their parents provide predictably positive operant responses to them. In this sense, parents shape their infants to continue to behave in the manner they desire. This type of conditioning works because infants' feelings are influenced by their parents' feelings. Infants will repeat or inhibit a particular behavior based on the feelings they perceive in their parents in responses to their behaviors. In a family that maintains a developmentally enhancing goodness of fit, this transactional shaping process goes both ways between parents and infant. Thus all members will learn from each other.

Skinner (1969) conducted experiments that showed that spontaneous behaviors in a person are a direct function of the environment's response to those behaviors. In illustrating this operant organizing principle, an infant is motivated to repeat behaviors that bring positive operant responses. Those behaviors are then considered to have been reinforced. Behaviors that bring negative operant responses are eventually suppressed. Actions that bring no responses are extinguished.

This view is quite different from Piaget's view that children become motivated to modify (through assimilation and accommodation processes) their behaviors based on the responses they receive from their internal or representational world (i.e., the pleasurable excitement associated with assimilating an experience and the pleasurable uncertainty associated with nonassimilation and the activation of accommodation processes).

Maturation and Development of Temperamental Characteristics

Temperament can be defined as the style in which infants express the following temperamental characteristics (Goldsmith et al. 1987):

1. *Activity,* in stimulating the environment
2. *Reactivity,* in responding to environmental stimulation
3. *Emotionality,* in terms of the thresholds of stimulation that generate each of their emotions, the behavioral style in which each emotion is expressed, the intensity of each emotion, and the time it takes to return levels of stimulation to within their optimal stimulation range and thereby achieve emotional self-regulation
4. *Sociability,* in terms of initiating social responses from others and responding to social communications

An infant's emotional style is how the infant expresses a particular emotion and recovers from it. For example, one 2-month-old infant might become angry more quickly and take much longer to calm herself than another infant of the same age. Also, the style in which infants express one emotion may not necessarily be the same style in which they express other emotions.

Researchers have found evidence indicating that infants' temperamental characteristics are present from birth and persist over time (Mitchell 1993). However, these characteristics also undergo maturation. Both innate and maturationally emerging temperamental characteristics operate as psychological stimuli that then interact with the social environment and ultimately lead infants to begin to construct representations of each of their temperamental traits.

Temperamental characteristics help to regulate infants' social relationships in that their style of actively engaging with and reacting to their parents can elicit, modify, or prevent many of their parents' social behaviors (Goldsmith and Campos 1982). For example, the source of an infant boy's excessive crying might traditionally have been attributed to inappropriate nurturing: either the parents were not protecting him from being over- or understimulated, or he was being stimulated through a modality that was displeasurable to him (e.g., his parents might have been rocking him at a rate that never matched his soothing rhythmic rate). With the discovery of temperament, this same infant would be viewed as possibly possessing a restricted optimal stimulation range, or at least preferring stimulation through sensory modalities to which his parents were not attuned. Alternatively, this infant might reach his upper or lower stimulation threshold more quickly than other babies, thus signaling his displeasure by crying. He might also need a longer duration of parental soothing behaviors in order to stop crying because his capacity for regaining emotional equilibrium is lower than that of other infants. The important point here is that, with the introduction of the concept that infants are born with differing temperaments, the temperamental characteristics of each infant's nature are now considered as his or her own contribution to how much or how little crying dominates his or her earliest socializing interactions with the parents. As Mitchell (1993) noted,

> One of the most important concepts emerging repeatedly from recent infancy and childhood research is the importance of "fit" between the baby's natural rhythms and thresholds and those of the caregivers. . . . The response to discomfort and/or frustration varies greatly from baby to baby, covering a wide range from fussing to listlessness to intense rage. (p. 364)

The belief that the love and special ministrations of an infant's biological mother were the only necessary ingredients for an infant to develop into a fairly self-confident older child has long been perpetuated (Kagan 1984). No other substitute for the mother's love was thought possible, including that of the biological father. Infants also were not thought to possess any special characteristics (e.g., resiliency versus susceptibility to stressful parenting or other environmental stresses) that would make it easier or harder for their mother to assist in their development. In this traditional view, all infants possessed a similar endowed physical and mental nature and hence were equally malleable to the parenting practices of a reasonably competent mother. It was inevitable, therefore, that the etiology of deviant infant and child behavior was believed to be faulty mothering behaviors, either overt or covert.

However, infant-mother pairs were found whose transactions began to challenge this prevalent belief. One type of infant that began to be noticed by developmentalists was the resilient infant who was doing quite well developmentally, despite being nurtured by a mother or father who was physically abusive or emotionally unavailable, or who had a serious psychiatric illness that interfered with normal parenting. A second type of infant recognized was the more susceptible infant who would do poorly developmentally, even though no evidence of abnormal parenting could be found. The discovery of these two types of infants caused developmental researchers to consider that there were individual differences in 1) infants' innate physical and mental nature, and specifically in their temperamental characteristics, and 2) the expectations of, and the demands made on, infants by their parents. These two considerations were formally articulated by Thomas et al. (1968) when they introduced the developmental concept of *goodness of fit.* They began to realize that how infants were nurtured did not solely account for the differences in their behaviors. They also noted that, during one phase of the infant's life, parents and their infant would engage in behaviors that evolved into a goodness of fit that was developmentally enhancing, whereas, during a later phase, their behaviors would lead to a fit that was developmentally inhibiting.

Although developmentalists now accept that temperamental characteristics are an aspect of infants' physical and mental endowment, definitions of temperament have been problematic. Different definitions of temperament abound, and whatever definition is used affects the choice of what measures are used to operationally define and measure temperament (Goldsmith and Campos 1982).

Most developmentalists advise against a single-instance assessment of temperament. Discontinuity as well as continuity can be found in the expression of temperamental characteristics, as in other mental abilities and surface behaviors. Differences noted at any one age may reflect differences in the rate of maturation rather than in temperament, and the meaning of a particular response can change markedly in the course of a single year (Dunn 1981). Temperamental characteristics can be modified by various factors, including the environment (Dunn 1981). Kagan (1984) also noted that "each child's temperament leads him or her to impose a special frame of reference, thus making it difficult to predict the consequences of a particular home environment" (p. 70). (Here, "frame of reference" refers to the particular constellation of temperamental traits possessed by the child that engages the parents in unique transactions, the result of which is hard to predict.)

In the earliest formal research on temperament, Thomas and Chess (1977), beginning in 1956 and continuing to the present, launched a longitudinal study of a group of 133 infants born into white, middle-class, mostly professional families in New York City. From 1966 to 1980, Korn and Gannon (1984) studied another cohort of 98 infants born into Puerto Rican, working-class families. In both studies, temperament was defined as the style of an infant's reactions to his or her environment, but did not include the infant's emotions generated in specific stimulating situations or how an infant's styles of emotional and behavioral response to stimulation might vary as his or her specific emotions varied. Campos et al. (1983), in reviewing these studies, noted that, although these researchers believed that infants with a low threshold for crying would also have a low threshold for other emotions (e.g., anger), some infants might have a lower threshold for crying but a high threshold for anger. Thomas and Chess focused on 10 categories of temperament: activity level, rhythmicity, approach-withdrawal, adaptability, threshold, intensity of emotional response, quality of emotional states, distractibility, ability to complete a task, and attention span–persistence (see Table 3–4). From these were derived three topological characterizations of infants: easy, difficult, and slow to adapt (Chess and Thomas 1989; Thomas and Chess 1977; see Table 3–5). The infants' temperamental reaction patterns were evaluated primarily through parent and teacher report, not by direct observations of these infants.

Chess and Thomas (1989) found that, for some infants, the label assigned to them predicted and correlated highly with the traits they showed as young adults, whereas for other infants, the adult correlation was poor. Nevertheless, Chess and Thomas reported that the child viewed as being difficult at age 3 years tended to exhibit those same traits as a young adult. Carey (1986) cautioned that if an infant's difficult temperament is not identified by the infant's parents and then taken into account by them in modifying their parenting style with their infant, then there may emerge a developmentally inhibiting fit between the infant and the parents, often resulting in the development of psychiatric difficulties in the infant.

Anna Freud's research based on her work with orphans she took into her London nurseries during World War II (A. Freud

Table 3–4. Phenomenological categories of infant temperament action and reaction patterns in Thomas and Chess (1977) and Chess and Thomas (1984, 1989) studies

Activity level—Quantity, quality, and proportion of active to inactive periods

Rhythmicity—Regulation of irregularity of biological functions (e.g., hunger, sleep, wakefulness, excretion)

Approach-withdrawal—Assertiveness in approaching unfamiliar or unexpected situations versus inhibition and withdrawal

Adaptability—Time duration of achieving adaptation to a stimulating experience

Threshold—Minimum strength of stimulus needed to evoke a response

Intensity of emotional response—Behavior intensity of emotions as observed in various situations

Quality of emotional states—Presence of pleasurable emotions (e.g., joy, excitement) versus displeasurable emotions (e.g., fear, anger)

Distractibility—Degree to which extraneous stimuli alter behaviors

Ability to complete a task—Attention span and persistence at a task

Attention span–persistence—Ability to focus attention on a novel stimulus and persist at attempts to achieve mastery despite distracting stimuli

1955/1968) predated the data reported by Thomas and Chess (1977). She categorized the orphans into three groups similar to those of the Thomas and Chess clusters. The "favorites" of the foster parent caretakers were children who were easy to get along with and were lovable and friendly. The second group were the "wanted to be close" group who were shy and turned to other children for closeness before they turned to available adults. The last group were the "difficult to reach out" children. They were easily angered and had a low tolerance for any frustration.

In a Canadian study on the effect of parenting style and parental attributions toward infants and the overall development of children with "difficult" temperaments, Maziade et al. (1985) focused on two groups of 7-year-old children; one group in which the children were considered to be "difficult" and another in which they were considered to be "easy." The "difficult" children were characterized as such based on their low adaptability, withdrawal from new stimuli, intensity in emotional reactions, negative mood, and low dis-

---

Table 3–5. Topological characterization of temperament: major constellations

Easy infant
  Is biologically regular
  Displays predominantly positive mood
  Approaches new situations
  Adapts easily to environmental change

Difficult infant
  Is biologically irregular
  Displays predominantly negative mood
  Often withdraws from new situations
  Slowly adapts to environmental change

Slow-to-adapt (or warm up) infant
  Is mostly biologically regular
  Displays predominantly positive mood, but is slow in generating such a mood
  Initially withdraws from new situations, but will adapt slowly

---

Source.   Thomas and Chess 1977.

tractibility. These children and their socioeconomic status were evaluated at age 7 years and again at age 11 years through home observation, structured interviews with the children and their parents, and teacher questionnaires. Results at age 11 years showed that there was an association between developmentally inhibiting family functioning and the development of psychiatric disorders within the children in the difficult group. In reviewing the results of this study, the authors stated,

> There is a trend in our data suggesting that the risk for temperamentally difficult children increases if parents show little consensus and if family rules and demands are not clear or lack firmness or consistency. Conversely, almost no family with superior functioning in terms of behavior control was associated with psychiatric disorder in difficult children. This suggests that a higher than average quality of parental behavior control may be a protective factor against the risk associated with difficult temperament. (Maziade et al. 1985, p. 945)

Kagan (1984, 1989) has also noted another temperamental characteristic that seems to persist from birth through late childhood: the tendency to display an "inhibition to the unfamiliar" (more commonly known as shyness, caution, or timidity) on the one hand, or sociability, boldness, or fearlessness on the other. He hypothesized that this tendency to either favor or lack inhibition to the unfamiliar could persist through childhood because of its possible basis in a child's biological makeup. Kagan (1984, 1989) also observed that parents can encourage their temperamentally timid infant or child to be less fearful in approaching unfamiliar people and situations. Thus, although inhibition to the unfamiliar may be viewed as a risk factor, parents' nurturant behaviors can overcome the risk. *Risk factor* here is defined as a characteristic of the child—in this example, an aspect of the child's temperament—that would predispose the child to developing abnormally (e.g., predisposing the child to develop a faulty attachment relationship with his or her parents).

It is clear that an infant's or child's temperament and the parenting environment combine in a transactional process that has the potential to become either a developmentally enhancing goodness of fit or a developmentally inhibiting poorness of fit. Whether the fit is developmentally good or bad depends on whether or not it enhances the infant's or child's progress within his or her social environment. When the developmental taskings and goals of the family environment match those of the social environment, we would say that a goodness of fit within the family produces a goodness of fit in society. However, the opposite can also occur. For an example of a poor fit, I return to the longitudinal studies of Thomas and Chess and Korn and Gannon. Korn and Gannon, working with Chess and Thomas, selected children from Chess and Thomas's white, middle-class sample and children from their own Puerto Rican, working-class sample who manifested the temperamental characteristic of low regularity in sleep-awake cycles. The parents from each socioeconomic group were subsequently found to differ in how they viewed their infants. Korn and Gannon (1984) reported that, until these children reached age 5 years, children from Puerto Rican families would be allowed to go to sleep and awaken at any time they desired. Within the family environment, this temperamental characteristic did not interfere with a goodness of fit between child and parent. Further, it did not predict the presence of problem behaviors in these children's adaptation to their home environment. In persisting from infancy to at least age 5 years, this temperamental characteristic became a developmental continuity for these children. However, the goodness of fit in the family that was present in the first 5 years of life produced a poorness of fit in their society when these children started school at age 6 years. At that time, they began to develop adjustment problems, including not being able to perform well in school because of insufficient sleep and often arriving late for school.

In the white families, however, the parents' strong demand that their low-rhythmicity children follow a rhythmic sleep pattern predicted problem behaviors within the family environment (i.e., rebelliousness when these children were made to go to sleep and arise at specific times) from infancy through the first 5 years of life (Chess and Thomas 1986). However, because of these children's adaptability and their parents' demands, their low rhythmicity tended to be discontinuous for most of them. A goodness of fit developed between these children and their family by about age 5 years when the children fully adapted to their parents' demands about their sleep schedule. This behavior in turn produced a goodness of fit between these children and their society when they went to school: their sleep patterns fit their school schedules.

In summary, temperamental characteristics, as innately present and maturationally emerging aspects of infants' mental nature, develop in the context of the socializing parental environment. By age 18 months, when infants develop an objective awareness of their own temperamental characteristics, they begin to become consciously aware that their parents support some of their temperamental traits and want them to change others.

Maturation and Development of Emotions

■ Role of Emotions

Infants are capable of generating several distinct emotions in response to sensory stimuli. Their primary emotions are joy, fear, anger, sadness, disgust, and surprise. These emotions are characterized both by their early appearance and by having prototypic and universal facial expressions (M. Lewis and Brooks-Gunn 1979). An example of the facial expression of joy is shown in Figure 3–2, and of surprise, in Figure 3–3.

Whether a pleasurable or displeasurable emotion is generated is determined by the level of exteroceptive (external) and proprioceptive (internal) stimulation received by the infant. The self directs its ego to generate mental activity and surface behaviors according to the stimulus principle. The ego's barometer is the infant's unique stimulus threshold to each stimulus modality: stimulation within the infant's optimal stimulation range generates a pleasurable emotional state, and stimulation that exceeds or falls below this range or stimulation that is within a stimulus modality not well accepted by the infant will generate a displeasurable emotional state. Emde

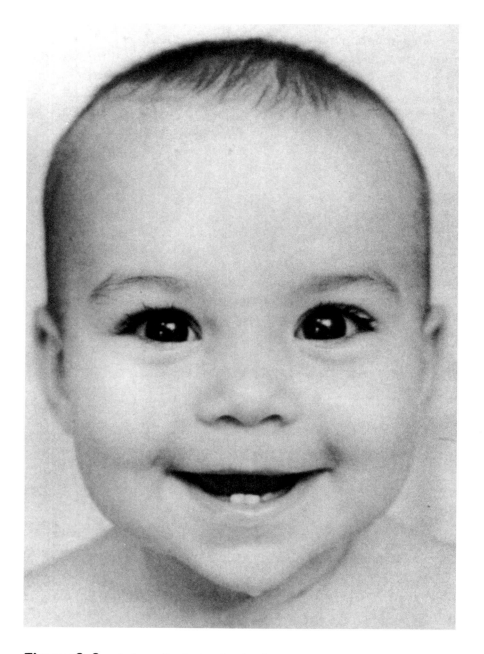

Figure 3-2. Infant displaying look of joy.
Source. Photograph by Florence Sharp; used with permission.

(1983) noted that, through this process, infants are preprogrammed to monitor their experiences according to what is pleasurable and displeasurable. Within the biopsychosocial model, the

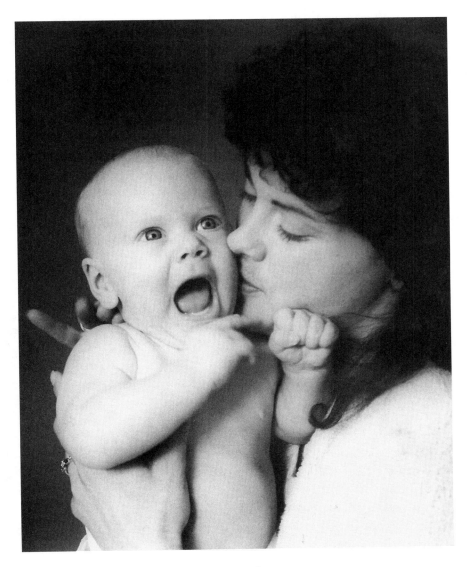

Figure 3–3. Infant displaying look of surprise.
Source. Photograph by Florence Sharp; used with permission.

infant is becoming motivated to seek to repeat emotionally plea-surable experiences—especially those that generate competency pleasure—and to avoid those experiences that generate displea-surable emotions.

Emde postulated that infants are innately endowed with an af-fective self that, like other aspects of the self, develops silently dur-ing the pre-self-aware phase of life (i.e., prior to age 18 months). According to J. B. Miller (1991), the first 18 months of life is the

> beginning of a sense of "self" that reflects what is happening be-tween people. The infant picks up the feelings of the other per-son, that is, it has an early sense that "I feel what is going on in the other as well as what is going on in myself." . . . [The infant] experiences a sense of comfort (i.e., emotional self-regulation) only as the other is comfortable, or, more precisely, only as they are both engaged in an emotional relationship that is moving toward greater well-being. . . . In this sense, the infant, actively expecting an effect on the relationship, begins to develop an in-ternal sense of itself as one who changes the emotional interplay for both participants . . . for good or ill. (p. 78)

As self-awareness is attained after age 18 months, infants' affec-tive selves continue to develop, lending a continuity to their expe-riences in the face of all their changes. This "affective core" is the means by which they come to understand others through under-standing their feelings (J. B. Miller 1991). The representations in-fants construct of their emotional experiences become future ingredients of how they eventually define themselves. Kagan (1984) postulated that emotions are one of the sources of evidence on which the concept of the self rests.

In developmental research, emotions are the aspect of the life experience that has been the most difficult to describe. As with temperament, different definitions abound as to what an emotion is, and the subsequent definition determines the choice of what measures are used to identify and quantify emotions. Emotions are frequently generated by the stimulation of infants' innate needs, but emotions can also come before or coincident with stimulation of an innate need. It would appear that a basic aspect of human nature is the production of a number of discrete, preadapted emotions that subsequently develop through interaction with the environment.

Freud tended to view emotions as the qualitative aspect of instinctual wishes. Because he postulated that instinctual wishes derived from innate and biologically maturing drives, he viewed emotions as evolving biological structures. This biological model of emotions (Demos 1982) would thus place the emotions within the domain of the brain (see Chapter 1), which I describe as the biological referent domain from which each person's mental nature derives. What the biological model of emotions does not address is how biological emotional structures find expression within the mental domain.

Interest in how emotions are experienced within the mental domain has led researchers to postulate a psychosocial model of emotions (M. Lewis and Brooks-Gunn 1979; M. Lewis and Michalson 1982). This model is in essence a biopsychosocial model of emotions: Infants must construct representations of their emotional experiences and store this knowledge within their long-term memories. These memories, as psychological stimuli within their representational world, then influence their perceptions of their current experiences involving the social world. Parents must first teach their infants to recognize how an outside event (an emotional elicitor) stimulates an inside reaction (an emotional state), and how this produces a physically observable reaction in them (an emotional expression). The latter is correctly identified and communicated to infants by their parents through actions (or, if the infant has become verbal, in words). This is how infants construct a representation of each of their emotions (an emotional experience). For example, a 3-year-old girl goes with her father to the beach for the first time. While holding her father's hand, she walks to the edge of the water. A wave then knocks her over (an emotional elicitor). Her father tells her, in seeing a look of fear on her face (an emotional expression), "The wave knocked you down and made you afraid" (an emotional state).

Eventually, infants slowly construct a memory bank of perceptual representations of their different emotions and how they expressed them and how their parents responded to them. In this way, their inner world of emotional representations is constructed and developed. As Stern (1985) expressed it, "For each separate emotion, the infant comes to recognize and expect a characteristic constellation of things happening" (p. 89). The "things happening" most often involve the things that people do or do not do when infants express an emotion. Infants thus develop a sense of themselves within the context of a relationship with another. "Being in relationship, picking up the feelings of the other, and attending to the 'interaction between' becomes an accepted 'natural-seeming' way of being and acting" (J. B. Miller 1991, p. 84).

■ Parents' Interpretations of Their Infants' Emotions

Infants' emotions are open to interpretation by their parents. They are also strongly influenced by their parents' aspirations, beliefs, and projections of their own feelings, given that pre-self-aware infants do not possess an objective sense of being separate selves in a world of parents and others. As Shapiro and Hertzig (1988) expressed it,

> Emotional experiences require a sense of self—an "I" to evaluate changes in "me"—as well as the cognitive [conceptual thinking] capacity to perceive, discriminate, recall, associate, and compare. From this perspective, the very young body's emotional expression tells us little of his or her emotional experience. Nevertheless, parents and others respond to the infant's emotional expressions as if they were reflection of subjective experience. By interpreting and evaluating emotional expression, the social environment provides the rules by which children come to learn, to evaluate, and interpret, in other words, to experience their own behavior [and emotional] states. (p. 108)

For example, W. Johnson et al. (1982) reported that mothers believed their 1-month-old infants expressed the following emotions: fear (58%), sadness (34%), surprise (74%), joy (95%), and interest (99%). In an earlier study (F. Johnson et al. 1980), mothers attributed an even greater range and degree of emotions to their 3-month-old infants: interest and joy (100%), anger (86%), surprise (69%), and fear (69%). However, as Stern (1985) noted,

We simply do not know if infants are actually feeling what their faces, voices and bodies so powerfully express to us, but it is very hard to witness such expressions and not make that inference. (p. 66)

Perhaps parents' "seeing" emotions within their infants, and interpreting those emotions according to their own representational world, is a necessary nurturant ministration for infants to mature and develop their emotional life. Certainly there is a growing body of observational data that documents infants' perceiving their parents' emotional states and using this information to acquire knowledge about themselves, their parents, and the inanimate world.

■ Infants' Ability to Perceive Others' Emotions

By age 2 months, infants appear to be quite sensitive to their mother's emotional states. In one study, Cohn and Tronick (1983) had mothers of 3-month-old babies compose their face into a depressed look, talk to their infant in a monotone voice, and show minimal body movement. In response, the infants showed much more gaze aversion, protest behavior, and crying than when the mothers behaved normally. Beebe and Sloate (1982) reported how a 3-month-old infant, after repeated smiling at his mother only to receive a blank stare in return, eventually began to avoid gazing into his mother's depressed face.

Infants' own emotional response to these perceptions are added to what they perceive of their parents' emotional responses. For example, what stops infants from crawling off high surfaces is not their fear, learned from having experienced other falls, but their parents' emotional reactions to their near falls (Campos et al. 1983). Thus another's emotion becomes a crucial organizer for infants as they construct knowledge about the inanimate world.

Emde (1983) noted that pre-self-aware infants are able to perceive emotional information emanating from their parents and use this information for emotional referencing. This ability to engage in emotional referencing propels infants to spontaneously seek and actively scan their parent's face for emotional information as they assertively seek a novel stimulus. When a parent's face expresses fear, the majority of infants will cease to pursue that stimulus; on the other hand, when a parent's face expresses happiness, the majority of infants will be encouraged to continue to explore the stimulus.

It appears that, although infants' emotions regulate their expression of their innate needs and resultant surface behaviors depending on whether a behavior generates pleasure or displeasure, they are not sufficient to regulate infants' mental activity and resultant surface behaviors. This is where emotional referencing comes into play as another "self-regulatory process in a situation of dynamic social interchange" (Emde 1983, p. 170). In my view, this statement refers to infants' ever-present need to use their parents' emotions to help them regulate their levels of stimulation so that they remain within their optimal stimulation range. As Stechler and Kaplan (1980) noted,

> There are plenty of moments when different need states are mutually incompatible (e.g., hunger and fatigue), but whichever one is ascendant will govern behavior. (p. 93)

What often determines which state becomes ascendant is the infant's perception of the emotional state and behavior of the parents. The infant is then able to use these perceptions to choose behaviors that stimulate the parents' approval and their pleasurable emotional signals and avoid behaviors that engender their parents' disapproval and their displeasurable emotional signals. Take for example the case of Nancy, an infant girl whose parents, although primarily loving toward her, had been periodically observed in their socializing of their infant to feel compelled to prohibit, scold, or spank her:

> [At the age of 6 months, Nancy was] progressing smoothly in her development, as being able to maintain her own direction of interest and to adapt readily to a variety of external cues. She was very responsive socially, but, at the same time, very selective as to which stimuli she responded to. She was able to block out or accommodate to a range of intrusions.

At the age of 9 months, she refused to take a nap and was spanked by her father. She responded with compliant behavior. Thereupon, she showed highly differentiated behavior toward her father. She could observe a frown on her father's face and become upset. She did not, however, make attempts to avoid her father but made . . . active efforts to engage him and to get him to smile—at which point she relaxed and joined the game. . . . [She showed] early evidence of her awareness of different affects and her active searching for ways to influence events so that she could end with a pleasurable affect. . . . Although Nancy responded to her father's frown with distress, with non-pleasure, she nevertheless persisted in maintaining contact with him until she could change his behavior and eventually produce a pleasurable situation for herself. . . . Her experiences inform her that she can influence events . . . [and] make a difference in her interpersonal world. (Stechler and Kaplan 1980, pp. 95–96)

As early as age 9 months, this normally progressing infant girl had begun to store representational memories of her assertiveness in taking the initiative, of her own emotions, of her parents' emotions and behaviors, and of her ability to bring about both a pleasurable and displeasurable emotional state in her parents. The authors continued to observe Nancy and noted how, when she was age 1 year, she regulated her own initiated actions to avoid causing displeasurable emotions in her parents:

[Nancy] has a wish, carries out her own plan on her own initiative, and then meets up with the forbidden parent. She then reduces the impulsive quality of the response and checks the result with the parent to see what the change in her behavior produces in the parent's reaction. . . . On any number of occasions, her behavior increasingly reflected a choice: when, in an empathic climate, she was presented with the necessity to choose between a behavior that reflected the pursuit of the desire versus that which constituted an alliance with the parent, she chose the latter. (Stechler and Kaplan 1980, p. 97)

Within the first 18 months of life, this infant girl had become regulated and organized by the active emotional interplay between herself and her parents. In addition, this self-regulation was experienced by her as a subjective feeling of control. Eventually, Nancy began to perceive a conflict between her need to explore novel stimuli and her parents' need to inhibit such behaviors in her. In the following scenario, Nancy and her mother had just arrived at a new office playroom where Nancy was to undergo some developmental testing. Nancy apparently perceived the testing cubes in the office as novel stimuli and evidenced joy while throwing them onto the floor.

> She got deliberate about it [i.e., the cube throwing] and with considerable vigor threw a cube down on the floor. . . . Mother expressed annoyance, then started a series of prohibiting "uh, uhs," calling out her [Nancy's] name with increasing loudness. There was a response in that Nancy did restrain herself, then looked searchingly at mother, followed by an abortive attempt to throw the block. She was poised to drop the cube, again looked at mother, and finally let the cube just slip out of her hand. She was now much more tentative, did not actually throw the cube, and kept checking back for mother's reaction. (Stechler and Kaplan 1980, p. 98)

At the point when Nancy was "poised to drop the cube" but did not drop it immediately and instead delayed her action by looking at her mother, Nancy was beginning to exercise self-inhibition. What motivated this inhibition was her desire to receive a pleasurable emotional response from her mother. In Nancy's inhibiting her own innate assertive needs, she was beginning to identify with and learn the behaviors she saw her mother do herself.

In their observations about Nancy, the authors wrote:

> We witness the struggle between the wish to express, to act upon the desire, versus the wish to please and remain on friendly terms with the parent. Nancy develops the capacity to resolve this conflict in the direction of an inhibition or modification of the desire, she takes a step in the direction of identifying with her parents and aligns herself as being opposed to the wish. We especially emphasize those solutions which imply the capacity to compromise, to find new solutions. . . . She now creates a previously *never existing behavior;* e.g., the slow release of the

cube is a creative solution to the incompatibility. This synthesis leads to mastery. (Stechler and Kaplan 1980, p. 100; italics in original)

Nancy's creative solution of her conflict, therefore, led to a sense of mastery and competency pleasure that enabled her to re-achieve emotional self-regulation (i.e., regulation of maintaining her level of stimulation within her optimal stimulation range). When self-awareness began to emerge in Nancy at about age 18 months, she already had constructed representations of her experiences with external conflicts and her achievements and failures at attaining mastery. Consequently, she immediately had a sense of having at her disposal various ways of maintaining self-regulation of her emotions. Because of this, she, as a typical objectively self-aware 18-month-old toddler, would not become excessively over-stimulated in becoming consciously aware of possessing innate needs, emotions, memories, and so on as a separate person in a world of others who possess the same characteristics.

■ Anger

One controversial emotion needs to be discussed: anger. Earlier in this chapter, I discuss the view held by Freud that infants were born with an innate aggressive instinct or death instinct that was the source of their destructive rage or hostile aggressiveness. Mitchell (1993), in reviewing Freud's hypothesis about the existence of a death instinct, noted the following:

> Freud regarded aggression as an indigenously arising, continuous pressure demanding discharge. There is a need to harm and destroy, which often finds frustrations to serve as a rationale; but if there are no causes to be found, no rationales, the need for the discharge of aggression may overrun the defensive controls that ordinarily hold it in check, and aggression emerges spontaneously. (p. 354)

Along with many developmentalists (Kohut 1971; Lichtenberg 1989; Parens 1979; Stechler and Halton 1987), I find it difficult to attribute to the human infant an innate compelling need to destroy others. Instead, I see infants' aggression as a reaction to a perceived threat that will overwhelm their capacity to maintain stimulation within their optimal stimulation range. Once the source of stimulation that is causing the highly displeasurable emotions is fought off or eliminated in some way, the aggression ceases.

Stechler and Halton (1987) differentiated between infant assertive behaviors and infant aggressive behaviors:

> Assertion derives from the universal tendency to be active, to seek stimuli, to generate plans, and to carry them out. It is a self-activating system and is generally associated with the positive affects of joy, interest, and excitement. Aggression derives from the equally universal self-protective system. This system, however, is reactive in the face of a perceived threat and is associated with the dysphoric affects of anger, fear and distress. . . . Our position . . . is that aggression is part of a primordial self-protective system and as such will become manifest only in reaction to a perceived threat. (p. 821)

Less psychologically aware parents can misinterpret their infant's assertive behaviors as manifestations of aggression. If reacted to punitively,

> the child in turn feels threatened and becomes self-protective. The result is a contamination between assertion and aggression. . . . If assertions are frequently blocked, and contamination may be extensive, it may appear as if an aggressive instinctual process is present. (Stechler and Halton 1987, p. 821)

In other words, the infant may appear to have a driving need to hurt and even kill others, hence possessing a "death instinct."

In the process of the infant's normal development, parents view their infants as inherently lovable and treat them with more love than anger. There is little evidence suggesting that a lovingly nurtured infant becomes a child dominated by aggressive wishes and fantasies and angry and hateful emotions. Instead, observational and longitudinal data suggest a correlation between parental aggression toward a child and that child's viewing himself or herself as an aggressive person and not seeking or giving love. Often parents' aggressive treatment emanates from one or both of the parents' faulty belief that their infant is overly aggressive and constantly wishes to attack them. In such a transactional process in which infants' normal assertive expression of their needs and feelings is viewed by their parents as an expression of their destructive, aggressive tendencies, it is no wonder that, as early as infancy, these children begin to construct representations of their assertive wishes and behaviors as aggressive, hostile wishes and behaviors. Their representational world becomes filled with long-term memories of experiences with their parents and others that are characterized by something akin to "I hate people," or "I hurt people because I'm bad," as did the boy in the following case example:

> A physically and emotionally abused 10-year-old boy I was seeing in therapy told me, "When I was little, my mother told me I was bad like my father who went to prison. I know I'm mean and that I hate people."
> On one occasion in a family therapy meeting with his mother and a younger sister, this boy produced an injured bird that he had carefully shielded within his pocket. He stated, while showing the injured but still alive bird that he held gently in his hands, "This bird was left, and I want to take it home and help it fly again." His mother thereupon turned to me and instead of positively mirroring her son's assertive behavior, she projected her own self-hatred onto him in a piece of negative mirroring and said, "See what I have been telling you? He doesn't care about anyone but himself. We have a small apartment and a bird will only make messes and cause me more work. He is basically selfish and mean; I saw these traits in him when he was an infant." Without the boy's saying a word, his facial expression turned into an expression of hatred, and he quietly placed the wounded bird on the floor near one of the walls of the room. Suddenly, he pushed a desk up against the wall, instantly crushing and killing the bird. While I looked at him in a moment of shocked disbelief, he said to me, "She's right. See how really mean I can be? I don't care about anybody."

In summary, emotions are infants' main organizers for achieving 1) energy mobilization (i.e., mobilizing their mental energy to assertively seek new experiences, repeat previous experiences that generated pleasurable emotions, and avoid previous experiences that generated displeasurable emotions), 2) self-regulation (i.e., maintaining stimulation within their optimal stimulation range), and 3) social adaptation (using emotions in the pre-self-aware, pre-verbal stage to communicate with their parents [Cicchetti and Schneider-Rosen 1986]).

Development of the Self and Object Relationships

■ Developing a Sense of Self-Value While Engaged in Transactional Relationships With Others

One important social function parents fulfill is to instill within their infants a sense of self-esteem. This self-esteem is developed in a nurturant arena in which infants are given the physical space and an interesting and novel environment in which to perform and produce. While the parents are fulfilling this and other social functions, they are operating as selfobjects.

Kohut and Wolf (1978) defined *selfobject* as an object that is experienced as part of oneself and that one expects to control in the same manner in which one controls one's own body and mind. (The term *object* refers to a person's internal representation of a certain person or phenomenon, which is actually an amalgamation of the various images that person has formed of the person or phenomenon during his or her past experiences with it.) Pre-self-aware infants perceive their parents as being both separate objects and a part of their self-absorbed experience, that is, as selfobjects. Lichtenberg (1989) described the selfobject experience as

A particular affective state characterized by a sense of cohesion, safety and competence. . . . At each period of life there are specific needs, and when these needs are met, the result is that of a selfobject experience. When these needs are not met, the individ-

> ual experiences a sense of disturbed cohesion . . . [such as] when a distracted friend fails to [positively] mirror one's greeting. . . . Need satisfaction is fundamental to the maintenance of self-cohesion and is the source of selfobject experience. (p. 12)

The validity of the assumption that infants can relate to their parents as selfobjects and never experience them concurrently as whole objects—or that parents can relate to their infants only as selfobjects—is currently being debated by developmental researchers. As Kohut seemed to define it, when pre-self-aware infants begin to construct representations of their parents in their selfobject functioning, these selfobject representations are the only representations that exist within their inner world prior to age 18 months.

In my view, infants relate to each parent as both a selfobject and a whole object, and both selfobject and whole object representations develop concurrently within infants' inner worlds. For example, Coen (1981) observed that, in general, the concept of the selfobject "tends to obfuscate the subject's relation to the object. The subject's attitudes, representations, feelings, and valuations of the object tend to be neglected" (p. 398). In this statement, Coen was suggesting that, when pre-self-aware infants manifest a need that involves their parents' providing a selfobject function that they are unable to provide for themselves, they are entirely focused on their need at the moment and do not sense the parent as a whole object. However, their beginning representations of their parent as a whole object exist even during these situations. It would appear, therefore, that infants perceive their parents—the supporters and developers of their sense of value and self-esteem—as both selfobjects and whole objects.

Wolf (1993) illustrated the difference between when an infant, child, or adult engages in an object relationship with another and when the individual is relating to another as a selfobject:

> When my watch misfunctions I take it to a watch repairman, who either fixes the watch or fails to fix it. Neither my self nor my subjective awareness of myself are involved. I may like or dislike the watchmaker. . . . I may love or I may hate the manner

in which he deals with me: all these are aspects of an object-relationship. But let us suppose he wants me to come back once a month to adjust my watch more precisely, and on my visits to his shop we talk of all kinds of things, person-to-person, not just about the watch. Gradually I notice that I am beginning to care how he thinks and how he feels about me: the object-relationship, in part, has taken on some aspects of a selfobject relationship. My feeling of well-being is influenced, if ever so slightly, by my relationship with the watchmaker. I feel good if I experience him as positively responsive to me—my self [esteem] is enhanced. On the other hand, if I experience his response as lacking or desultory, then my self [esteem] is diminished . . . and I do not feel so good about myself. . . . The intensity of selfobject experiences also ranges widely: from slight to the deeply involved ones that are characteristic of relationships with significant others, such as parents, spouses, children, friends and lovers. (p. 677)

Normally developing infants and children are thought to need their parents to function as both idealizing and mirroring selfobjects (Kohut 1971, 1977; Kohut and Wolf 1978). Eventually, children learn to perform these mirroring and idealizing social functions for themselves. However, when parents fail to provide these functions in early life, children can grow up with serious deficits in their ability to provide these functions for themselves.

As *idealizing selfobjects,* parents fulfill their infants' need to idealize and otherwise view their parents as all-powerful and perfect. For infants to become consciously aware of the need to idealize their parents, they must achieve self-awareness (at about age 18 months) and have experiences in which they begin to learn that they are vulnerable to abandonment and injury. It is then that self-aware infants turn to their parents with the need to view them as all-powerful and all-protective. (This idealization is discussed further in Chapter 4.)

As *mirroring selfobjects,* parents fulfill their infant's need to receive acceptance and admiration for his or her performances, something that pre-self-aware infants cannot provide for themselves because they are unable to recognize their own competencies. Infants then incorporate this parental acceptance and admiration into their gradually developing self-representation. If infants do not receive this acceptance and admiration (e.g., if they are not given tasks that are within their innate and maturing abilities to perform for which they can then be admired), they will not begin to establish a sense of self-value. Parents develop their infant's sense of value and associated self-esteem through providing admiring and accepting mirroring responses of their infant on two bases: an intrinsic, unconditional, or non-performance-related basis and a conditional, performance-related basis (see Figure 3–4).

Parents usually perceive their newborn as invaluable. Despite how the infant looks or despite his or her gestational age or gender, proud parents exclaim, "Isn't my baby just wonderful!" Sensitively aware parents do not say, for example, "Well, our baby boy hasn't shown us his level of assertiveness, or whether he has an easy or difficult temperament, so we'll have to reserve our judgment until he begins to perform." Before infants have any conscious ability to understand any concept of value, they subjectively experience a sense of esteem when they gaze into their parents' eyes and, despite

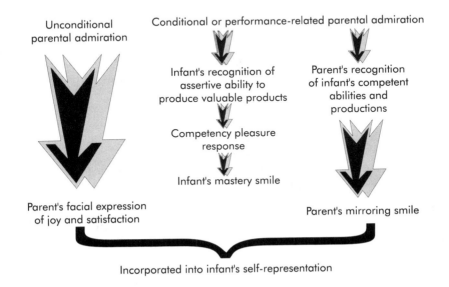

Figure 3–4. Sources of infants' developing a sense of self-value.

how they are functioning at the moment, see a gleam of satisfaction, admiration, and joy. This *non-performance-related positive mirroring* from their parents becomes the crucial social stimulus involved in infants' development of self-esteem.

The second source for infants' sense of value is *performance-related positive mirroring* responses from their parents. Parents give these responses when they observe their infant's expression of competency pleasure and when parents spontaneously respond to their infant's pleasing behaviors prior to their infant's evidencing any competency pleasure. When infants are able to master a novel stimulus or effect an interesting change in their environment in an assertive manner (e.g., when an action by the infant [such as kicking a foot] causes a response in the environment [such as causing a hanging toy to move]), they are likely to display a smile, designated as a *mastery smile.* This innately developing smile tends to be generated whenever infants experience competency pleasure and does not require an audience. However, parents usually are quite happy to see a mastery smile on their infant's face and are quite willing to respond with a performance-confirming, positive *mirroring smile* of their own. Each mastery smile and complementary parental mirroring smile fuels the infant's development of a sense of value and associated self-esteem. In forming memories of these mirroring smiles, the infant then begins to look for a positive mirroring smile in his or her parents after he or she experiences a mastery smile of his or her own.

Another source of performance-related acceptance and admiration is when the parents produce a spontaneous smile in response to their infant's behaving in a manner that the parents believe is necessary for the infant's socialization. Infants take pleasure in perceiving that their behaviors can produce pleasurable emotions in their parents.

Parents' provision of performance-related positive mirroring must involve their use of empathy in assessing when to positively mirror their infant's competency pleasure and when to emotionally signal that their infant is beginning to engage in a potentially displeasurable or dangerous situation. For example, a 6-month-old boy may evidence a mastery smile as he begins to crawl away from his mother. The infant also engages in emotional referencing by periodically looking back at his mother's face. The mother, according to Kohut and Wolf (1978), must provide an empathically attuned, selfobject mirroring function in reflecting her infant's competency pleasure in demonstrating his crawling ability—as indicated by the infant's mastery smile—and at the same time be attuned to the infant's stimulation level. If the infant is feeling a joyful excitement, the empathic mother mirrors back her joy and the infant begins to construct a joyful perceptual representation of this and later assertive crawling experiences. If, however, the infant is beginning to experience too much stimulation (e.g., he begins to notice the growling family dog near where he is crawling), the empathically attuned, selfobject functioning mother senses her infant's beginning displeasurable emotional state and mirrors back her emotional concern. She visually signals with her eyes and facial expression her concern (an emotional signal) or through a hand signal motions her infant to return. Alternatively, she goes immediately to pick him up. In providing this response to her infant's stimulation level, the mother uses her empathy to perceive when her infant is becoming overstimulated, signals her distress, and acts in a way to assist her infant in regaining the pleasurable emotional state that initially was associated with his crawling. In providing this stimulus-regulating function, the mother operates as a selfobject who is also very slowly fostering the development of her infant's own capacity to provide this stimulus-regulating and emotional-regulating function for himself.

A question that is currently being posed by developmental researchers is, What constitutes a normal degree of empathy? At what point do parents empathically fail their infants by not providing functions that they cannot yet provide for themselves on the one hand, and providing functions that their infants should be beginning to perform for themselves on the other? The answer given by Kohut is somewhat confusing. At one point in his book *Restoration of the Self* (1977), Kohut stated that parents who cling to their infants when they should be sending messages to them that they should begin to become more autonomous are empathically failing their infants as mirroring selfobjects. Alternatively, Kohut also stated that, if parents encourage their infants to behave in a manner that is too autonomous of the parents' caregiving before they are ready, then the parents would also be empathically failing their infant. In my view, being properly empathic as a parent is an ideal for which psychologically attuned parents should strive. Thus in achieving empathy for their infant, parents demonstrate their own competency as a parent. This competency affects the infant's sense of value and associated self-esteem because the transactional process through which infants and parents develop a goodness of fit is also a reciprocal process of positive self-esteem nurturance; that is, the infant's performances and productions become a source of every parent's self-esteem.

In certain abnormal situations, an infant can become the only source of a parent's self-esteem. For example, if a mother judges that her infant is not performing according to some rigidly held standard, the mother will experience a sudden depletion of self-esteem in believing she has failed as a parent. She will mirror her displeasure in various communications to her infant. The mother then may rid herself of the depleted self-esteem she feels from what she judges to be her infant's deficient behaviors through projecting her negative self-esteem onto her infant and beginning to view the infant as being the who has failed, not herself. She may then regard her infant as inferior or retarded, or may react toward her infant with anger, shame, or both. Alternatively, if she views her infant as willfully refusing to perform at the level she expects, she may begin to attribute the infant with having malevolent motives toward her that the infant does not truly possess. Such an infant will begin to see a look of contempt reflected in her eyes. This process was operative in the following case example:

A single mother grew up believing that she would be accepted by her mother and all women in positions of authority only if she performed perfectly. Consequently, she approached her infant daughter with the expectation that she also should perform perfectly. When her daughter was age 14 months, the mother changed baby-sitters from the one her daughter had had since age 1 month. Her daughter reacted by crying and fretting. When this crying persisted for 3 days, the new baby-sitter told the mother that her daughter was much less well-behaved than the other two infants she cared for. The mother at first felt ashamed and became critical of herself. Then she projected this self-criticism onto her infant and subsequently became quite angry at her.

In this example, the mother may be viewed as using her infant daughter as a selfobject because she sought to have her daughter fulfill functions that she was unable to provide for herself. The mother was unable to maintain her own self-esteem relatively independently of the criticisms of others and so needed her daughter to perform perfectly in order to maintain it. The needs and feelings of her daughter were neglected in this interactive, not transactive, process. The mother did not perceive her infant as a separate other but as a selfobject that she needed to control, as if the daughter was an extension of herself. When a parent views his or her child as a selfobject, the individual separateness of the object (the child) is not within the parent's conscious awareness.

■ Developing a Sense of Separateness

In addition to parents' wanting to instill a sense of value in their infants, they also want to instill a sense of separateness. Awareness of both qualities develops concurrently while infants are engaged in transactional relationships with each of their parents. These transactions include the following:

In transactions related to infants' innate needs. As parents respond to their infant's maturing innate needs, emotions, temperamental characteristics, and cognitive competencies, they help their infant have a dawning awareness of where his or her behaviors interface with their own behaviors. Positive parental mirroring of an infant's sucking behaviors, for example, assists the infant in gradually developing a sense of separateness and a concurrent awareness of his or her parents as separate individuals. When parents mirror their approval of their infant's competency in demonstrating healthy sucking behaviors, they begin to teach the infant that this sucking behavior is part of an innate need possessed by them. Eventually, by age 3 years, children are able to say "I want to eat," not "My mother wants me to eat, I never like to eat."

Infants discover their true selves when they begin to construct representations of their innate needs, emotions, temperamental characteristics, and cognitive abilities as belonging to themselves as opposed to possessing false representations that result from their being taught that these come from, or belong to, their parents. When parents foster the development of a false self within their infant, the infant begins to live "a fake life built on reactions to external stimulation" (Winnicott 1965). Nancy, the 1-year-old girl mentioned above, was developing a true self as evidenced by her continuing to learn that her innate needs were her own, that she could use her emotions and the emotions of her parents to determine if she was pleasing or displeasing her parents, and that she could inhibit her method of gratifying a need that was displeasing her parents to arrive at new creative ways to gratify the need.

In low-stimulation, everyday caretaking activities with parents. Another set of experiences that lead to infants' development of a sense of separateness while engaged in relationships with their parents are those that take place when infants are relatively quiet and unstimulated. Pine (1985) identified a range of these everyday experiences: touching, rocking, seeing, smiling, and sucking. He noted that these low-key pleasures can add a sense of quiet bodily and receptor pleasure to an infant's ongoing self-experience. These quiet pleasures, which often occur as infants are being ministered to and interacting with the body of their mother and father, become the background to the child's life. Such background experiences also contribute to infants' developing a sense of having a separate body that produces separate behaviors.

Through bodily contact.   Another set of experiences that helps an infant experience a sense of separateness while being engaged in transactional relationships with his or her parents involves the infant's body wholeness. *Body wholeness* is the term used to describe each individual's "sense of being a nonfragmented, physical whole with boundaries and locus of integrated action" (Stern 1985, p. 71). These boundaries are conveyed by each individual's skin and sensoriperceptive organs (Mahler and McDevitt 1982).

Once again, parents will influence what kind of representations their infant forms of his or her body. One way in which parents' emotional reaction to their infant's body is communicated is how parents handle their infant's skin. This handling becomes an important source of the sensations and perceptions the infant uses to construct representations of his or her body's boundaries and wholeness. Once when I was visiting a family, I was amazed to see the mother suddenly put her 2-month-old infant boy in his crib so she could put on a pair of rubberized gloves. She then picked up her son and said, "I felt he was wet and I know that body products are very damaging to a mother's skin. I always use these gloves whenever I change him." As a result of her actions, that infant sometimes felt rubber and at other times, when he had not urinated or defecated, would feel skin.

The sense of body wholeness involves infants' eventual slow construction of a body image. From birth to about age 18 months, infants can subjectively sense and perceive their body and bodily processes and then form and store representations of them. However, they do not yet have a conscious, objective awareness of possessing their own body in a world of other bodies; they have only a self-absorbed or subjective awareness of their body's boundaries and wholeness. Without an objective awareness of having a body in relation to their parents, infants are strongly influenced by their parents' perceptions of their (the infants') body and body processes.

Through parental responses to infants' gender. Another set of experiences that affects how infants "color" their sense of separateness involves how their parents perceive the gender-related parts of their body (i.e., their external genitalia). Parental responses to their infant's gender will begin to help the infant discover and own his or her gender.

When infants become able to view themselves as an objective self (at about age 18 months), they will construct an early gender representation. This early *gender identity* is the conception they construct of their being a member of the male or female category. As they grow older, they will learn what it means to be male or female within their family, and eventually will define for themselves gender role behaviors in discovering what it means to be masculine or feminine.

The biopsychosocial stimuli present during infancy that become the ingredients for a child's beginning gender identity at about 18 months of age are 1) the child's sex chromosomes, originating in fetal life (biological stimuli); 2) the parents' proper gender assignment at birth in labeling their infant a male or female (social stimuli; even though parents may give the correct assignment at birth, they may unconsciously be acting out a wish to have the opposite gender child [e.g., they may dress their infant boy in girl's clothing and give him a quasi-feminine name, such as Marion]); 3) the parents' attitudes and beliefs about the infant's gender (social stimuli); 4) the infant's experiences with his or her own body (biological stimuli) (Stoller 1968, 1985; P. Tyson 1994); and 5) the infant's innate need for sensory and sexual emotionally pleasurable stimulation and gratification that propels the infant to manipulate his or her genitalia (psychological stimuli).

Parents' attitudes about their infant's gender are communicated in the way they value their infants when they demonstrate the biological gender with which they were born. Usually parents admire and support those activities of their infant that are appropriate gender role behaviors. Thus, although empathically attuned parents may respond by communicating their admiration, acceptance, or empathic guidance, less-attuned parents may respond by communicating their disinterest, displeasure, or even contempt. Often the parent who responds with negative mirroring to an infant's perception of his or her gender is the parent whose own parents created an atmosphere within the family, or exposed the child to experiences outside of the family, that made the parent's gender a childhood burden, as in the following example:

> A mother had been sexually abused by her father from approximately ages 9–19 years; at age 19 years, she left home to marry her husband and "escape" her family. Her mother had died when she was age 10 years.
>
> When this woman bore a son at age 26 years, she began to dress him in her older daughter's clothing, saying, "He always looks cuter in them." She did not become aware of the real mo-

tivation for her behavior until she entered psychotherapy when her son was age 5 years. At about that time, her son had told his pediatrician that he wanted an operation to "make him a girl." The mother only then began to slowly and painfully become aware of her long repressed rage toward her own father, related to her unconscious traumatic memories of being repeatedly sexually abused by him. Her rage at her father for taking advantage of her being a girl had been transferred to all men, and she had become quite uneasy in gazing on her son when he was born. By dressing him as a girl, she could nurture him, as she stated it, "without feeling a strange kind of anxiousness." Through psychotherapy she became aware that this "anxiousness" resulted from her anger and her wish to hurt her infant whenever she gazed on his penis. All through her son's first 5 years of life, she had transferred her own rage toward her father's penis onto her son's penis.

In addition, this woman had always been afraid to look at or touch her husband's penis because of her wish to injure it. She did not take pleasure in intercourse and had never had an orgasm during sex with her husband. Her husband ignored her inhibitory behaviors during sex and her dressing their son as a girl, as he tended to ignore all parenting activities related to his son. He had had a distant and hostile relationship with his own father and presently had few male friends. He was quite unable to access any degree of empathy for his son, and in hearing his son at age 4 years tell him that he wanted to be a girl, dismissed it as a joke.

By having a chance to raise a son, both of these parents were being offered an opportunity to restructure their own representational worlds of past painful memories. However, neither was able to avail himself or herself of that opportunity. They were unable to give their infant son the empathically generated positive mirroring he needed to construct an appropriate masculine gender identity. Hence, by age 5 years, their son tended to believe that he truly was a girl trapped inside a boy's body. In a playroom psychiatric interview, he stated, "You know I have a penis but I want a vagina; I'm really a girl inside." He was saying, in effect, that although his outside "said" that he was a member of the category "boy," what he had constructed of his experiences in his family and incorporated within his gender identity was that he was a girl within his inner or representational world.

In summary, infants, during their pre-self-aware phase, have many experiences involving their gender. Their representations of these experiences become the forerunners of their future gender identity.

Parents' perceptions of their infant's body and body processes will always be colored by their already well developed representational world of needs, beliefs, and fantasies. Pre-self-aware infants and their parents, therefore, transact within an intersubjective field (Trevarthan 1980). Psychologically attuned parents are able to objectify their transactions with their infant—in recognizing their operating as separate objects from their infant—but, from the point of view of the infant, this initial field of transaction with the parents is a completely intersubjective one. Stern (1985) noted that intersubjectivity "concerns the mutual sharing of psychic states" (p. 144). When such mutual sharing takes place, sometimes a parent—and always the pre-self-aware infant—imbues the other with his or her own subjective feelings, perceptions, and beliefs. A mother, therefore, who says "I'm so happy and so is my baby" before empathizing with whether her baby is in fact happy at the moment is relating to her baby in an intersubjective manner.

Parents differ in their ability to be aware of the influence of their representational worlds on their perceptions of their infant. Some parents have a well-developed self-awareness and are able to use their introspection and empathy to explore their fantasies and beliefs about their perceptions of their infant's body and gender. Other parents are not able to do this. For example, the mother who wore rubber gloves when changing her infant did not appear to realize how bizarre it was to believe that body products could "damage" her skin. If this mother remained as her son's only caretaker, then, by age 3 years, he might perceive his own bowel and bladder contents as injurious substances that he should never come in contact with. He might then believe that, because this poisonous substance was produced by his body, his body was bad, his entire self was bad, and his mother had correctly perceived his "inside badness." Although all children must learn that their feces and urine are unclean substances that must be discarded, they are not viewed by normal 3-year-old children as bad body products. Far more often children tend to believe, as do their parents, that their urine and feces are good body products that allow them to stay healthy as long as they are disposed of correctly.

■ The Attachment Relationship

An *attachment relationship* is the specific relationship that forms between infants and their parents in a specific context (Bowlby 1958, 1969, 1988; Main 1993; Rothbard and Shaver 1994). The *attachment context* is one in which infants are completely dependent on the specific behaviors of their parents for survival. In this mutually activating and stimulating relationship, socializing transactions occur between infants and their parents.

The goals of the attachment relationship are 1) to ensure the infant's maturational survival and 2) to ensure the infant's development as a socialized member of the society in which he or she is being nurtured. The first goal can be attained without the attainment of the second—that is, survival can occur without socialization—but the result is often a child who can survive only in an isolated environment. Thus one reason it is necessary to understand the "ingredients" of a good attachment process is to ensure that a child is not only growing, but growing up and developing as well.

In one recently publicized case, a 3-year-old boy was found who had been confined to his house since birth. He had not had normal socializing exposure to other adults and children, had not been afforded the stimulation of leaving his home, and had been relegated to spending his life in isolation from all other humans except for his parents. The local child protective agency was asked to evaluate the family. The parents of the boy questioned, "What is all the fuss about? We give him food and shelter, but he is better off not being exposed to the outside world. He'll only discover that people are out to hurt you; you can't trust people, so it's better to avoid them." These parents were ensuring his physical survival, but not his social and psychological development. They were instilling within him their own abnormal or pathogenic belief that people are treacherous.

In reviewing this boy's situation, developmentalists would agree that the parents possessed an abnormal belief that their son's socializing with others would lead to his harm. However, the same developmentalists would also agree that, if the parents had not provided some critical level of family stimulating interaction for their son, he would not have survived. Feeding and clothing without a certain critical amount of socializing interaction can predispose an infant to death.

In a classic study, Rene Spitz (1945), one of the first psychoanalysts to observe infants directly and systematically, evaluated a group of 91 infants in a foundling home who had been left at the home after having been breast-fed by their mothers up until age 3 months. Following weaning, the infants had little interaction with their foundling home caretakers other than when they were being fed. Thus these babies were not stimulated by others and, while lying in their cribs all day, were not given an opportunity to assertively seek novel stimuli. By age 18 months, 32 infants had died from a variety of physical ailments while manifesting an emotional state of profound withdrawal and apathy. This emotional state, associated with the abrupt separation at age 3 months from a breast-feeding mother, was the syndrome Spitz labeled, *anaclitic depression* (with "anaclitic" describing a relationship in which one person is totally dependent on another, as were these infants during the first 3 months of their life). These anaclitically depressed infants had seemed to lose interest in their environment. Their profound withdrawal and apathy predisposed them to succumbing to rather minor infections. Of those who survived, only 8% were walking at age 2½ years, and a large number were severely developmentally retarded at age 4 years.

Although Spitz's study suggests that transactional socialization is necessary to ensure infants' physical survival, later studies have addressed whether this socialization can be provided by multiple caretakers or must be provided by at least one constant caretaking person for at least the first 2 or 3 years of a child's life. Tizard and colleagues (B. Tizard and Hodges 1978; B. Tizard and Rees 1975; J. Tizard and Tizard 1971) studied children institutionalized from before age 4 months until age 8½ years. By then, the children either were still in the institution or had been adopted, placed in foster homes, or returned to their natural mothers. Campos et al. (1983), in reviewing this longitudinal study, reported that, in these generally high quality institutions, the caretaking strategy was designed to prevent children from forming strong attachments to particular nurses. By the time the average child was age 4½ years, he or she had been cared for by about 50 different nurses.

In comparing these children with a control group of children of similar ages, Tizard and colleagues found that, at age 4½ years, the continuously institutionalized children showed marked attention-seeking behaviors, poor peer interactions, and a clinginess to adults that was indiscriminate and pressured. They showed no particular preference for any caretaker, and did not seem to react to the absence of any one person in their life. They did not show any feelings of caring for any other person—adult or child. The majority of those children who had been returned to their natural mothers after age 4½ years had severe behavioral disturbances (much greater as a group than all the other groups, including the continually institutionalized children). It was noted that the quality of socialization experiences provided by the natural mothers on the return of their child was primarily threatening and emotionally indifferent. A great number of these mothers admitted to not caring for their children, regularly threatening to return them to the institution, and seldom, if ever, playing with them.

The results of this study can be interpreted as indicating that either too many caretakers or a single unloving and emotionally uninvolved caretaker who does not protect or value the child can produce a child who has learned how to survive but may never become motivated to assertively seek pleasurable interactions with significant others. We can assume that the institutionalized children in Tizard's study constructed a common conceptual belief about their innate need to engage in emotionally pleasurable interactions with others along the lines of

> I never learned that anyone belonged to me, and I never belonged to anyone. It's better to never trust or like anyone too much, because they will not be there if something happens and you need them. I'll just take what I can get from people, but I will not give anything to anybody.

This would be a way for these children to give meaning to their abandonment by others in order to achieve some sense of control over their emotionally painful feelings about their abandonment. As Rochlin (1965) noted,

> The belief that there will be someone who cares provides a measure of relief from the fears of being abandoned as worthless. (p. 454)

As each institutionalized child eventually learned that children usually belong to their parents, and specifically to a mother, the institutionalized child would realize that he or she had been left behind.

Results of the studies by Spitz, Tizard and colleagues, and Rochlin support the view that infant development is optimized by an ongoing, uninterrupted attachment relationship with a biological or adoptive mother or another primary caretaking person for at least the first 3 years of the infant's life. Fraiberg (1969), a child psychoanalyst, echoed this view, suggesting that infants need the single and full-time involvement of their mother for approximately the first 3 years of their life. She noted her concern that many infants were being exposed to too many caretakers during the first 3 years of life, which could possibly teach these infants that attachments were fleeting and should be avoided in later life.

Another developmentalist, Bowlby (1969), set out to prove that infants' motivation to attach to their mothers was fueled by more than their mothers' provision of food and shelter. (He defined "mother" as not only the biological mother but any man or woman who assumed the bulk of an infant's caretaking.) Bowlby, in essence, disavowed the traditional view that the infant was passive, sought no stimulation, and was not oriented toward socialization.

Bowlby turned to ethological research for biological proof of his postulates. From animal research data, he learned that a special type of learning, designated as *imprinting*, exists in many mammalian species. Imprinting occurs when specific experiences take place during critical phases in the life cycle of the animal. Once imprinted by a member of the animal's species, the animal forever prefers and acts in a special manner toward his own species. Bowlby cited work by Goodal, who observed that, in order for an infant gorilla to develop a selective seeking response to the mother and other adult gorillas, the mother must, during the first 8 months of the infant's life, seek and hold the infant gorilla. This is when imprinting takes place. Up until age 8 months, whenever the mother leaves the infant gorilla, he or she does not respond nor physically seek the mother. After age 8 months, however, if the infant gorilla has been imprinted, when the mother leaves the infant gorilla responds with reaching, following, and selectively seeking his or her mother over any other adult gorillas in the area.

Bowlby also cited work by Harlow (1960), who studied infant and mother rhesus monkeys. Harlow demonstrated that the primary reason for infants' attachment to their mother was their need for tactile stimulation rather than food. In Harlow's study, infant monkeys removed from their mother at birth were fed alternately from a wire monkey and a cloth monkey. The results of these experiments showed that contact comfort alone led the monkeys to become attached to the cloth monkey, whereas food comfort could not entice them to become attached to the wire monkey.

When Bowlby applied ethological theory in extrapolating data from Harlow's and Goodal's experiments to human development, he postulated that biologically preprogrammed or innate behaviors exist in both infants and parents (specifically the mother) that predispose both to develop an attachment relationship.

Some of the findings in the kibbutz communities in Israel have been interpreted as supporting Bowlby's idea that there exists an innate need in the biological mother to attach to her infant (Henry and Stephens 1977). Kibbutzim are collective communities in which infants are cared for during most of the day by assigned caretakers while their mothers and fathers work in full-time employment outside of the home. In living within the kibbutz, women are freed of traditional housewife and household chores and are given as much independence as men in choosing a career. What was observed during the first 20 years of the existence of the kibbutz communities was a gradual increase in the number of women seeking jobs that allowed them more attachment-enhancing time with their infants. This selection phenomenon could be interpreted as demonstrating the presence of a biological need within a mother to attach to and interact with her infant.

In his three-volume work on attachment, separation, and loss,

Bowlby (1969, 1973, 1980) emphasized that, although infants have basic needs for food, warmth, and protection to sleep, the most crucial basic need is the need to attach to at least one caretaker. (I express this as the innate need to engage in emotionally pleasurable interactions with others.) He postulated that infants possess innate attachment behaviors that "release" caretaking behaviors in the mothering person. Hence infants actively reach toward and cling to their mothers, and mothers respond with actively holding and cuddling their infants.

Thus Bowlby agreed with Fraiberg that infants are biologically predisposed to form a primary attachment relationship with one individual. That individual, usually the biological mother, has to produce predictably reliable and responsible caretaking behaviors for a developmentally enhancing, goodness-of-fit attachment relationship to occur. Bowlby termed this relationship a "secure attachment" (1973, 1988). He described securely attached children as being

> confident that their parent (or parent figure) will be available, responsive, and helpful should they encounter adverse or frightening situations. . . . They feel bold in their explorations of the world . . . [and] this pattern is found to be promoted by a parent (in the early years, especially the mother) being readily available, sensitive to her child's signals, and lovingly responsive when he or she seeks protection and/or comfort and/or assistance. (Bowlby 1988, p. 4; parentheses in the original)

■ The Triadic Attachment Relationship

If an infant is provided with at least one constant caretaker for the first 3 years of his or her life, could and does he or she attach to both parents during that same period? In the more traditional dyadic model of the infant attachment relationship, the mother was the only caregiver and attachment object for the infant. The father was viewed only as the mother's supporter, which left the mother better able to establish an exclusive attachment relationship with her infant. Children were also thought to have little, if any, influences on their siblings. Similarly, infants were viewed as responding only to their father and siblings sometime near age 2 years.

Father engrossment. As developmental researchers began to ask fathers what they felt and experienced around their infants, they found that fathers, both those who were overworked and unavailable and those who spent a great deal of time with their infants, all talked about an emotionally rich quality of interaction with their infants that heretofore had been thought to be absent (Lamb 1976, 1981a, 1981b). In addition, Lamb's studies revealed that many fathers were spending more time with their infants than they recalled their own fathers had spent with them during their infancy. Based on these results and those of other studies (Herzog 1982, 1984), the older dyadic model has been gradually replaced by a newer triadic model that addresses the attachment relationship as taking place among the mother, father, and infant.

In a review of infant-mother deprivation studies (i.e., where the mother was unavailable, unable, or unwilling to exert energy into establishing a developmentally enhancing attachment with her infant), Herzog (1980) found that, in some cases, the disruption of the attachment bond came primarily from father detachment. These were cases in which infants (both male and female) had become attached to their fathers and then the fathers had abruptly left the family. This abrupt separation caused the infants to withdraw and show less attachment interest in their mothers. The fathers' leaving also caused the mothers to become less responsive and less motherly toward the infants. In the older dyadic view, this emotionally displeasurable mother-infant dyad might have been viewed as being caused entirely by the mother's faulty attachment behaviors.

Within the last 15–20 years, certain new sociological phenomena have affected fathering behaviors toward their children:

1. An increase in two-career families, which makes it imperative that infant caretaking behaviors be shared by both parents. In these families, infants often show good attachment relationships and actively seek interaction with both parents.
2. An increase in single-parent families where the father is the only parent. Once an unheard of consequence of child custody hearings, courts now routinely consider rewarding fathers custody of their children when the mother is judged incompetent as a parent.

3. The choice by a husband and wife for the wife to be the gain-fully employed parent outside of the home and the husband to be the full-time infant caretaker within the home.

During the first 6 months of an infant's life, the father's attachment to him or her is both similar to and different from that of the mother. A father assumes indirect and direct caretaking roles with his infant. In his indirect role, a father helps to relieve the mother's stresses and supports the mother in becoming attached to their infant, relieving her of the worry that her attachment to their infant would interfere with her relationship with him. In his direct nurturant role, a father offers a qualitatively different experience for his infant than what the mother usually provides. A father provides more physical, spontaneous interactions as well as more novel and complex behavioral interactions (Parke and Tinsley 1981). For example, whereas mothers typically contain and soothe their infant, thereby modulating their infant's level of stimulation, fathers typically approach their infant in ways that heighten stimulation. Fathers talk at a faster pace in a louder voice and in more staccato-style speech than mothers, who talk in a slower and more rhythmical, musical, and repetitive manner (Greenspan 1981). Thus, as Neubauer (1985) stated,

> The mothers held the babies more frequently to comfort them—the fathers to play with them and to stimulate their explorations. It will depend on the infant's disposition which of these experiences they prefer or which they will seek at different times during the day and at different stages of development. (p. 167)

Traditionally it was believed that mothers were more biologically preprogrammed to sensitively respond to their infant's reflexive, perceptual, emotional, temperamental, and other behaviors. Greenberg and Morris (1974), however, found that fathers develop unique bonds to their infant within the first 3 days of the infant's life. They labeled this strong emotionally positive bonding experienced by fathers as *engrossment.* An engrossed father experiences feelings of elation, preoccupation, absorption, and interest in his infant. They noted that engrossed fathers also reported a strong desire to look at, feel, and stimulate their infant.

Engrossment has been hypothesized as a preprogrammed maturational potential that facilitates a father's biological preparedness to enter into an attachment relationship with his infant (Greenberg and Morris 1974). Perhaps engrossment is the result of a genetically induced process brought about by men's experiences as fathers. If so, the structural genes that mediate the phenomenon of father engrossment may be activated by environmental factors. It is interesting that many men will attest to an awareness of being changed by their caretaking activities with their first child; many communicate a new sense of commitment to fatherhood that they did not sense prior to the birth of their infant.

Two factors influence the development of engrossment in fathers: 1) cultural permission to manifest the characteristics of engrossment (a social factor) and 2) a father's conceptual beliefs and fantasies about what constitutes a man's role with his infant (a function of the father's representational world) (Zelago et al. 1977). It would seem necessary for fathers to place themselves in a caregiving social context in order for their caretaking competency to mature and develop. Lamb (1981a, 1981b) made systematic home observations of infants interacting with their mothers and fathers. He studied the question of whether there existed differences in caregiving competencies based on the parent's gender. He concluded that there were no biologically based gender differences between fathers and mothers in their responsiveness to their infant and that any behavioral dimorphisms that had emerged were in response to societal pressures and expectations.

The following summarizes recent findings concerning shared father-mother attachment to their infant:

1. Infants can form multiple attachments; the strength of the attachment to each parent is a function of the quantity and quality of transactions with each parent.
2. A lower quantity of quality care provided by a parent is more important than a higher quantity of poor quality care. For example, infants and mothers, as well as infants and fathers, become bored with each other if they are involved in an activity that has become displeasurable because of its monotonous predictability.

3. Fathers can fulfill attachment roles. Data now exist that demonstrate a stronger attachment between the infant and the father when the mother spends less time with her infant, such as in families where the mother is the primary economic provider and spends more time out of the home than the father. Also, Chused (1986) noted that,

> When mothering is inadequate or provided intermittently, a dyadic relationship with the father can provide the continuity and the nurturance that is necessary for the successful navigation of infancy and early childhood. (p. 435)

4. In two-career families, when the husband has supported his wife's pursuit of a career, their daughters will often grow up believing that the female role presents an opportunity to develop both career and motherly ambitions.

5. There are data that document the effects of father-infant deprivation. Herzog (1980) studied a group of 2½-year-old children who were brought to a child psychiatry clinic because they woke up screaming each night. All these children had lost their fathers between ages 18 months and 2½ years. After their father's departure, they had begun having nightmares associated with awakening and screaming. Their mothers had great difficulty in soothing them once they were awake. In Herzog's view, these infants were reacting to the sudden disruption of the attachment bond they had established with their fathers.

Maternal bonding. As noted above, no longer do developmentalists assume that the only early step on the "path" to normal development is an infant attaching to his or her full-time biological or adoptive mother in the home environment. However, regardless of whether the mother stays at home to provide the primary caretaking functions that her infant requires, or enters into full- or part-time regular activity outside of the home, the question remains of whether it is important for a mother to be with her infant for at least 4–5 hours/day for at least the first 1–2 months of the infant's life. Before addressing this question, I first look at mother-infant bonding at birth.

Influenced by researchers such as Bowlby (1980), developmental researchers have directed their attention toward investigating whether bonding does take place between a mother and her infant in the period immediately following birth. *Bonding* is defined as "the establishment of a long lasting, affectionate attachment of a mother toward her infant as the result of the mother's skin to skin contact with her newborn during a hormonally sensitive period lasting for a few hours after birth" (Campos et al. 1983, p. 820).

Klaus and Kennel (1976) studied bonding in 28 first-time mothers placed in two groups: a control group and an extended-contact group. The extended-contact group of mothers had 16 extra hours of contact with their infants during the first 3 postdelivery days compared with the mothers in the control group. The mothers in the extended-contact group were given their nude infants for 1 hour within the first 3 hours after birth, and then for 5 extra hours each afternoon of the 3 postdelivery days. The results of the study revealed that, 1 month after giving birth, the mothers in the extended-contact group showed more soothing caretaking behaviors, made more eye-to-eye contact, and engaged in more fondling with their infants than did mothers in the control group. Seen 2 years later, the mothers in the extended-contact group engaged in more lengthy language interactions with their children, and their children, in turn, showed a greater variety of verbal interchanges with their mothers than did the control infants. However, researchers in later studies (Grossman et al. 1981; Siegel et al. 1980) have shown that the effects of early bonding are not necessarily extended past age 1 year.

The Klaus and Kennel (1976) study had a significant effect on hospital care in the late 1970s. Prior to the study, mothers and their infants were often brought together only for feedings. Undoubtedly, many an infant was wide awake in the nursery, perhaps visually searching for his or her mother, while the mother was in the maternity ward wondering what her infant was doing. Following the study, mothers and babies were kept together for as much of the postpartum period as hospital routine would allow.

I recall one mother I saw in therapy who was pregnant with her seventh infant. She and her husband were lamenting their stressed financial condition. They had been married 7 years and had six children. After several interviews, the mother revealed to me a combined conceptual belief and fantasy she possessed about motherhood. With much embarrassment, she stated,

> I know it's not supposed to be normal, but I love and need to have a baby to fondle and hold close, especially right after they're born. When each of my babies began to crawl away from me, though, I began to feel abandoned. That's when I lose a lot of interest in my baby, and I start to wish to become pregnant again. I don't know why I feel so strongly about this.

Whenever she yearned to become pregnant again, her husband had always become "seriously worried" that, if he did not support her belief, she would become depressed, so he continued to support her wish and cooperated in making her pregnant again.

Perhaps in a bonding study, this mother would appear bonded to each of her infants, but this close bonding would eventually come under the "shadow" of her pathogenic belief that the emergence of her infant's ability to crawl was an indication of her infant's wish to crawl away from and eventually abandon her. This mother would not be able to establish an attachment relationship that had any degree of secure continuity until she, through psychiatric help, could understand the irrationality of her belief that her infant's desire to assertively explore his or her social world through crawling was a sign of the infant's desire to terminate all attachment with her. This mother had been automatically abandoning her infant before, as she believed, her infant would abandon her.

Maternal attunement. An aspect of the early relationship between an infant and more psychologically aware mother is captured in the term *maternal attunement* (Emde 1983; Stern 1985). This phenomenon is similar to father engrossment in that its etiology is thought to be based in a genetically induced, preprogrammed capacity in the mother that is released through the nurturing experience. *Attunement* is defined as the ability in the mother to tune in to her infant in a form of behavior that is more similar to matching than to imitation (Stern 1985). An example given by Stern captures the essence of an attuned maternal response:

A 9-month-old boy bangs his hand on a soft toy, at first with some anger but gradually with some pleasure, exuberance, and humor. He sets up a steady rhythm. Mother falls into his rhythm and says, "kaaaaa-bam, kaaaaa-bamm, kaaaaa-bamm," the "bam" falling on the stroke and the "kaaaaa" riding with the preparatory upswing and the suspenseful holding of his arm aloft before it falls. (p. 140)

This mother was able to distinguish her infant's needs from her own, as well as monitor the stimulating aspect of her behavior in reference to her infant's response. These abilities show that the mother was able to perceive her son's surface behavior relatively free of serious distortion emanating from the influence of her representational world.

In Chapter 2, I emphasize that parents view their infants through the "filter" of their own conscious and unconscious beliefs, aspirations, and wishful fantasies. Hence what a mother actually chooses to become attuned to will be influenced by her representational world. Stern (1985) noted that these "selective attunements" are one of the most potent ways that parents can shape the development of their child's subjective and interpersonal life because, in essence, attunement is another form of teaching through operant conditioning. When a mother tunes in to an infant behavior—responding with positive mirroring and other supportive behaviors—she is rewarding that infant behavior and reinforcing its repetition in the future. At the same time, she is functioning as a selfobject for her infant.

Beebe and Sloate (1982) identified the following attunement transactions:

- *Mutual gaze*—At birth, infants show visual preference for patterns and are capable of following a bright light with their eyes. By age 7 days, eye-to-eye contact between infant and mother is observed, with the development of selective visual gaze for the mother's face. From birth through approximately age 2 months, the depth of visual focus in the infant is approximately 13 centimeters, which is the approximate distance from the mother's breast to the mother's face. Hence infants are innately endowed with the perceptual capability to focus on their mother's face while feeding at the breast.

- *Maternal play stimulation*—A good early maternal attunement is also indicated by a regular rhythm in the mother's vocal, facial, and kinesthetic interaction with her infant. The attuned mother is tuned in to her infant's specific attention-inattention and activity-inactivity rhythmic cycles.

- *Facial emotional interchange*—From the first few days of life onward, an indication that a good attachment bond is developing is whether the mother and her infant seemingly exchange emotional glances. By the time the infant is age 8–12 weeks, this interaction culminates in the emergence of the infant's social selective smile (see below).

- *Soothing*—In the early weeks of her infant's life, a mother learns which soothing ministrations her infant responds to the best, in accordance with the infant's innate stimulation range and preferred sensory modalities for communication (e.g., soothing touch versus soothing sound). This function of the attuned mother is part of the social function parents provide in being predictable sources of stimulus modulation and protection in line with their infant's unique optimal stimulation range. Infants slowly learn, through their kinesthetic and emotional sensing of their mother, about their mother's unique optimal stimulation range. Accordingly, infants begin to be able to sense when their mother becomes tense in response to their rocking, and they will modulate their rocking until their mother becomes less tense. Mothers and infants in their attachment relationship help regulate the stimulation level in each other (Lichtenberg 1982).

■ Phases in the Attachment Relationship

Following engrossment and maternal bonding and attunement is the longitudinal unfolding of the attachment relationship (Ainsworth 1964; Ainsworth et al. 1978). This can be roughly divided into three phases:

1. Emergent social responsiveness (birth through age 2 months)
2. Discriminating social responsiveness (ages 2–6 months)
3. Active initiative in seeking proximity to primary caretakers (age 6 months onward).

Phase 1: Emergent social responsiveness. Although pre-self-aware infants have no conscious objective awareness that they are separate individuals in a world of other separate individuals, it has become increasingly apparent that infants are deeply engaged in and related to social stimuli (Stern 1985). Much of the actual surface behaviors that transpire between infants and parents in this phase have to do with infants' achieving homeostasis. (*Homeostasis* was defined by Greenspan [1979] as an infant's capacity to regulate states; form basic cycles and rhythms of sleep, wakefulness, and alertness; organize internal and external experience [e.g., habituate to stimuli, organize patterns]; and integrate a number of modalities into more complex patterns [e.g., developing self-soothing behaviors].) For example, while feeding or putting their infant to sleep, parents engage in social behaviors such as rocking, touching, soothing, talking, singing, and making noises and faces. These occur in response to infant behaviors that are mainly social, such as crying, fretting, smiling, and gazing. As Stern (1985) noted, "A great deal of social interaction goes on in the service of psychological regulation" (p. 43). Thus it appears that infants, even in their first 2 months of life, are transactional social beings—that is, they are equipped to react to and produce reactions in their socializing environment.

The view of the infant who is biologically prepared to engage in socializing interactions posits an infant that is endowed not only with an innate need to engage in emotionally pleasurable interactions with at least one other person, but who is also innately endowed with perceptual competencies and behavioral capabilities that enable him or her to be active in socially engaging with his or her parents. I believe that infants possess such an innate need for socialization from birth, and, based on this belief, I tend to see behaviors in the infant that are related to the presence of this innate need to engage in pleasurable social interactions with others.

In the last 20 years, developmentalists—in discovering infants' innate socialization behaviors—have labored to develop a way of assessing individual infant socialization competencies within the first 2 months of life. One such researcher is T. Berry Brazelton. The Neonatal Behavioral Assessment Scale (Brazelton 1989) is used to assess the behavioral and neurological status of infants from age 2 days to age 6 weeks by rating physiological organization (e.g., motor performance) and interactive behaviors (e.g., the infant's ability to be consoled by an examiner's soothing interventions). Behavioral clusters point to either a "normal" or an "at risk" infant (the latter being at risk for developing a faulty attachment relationship if the parents do not realize their infant's difficulties in being soothed when overstimulated and so on).

Phase 2: Discriminating social responsiveness. As with all their innate needs, infants must also discover, own, and construct a beginning representation of their innate need to engage in emotionally pleasurable interactions with others. Parents must permit this initial ownership lest their infant develop into a child who believes that he or she does not want to relate to people.

In a growing body of literature, written mostly from the psychoanalytic and psychodynamic perspective, researchers have posited that infants' innate need for others must be nurtured in the first 18 months of life so that, when they begin to manifest newly emerging assertive abilities, they will have taken into their representational world both a deepening sense of their need for emotionally pleasurable relationships with others and a growing sense that others can be trusted to provide nurturance, admiration, acceptance, and protection from most emotionally displeasurable life events. If they have not experienced such nurturance, admiration, and so on, they will begin to deny their need for such positive experiences. If pre-self-aware infants' attachment behaviors are either not responded to or responded to with negative mirroring, then their need to establish an attachment relationship can remain significantly underdeveloped. Such children will develop false selves in that they will falsely believe that their innate need for others does not exist.

Modern developmental researchers posit that, whereas infants are more engaged with social behaviors directly bearing on the regulation of their physiological needs (Stern 1985), at age 2 months a maturational discontinuity occurs: they begin to direct more of their attention to the outside world, and particularly become more sensorially and perceptually oriented toward perceiving their actions and the action of their parents. As Shapiro and Hertzig (1988) stated,

> The period between 2 and 7 months is perhaps the most exclusively social period of life. Babies are seen as liking people to pay attention to them, to talk to them, and to sing to them. The spontaneous behavior of adults—making baby talk and baby faces— are well matched to the baby's [innate] perceptual biases, with the result that the adult social stimulus is maximally attended to. (p. 109)

In addition, at this age, infants demonstrate a growing ability to discriminate between different stimuli, including discriminating among the various parental facial emotional expressions that help them to begin to learn self-regulation of their own emotions. Although they are not yet consciously and objectively aware of their developing perceptual discriminating ability, infants demonstrate an increasing ability to discriminate in their behavioral responses to their mother and father. In a properly developing attachment relationship, they become more able to seek and activate responses from their parents.

Part of infants' increased attention to their social environment comes from the changes in their sleep-wakefulness pattern that occur between ages 2 and 6 months. By ages 8–10 weeks, their quiet sleep doubles, with a corresponding decrease of REM sleep (Emde and Metcalf 1970). Consequently, they learn to sleep through the night to a significant degree (Parmalee 1974). When this occurs, they develop longer periods of alertness and focus more on their environment, particular on their primary caretaker and interactions between them (Schaffer 1984).

Infants' ability to raise their heads, which becomes manifest at age 2 or 3 months, also aids in this attention to the environment because infants can further control and direct their visual gazing. Stern (1985) observed that by controlling their own direction of gaze, they self-regulate the level and amount of social stimulation to which they are subject. They can avert their gaze, shut their eyes, stare past, become glassy-eyed. (p. 21)

Concurrently with their developing ability to regulate their stimulation level (and in concert with having parents who are empathically attuned to their regulatory cues), infants begin to show an increasing ability to attend to and perceptually discriminate their parents from others.

A major maturational advance signifying the development of infants' perceptual discrimination associated with a growing representation of their parents is the appearance of the selective social smile. This smile is given preferentially to the infant's parents or other significant caretakers, including siblings, with whom the infant has been involved since birth. This selective smile can emerge anywhere between ages 4 weeks and 12 weeks. The selective smile also indicates that the infant is capable of recognition memory (discussed above). A stranger's face will now be recognized as different from that of the infant's mother or father, and the infant reacts with wariness and will not smile as readily at the stranger. The selective social smile is considered an important sign of a healthy attachment relationship between an infant and his or her primary caretakers.

Many parents report how a smile from their infant can immediately become a social stimulus for them to engage in playful interchange with their infant. In this sense, the infant's social smiles make a significant contribution to the transactional attachment relationship. Viewed in another way, when parents "discover" their infant's smile, they become shaped by it—that is, the infant begins to teach the parents through operant conditioning principles. The parent behaves in a certain way and the infant rewards the parent with a smile. The parent's behaviors are thereby reinforced, and the parent will be motivated to repeat that behavior to receive the smiling "reward" once again. In another sense, the infant is also functioning as a selfobject for the parents. (I use "selfobject" here in Lichtenberg's [1989] definition that the infant's social smile causes his parents to experience a sense of cohesion, safety, and competence.) The parents feel positively mirrored by their infant.

The parents' self-esteem is nurtured and reinforced by their infant's social smile, which is bestowed exclusively upon them.

Infants and parents, therefore, spend much time during the period between ages 2 months and 6 months engaged in periods of prolonged mutual gazing. As Schaffer (1984) noted,

> Interactions come to take place primarily in the context of face-to-face encounters, in which the exchange of looks and gestures and vocalizations predominates. The main theme for adult and child now becomes the regulation of mutual attention and responsiveness. (p. 120)

Also, when an infant's selective social smile emerges, parents will often trigger a smile by speaking to their infant. Thus from earliest life, pre-self-aware infants begin to construct representations of their own smiling, their parents' smiling, their own and their parents' pleasurable emotions, and the auditory reception of spoken language. In a developmentally enhancing goodness of fit between an infant and empathically attuned parents, this second phase of the attachment relationship is characterized by the infant's selective smile and the infant's consistent orienting response to the voice of each parent. Specifically, the parents are quite proud of their ability to actively engage their baby by their verbalization of such syllables as "ah-goo" (Stern 1985).

Phase 3: Actively seeking proximity to primary caretakers. Near ages 5–6 months, there appears to be a maturational advance in infants' innate need to assertively explore their social environment for novel stimuli. At this stage, they become preoccupied with inanimate things. Schaffer (1984) noted that, during this stage, it is

> largely up to the adult to convert the child's object play into a social situation. It is as though the child can attend to only one thing at a time, person or object, and so, having familiarized himself with the parent in the early months, he now turns to the world of things and, even during a joint play session, devotes his attention mostly to toys rather than to the parent. (p. 124)

In Mahler's (1975) theory, at about age 6 months, the infant's *psychological birth* occurs. Although Mahler's hypotheses about the existence of prior autistic and symbiotic phases are no longer thought to be valid, her separation-individuation theory, applicable to age 6 months to about age 3 years, is still highly relevant.

According to Mahler (1975), infants first go through a *normal autistic phase* in which they have no awareness of separateness from their mother. They awake only when in need of food and body stimulation. Once these needs are satisfied, they enter a sleeping state. Mahler, in outlining this phase, which lasts from birth to about age 2 months, supported the more traditional point of view of infants as passive, asocial, and predominantly driven by the pleasure-seeking pressure of their instinctual wishes or innate needs. Thus an infant's mother was seen to provide the socializing pressure and to be the sole activator of the infant's forming an attachment relationship with her. In this autistic phase, an infant's goal is to maintain the degree of internal homeostasis that was present inside the uterus. The mother's role is to become a "protective shield" for her infant and reduce the inevitable displeasurable stimulations that "break through." Based on the growing body of infant observational research during the last 15–20 years—which documents the reflexive, perceptual, emotional, temperamental, cognitive, and behavioral capabilities of infants during their first 2 months of life—Mahler's autistic phase is no longer thought to be valid (Stern 1985).

Returning to Mahler's theory, the autistic phase is terminated at about age 2 months with a "cracking of the autistic shell." Now the *symbiotic phase* emerges. Having achieved a "dim awareness of the need-satisfying object" (i.e., the mother) and with their stimulus barrier no longer present, infants are protected from the threat inherent in the recognition of their separateness by constructing "a delusion of a common boundary" (Mahler et al. 1975). Mahler postulated that infants possess an ability to construct complex mental images. This ability is used by them to blot out an awareness of their separateness. This awareness, in Mahler's view, is intolerable to infants.

Neither this symbiotic phase nor the autistic phase are now believed to be valid postulates (Shapiro and Hertzig 1988). The actually observed phenomena that signify a symbiotic infant-mother interrelatedness have never been defined. This primarily is because symbiosis refers to a hypothesized intrapsychic phenomenon (i.e., an occurrence within the nontalking infant's representational world). Current knowledge, which points to a socially engaged, stimulus-seeking, reality-oriented infant, goes counter to Mahler's symbiotic phase "baby" who, from age 2 to 6 months, retreats from his or her beginning awareness of separateness by constructing an image of infant-mother connected symbiosis. (See Mahler 1963, Mahler et al. 1975, McDevitt and Mahler 1989, and Pine 1994 for a more detailed discussion of Mahler's early phases.)

Mahler noted that 6-month-old infants appear to look more alert and are more goal-directed in their assertive pursuits than before. These new behaviors, which for Mahler ushered in the separation-individuation process, appeared to Mahler as indicating the infant's *psychological birth,* a sort of infant "hatching." Mahler divided the separation-individuation process into three subphases: 1) differentiation, 2) early practicing and practicing proper, and 3) rapprochement.

The first subphase—*differentiation*—is so labeled because it signifies infants' beginning development of a sense of separateness from their mother. Infants also begin to differentiate where their body ends and their mother's begins, manifested in their pulling at their mother's hair, ears, or nose and putting food into their mother's mouth (Mahler 1975). As infants continue to assert themselves in exploring the environment, the experiences that ensue between their maturing needs and their parents' responses will lead them to construct representations of how the parents respond to their assertive interest in novel objects. I refer once again to the developmental equation:

> The infant's mental processing of the transactions among maturation advances in physical abilities (biological stimuli) plus maturational advances in innate needs (psychological stimuli) plus environmental responses (social stimuli) plus prior knowledge and learning (psychological stimuli in the form of memories and current thoughts and emotions) equals resultant new developmental changes.

These developmental changes will lead to potential new learning experiences. For example, a 7-month-old girl is sitting quietly in her mother's lap, when she suddenly sees an object and reaches for it. Her mother will follow her infant's eyes to the object and encourage her exploration of it by monitoring her infant's hands with her own hands. Through emotional referencing, the infant perceives the emotional excitement in her mother and uses it to spur herself on in exploring the object. She reaches for the object and immediately looks at her mother's face once again. She sees a smile on her face and hears, but obviously does not understand, a loving "What's that?"; thus she experiences a pleasurable feeling of joy as she senses her mother's support of her assertive wish to explore and learn. When an infant's assertive seeking of activity is empathically mirrored by an attuned parent, the infant learns that it is okay to begin to develop a subjective sense of being separate.

In mother-infant pairs between whom the attachment relationship is quite faulty, what is often observed is that the mother finds it intolerable to allow her infant to initiate any activity the mother does not initiate herself. Her motivation for this behavior comes from her representational world, which is dominated by pathogenic beliefs. In such a faulty attachment relationship, the infant's innate and maturationally emerging need to express an assertive interest in the world is never developed. The following is an example of this type of faulty attachment relationship:

> I was interviewing a mother with her 6-month-old son sitting in her lap. While the mother was talking, the infant focused his gaze on a brightly colored vase in the office. His mother was talking about how she and her infant often smiled at each other. Suddenly, she turned her infant to face her and smiled at him. However, her son's eyes did not leave the vase and the mother immediately became rather tense. She thereupon turned the infant's face until he was looking at her, with his face coming within inches of her face. He thereupon smiled at her and then quickly turned away to look once again around the office. The duration of his brief smile did not satisfy his mother, and she took her hand and quite roughly turned his head to once again face her. He squirmed, tried to look back at the vase, and, when the

mother roughly turned his face toward her, he looked angry as he tried to push her hand away. The mother then angrily stated, "See, this is what he does. He first ignores me then tries to hit me! He seems to want me only to feed him and change him; he is now becoming just as selfish as little boys grow up to be."

This woman's son, in looking back into her eyes after he assertively looked at the colored vase, could sense his mother's disapproval and anger. After many of these types of experiences, such an infant might begin to equate his assertiveness with being an aggressive act against his mother.

In a later interview, this mother told me how selfish her older brother had been as a child, and that she could never understand why her parents had allowed him to act selfishly while she was required to always help around the house.

This mother was transferring aspects of her relationship from someone in the past (i.e., her brother) onto someone in her present (i.e., her son). In this case, the facts about what occurred between this mother and her brother were less important than the representations of her childhood that she carried within her. In every transference reaction of parent to child, what is transferred onto the child is an object representation, with no awareness in the parent of the transfer. In this case, the object representation that the mother transferred onto her son was something like, "I got angry at my son (not my brother) because he is selfish and wants to do things his way."

Another behavior that emerges at ages 5–6 months is wariness of strangers. Traditionally this has been designated as *stranger anxiety* or *stranger distress* (Emde et al. 1979; Nachman et al. 1986; Sroufe 1977). At this age, infants experience a displeasurable emotional state that is manifested by a reaching out and seeking proximity to their mother or father whenever a strange face appears in front of them. As noted above, at about this age, infants begin to develop the cognitive ability to understand object permanence (Piaget 1950), an ability that becomes fully developed by age 8 months. Prior to the emergence of object permanence, infants can remember only people or things that are currently generating external stimuli. With the emergence of object permanence, the pre-self-aware infant is able to evoke a memory when the person or thing is not within the infant's immediate sensory field (Brody 1982). Thus, in responding with fretfulness and distress signaling behaviors to a strange face, the infant is revealing that long-term memories have been stored as visual representations within its visual cortex. These representations are recalled and actively used to compare a strange face with a familiar, "stored" face.

Parents will usually be able to observe, almost to the day, when their infant responded to a person other than themselves with a fearful emotional response. The "stranger" can even be someone the infant has seen quite often, such as a neighbor who has held the infant and played with him or her for long periods of time in the past. Once the infant begins to manifest stranger anxiety, the neighbor becomes a stranger to the infant. If a parent is holding the infant, the neighbor may successfully approach the infant if the neighbor does so slowly and does not attempt to pick up the infant suddenly. In addition, the infant's fretful and withdrawing response to a stranger can sometimes be overridden by the stranger's presenting a novel stimulus (e.g., a new toy). Safe in his or her mother's lap, the infant may slowly begin to explore the new toy. Infants' assertive need to explore their environment will persist in a protected physical attachment bond with a parent.

About a month or so after the emergence of stranger anxiety, at about age 8 months, infants manifest a new anxiety—*separation anxiety*—or, as it is called by Kagan (1979), *separation distress*. At this stage, infants show fretfulness, reach out toward or seek proximity with a parent, and cry when a parent leaves them. After a while, infants learn a new contingency: they begin to associate the occurrence of certain stimuli right before their mother or father leaves with their actual leaving; their new knowledge will cause them to react to these preseparation occurrences. For example, an infant girl will reach for her mother and begin to whimper when she sees her mother putting on her coat in preparation for leaving.

In manifesting separation anxiety, infants are becoming better able to use object permanence to stimulate their evocative recall of past memories, especially those events in which their parents left and the infant experienced some displeasurable feelings. As expressed by Kagan (1979),

The [infant's] enhanced ability to retrieve and hold a representation of past experiences is correlated with the ability to generate anticipations of the future: representations of possible events. . . . The 9-month-old child has a new capacity, best described as "the disposition to predict future events and to generate responses to deal with discrepant situations." The child, for the first time, tries to cope with unfamiliar experiences rather than just assimilate them. If the child cannot generate a prediction or instrumental response, he becomes vulnerable to uncertainty and, therefore, distress. If he can successfully generate the prediction, he may laugh. (p. 1050)

Fear is the response to a real and recognizable danger, and anxiety is the response to an imagined or fantasized danger. When a 6- to 8-month-old infant sees a stranger or sees his or her parents leave, it would appear that what he or she is experiencing is anxiety. No real danger exists for such an infant if he or she is engaged in an attachment relationship with parents who, for the most part, use their empathy to strive to protect him or her from physical dangers, from highly displeasurable levels of stimulation, or from threats of abandonment. If, however, an infant is part of a family in which he or she is repeatedly exposed to strangers that cause the infant to become painfully over- or understimulated or even physically hurt, or when an infant's parents leave and stay away for excessive periods of time or leave the infant unattended, then the infant would more truly possess, in time, high levels of stranger and separation fear.

Parents keep their infant's separation anxiety within a tolerable level of displeasurable stimulation in the following two ways:

1. *Alleviating their infant's anxiety*—Securely attached infants will explore their environment freely when they are with a parent. In addition, they can be readily comforted by their parent following separation (Bowlby 1969, 1988). A parent's ability to alleviate their infant's separation anxiety will depend on how well the parent is able to respond to the infant's unique temperamental characteristics. As I noted previously, these characteristics involve infants' different emotional thresholds, their capacity for self-soothing, their adaptability, and so on

(Thomas and Chess 1977). Most parents have learned what it takes and how long it takes to soothe their infant by the time he or she is age 8 months. Occasionally, however, a well-meaning parent's style of soothing his or her infant is a poor fit with the infant's temperamental style. In such a case, the parent may not be effective in soothing the infant, with the result that the infant would be less than securely attached to the parent.

2. *Shaping their infant's separation anxiety and associated behaviors*—A healthy attachment bond is fostered when parents respond, but do not overrespond, to their child's separation anxiety and associated behaviors. An abnormal overresponse would be when, once an infant begins crying in seeing the baby-sitter arrive, the mother holds the infant and eventually soothes him or her, but does not then turn the infant over to the baby-sitter and leave. In this case, the mother is experiencing too much of her own separation anxiety, and is anxious that her crying infant will not be able to eventually achieve a self-soothing state in the arms of the baby-sitter. This type of parental overresponse will teach the infant to cling to the parent and become overly anxious when left with a baby-sitter. This type of response from an infant usually signals a developmentally inhibiting attachment process.

Parents who are periodically and unpredictably hostile to their infant's separation distress—either through physically abusive behaviors or by not attempting to soothe their infant—increase their infant's attachment to them when a separation event is impending. The attachment is an unhealthy one, because this infant clings tightly to the parent when he or she senses the parent is getting ready to leave. The infant is not developing the ability to regulate his or her excessive separation anxiety. Hence, separation anxiety becomes a feeling that generates both avoidant behaviors (including fight and flight behaviors) and mental defense mechanisms, because the infant consciously avoids feeling an excessively high level of separation anxiety. This infant reacts to his or her own separation anxiety as if it is bad. Concurrently the infant views baby-sitters as people to be completely avoided. Obviously, this interferes with the infant's development of basic trust in people making up his or her social world.

In infants involved in a developmentally enhancing fit with their parents, the emergence of moderate levels of stranger and separation anxieties is an indication that they have become selectively attached. These anxieties motivate them to be assertive in taking the initiative to maintain physical proximity to their parent. By age 10 months, most infants have formed selective attachments to a small number of (usually three or four) specific people (e.g., mother, father, siblings, baby-sitters, other relatives, family friends), with the strongest attachment usually to the mother (Shapiro and Hertzig 1988).

Most developmentalists acknowledge that selective attachments can develop in the infant by age 1 year. Consequently, there has been an effort to define both the quality and strength of attachment, as well as the infant's style or pattern of attachment (as a reflection of the infant's temperament). Indeed, Kagan (1984) has taken the position that any attempt to measure the strength of the infant's attachment (through measuring the degree of separation anxiety present) is basically a measure of the infant's characteristic temperamental style of reacting to the novel and unfamiliar. Ainsworth et al. (1978) described a standardized procedure that is believed to provide a measure of the strength and quality of the infant's security of attachment. (For further reviews of this standardized procedure, see Main et al. 1985 and Sroufe 1985). It has become known as the *strange situation procedure.*

Kagan (1984) described the procedure thusly:

Infants between 9 and 24 months are observed in the unfamiliar laboratory room during brief periods—each about 3 minutes long—when they are with their mother, with a stranger, with the mother and a stranger, or all alone. The two key episodes are those in which the mother leaves the child, once with the stranger and once alone, and returns several minutes later to be reunited with her child. The child's immediate reaction to the mother's departure and his behavior upon her return are supposed to provide a sensitive index of the infant's quality of attachment. (p. 57)

Kagan (1984) summarized the results of Ainsworth et al.'s (1978) study:

> Children who show mild protest following the departure, seek the mother upon her return, and are easily placated by her are regarded as the most securely attached. Infants who do not protest maternal departure, and who do not approach the mother when she reenters, are regarded as less securely attached and labeled "avoidant." Finally, children who become seriously upset by the departure, and who—through seeking contact with the mother—resist her attempts to soothe them, are insecurely attached and are labeled "resistant." (pp. 57–58)

Bowlby (1988) phenomenologically described three principal patterns of attachment:

> The pattern of attachment consistent with healthy development is that of secure attachment, in which individuals are confident that their parent [or parent figure] will be available, responsive, and helpful should they encounter adverse or frightening situations. With this assurance, they feel [assertively] bold in their explorations of the world and also competent in dealing with it. This pattern is found to be promoted by a parent [in the early years, especially by the mother] being readily available, sensitive to her child's signals, and lovingly responsive when he or she seeks protection and/or comfort and/or assistance.
>
> A second pattern is that of anxious resistant attachment in which the individual is uncertain whether his or her parent will be available or responsive or helpful when called upon. Because of this uncertainty the child is always prone to separation anxiety, tends to be clinging, and is anxious about exploring the world. This pattern is promoted by a parent being available and helpful on some occasions but not on others, by separations, and, later, especially by threats of abandonment used as a means of control.
>
> A third pattern is that of anxious avoidant attachment in which individuals have no confidence that when they seek care they will be responded to helpfully but, on the contrary, expect to be rebuffed. Such individuals attempt to live their lives without the love and support of others. This pattern is the result of the individuals' mothers constantly rebuffing them when they ap-

proach her for comfort or protection. The most extreme cases result from rejection and ill-treatment or prolonged institution-alization. Clinical evidence suggests that, if it persists, this pattern leads to a variety of personality disorders, from compulsively self-sufficient individuals to persistently delinquent ones. (pp. 4–5)

Bowlby also noted that, in families where caregiving arrange-ments are stable, these patterns will tend to persist, at least until the child is age 5 or 6 years, citing studies by Sroufe (1983), Main et al. (1985), and Wartner (1986). Bowlby (1988) also acknowl-edged that, as a child grows older,

> clinical evidence shows that both the pattern of attachment and the personality features that go with it become increasingly a property of the child himself or herself and also increasingly re-sistant to change. This means that the child tends to impose it, or some derivative of it, upon new relationships. (p. 5)

Here Bowlby is addressing the phenomenon of transference, in which the child tries to achieve mastery of a new relationship by transferring onto it aspects of an old relationship that is now contained within his or her representational world as an object representation. Thus, for example, a securely attached boy will un-consciously transfer an internal emotionally pleasurable attach-ment onto his new first grade teacher and generate positive expectancies that this new external type of attachment will be a secure, emotionally pleasurable one.

A new attachment classification—*disorganized attachment*—has recently been developed (Main 1993; Zeanah et al. 1989). Chil-dren with this type of attachment appear to lack a strategy for dealing with the departure of their mother, or else they will sud-denly change their strategy. For example, such a child, upon the mother's return in the strange situation procedure, might show a concern in taking care of her but then suddenly begin to order her around the playroom. This child's separation anxiety is usually quite excessive, but it is difficult to assess what he or she is most anxious about.

There is presently no clear delineation about how the tempera-mental classifications of Chess and Thomas (i.e., easy, slow-to-warm-up, and difficult) and the patterns to attachment classifications of Ainsworth et al. and Bowlby (secure, avoidant, and resistant) and of Zeanah (disorganized) correlate. As I noted above, temperamental measures relate more to the style of attachment, whereas attachment classification measures relate more to the strength of attachment. Future research may reveal that different styles of attachment correlate with different strengths of attachment. Also, to date there has been no systematic study of infants who were labeled as poorly attached once these infants passed age 8 years, so it is not known how much of the behaviors associated with the avoidant or disorganized attachment classifications persist, or to what degree later developmentally enhancing life experiences can correct the effects of a faulty early attachment. As I note in Chapter 2, developmental researchers who stress the discontinuous view of normal mental development would argue that unexpected developments could correct the effects of a faulty attachment relationship.

Empirical longitudinal studies of infant-parent attachment classifications—involving both securely and poorly attached infants—and the quality of social relationships when these infants enter adolescence and adulthood are still quite meager. We know, however, that most children growing up in stable families are, by age 6 years, able to tolerate more separations from their parents than children growing up in families that are chaotic in terms of parental absence or inconsistent parenting. This ability to tolerate separation from the parents (and the anxiety these separations generate) comes from these children's having learned that separations are temporary and that their parents are reliable and reachable. These parental qualities become fixed within these children's object representations of their parents.

In essence, the axiom of normal mental development that emerges here is that a secure, selective external attachment leads to a child's construction and internalization of a good attachment, as stored in the child's mind as a representation of the original attachment relationship. In healthy development, new attachments continue to be secure, and the child is more prone to become an adult who values attachment and expects that new attachments will help him or her gratify his or her needs and wishes.

Between ages 6 months and 8 months, infants also begin crawling away from and back to their parents. The parents' goal is to help their infant experiment and learn that he or she can explore their social world without needing the parent to always be in close proximity. But psychologically aware parents usually know how far away they can be from their crawling infant. For example, when an infant boy begins to assertively crawl and explore his social world and comes upon a stranger, he will look back to his mother. If the mother is not immediately in his visual range, he will go and find her. After she soothes him, despite being anxious about the stranger, he will begin to explore again.

Mahler described the above infant boy's returning to his mother as "emotional refueling." In essence, the infant is engaging in emotional referencing by looking at his mother's face for emotional information. As an empathically attuned selfobject, the mother puts aside her needs for the moment and provides an important function the infant is as yet unable to provide for himself: she either admires his new crawling ability and imbues him with the strength of her own positive feelings or she frowns to indicate her concern about his crawling explorations. This parental emotional information also assists her infant in his own effort to regulate his emotions in order to try to keep them within a primarily pleasurable range.

Mahler's third subphase of the separation-individuation process is called *practicing proper.* This phase occurs between ages 10 months and 16 months. At age 10 months, infants are crawling, tracking contingencies, remembering and acting in a way to follow a plan, and achieving competency pleasure in seeing their intentions come true. At about ages 10–12 months, a new maturational advance in voluntary motor functioning takes place—the ability to begin walking. Hamilton (1988) described Mahler's subphase of practicing, in reference to walking, as follows:

> When upright posture is achieved, the child sees the world from a different perspective. Locomotion opens up new vistas before him. . . . The bright eyed tyro is full of himself, toddling from here to there, exploring and mischievous. His facial expression declares his delight in each new discovery. . . . In catch-me-if-you-can, the toddler catches mother's attention and dashes off. He

flees, certain he will be followed and swooped up in mother's arms and released. (p. 155)

Everything noted above in reference to infants' crawling and stranger and separation anxieties now applies to infants' walking. Walking away from parents will cause infants to experience stranger or separation anxiety and cause them to return to their parents to periodically emotionally refuel. In the future, infants will recall these walking-and-refueling sequences and, during periods of separation from their parents, will regulate their own stranger and separation anxieties by soothing themselves.

Maturation and Development of Adaptational Capabilities
The Innate Need to Signal Distress

Infants use some of the same behaviors in their assertive exploration of their environment as they do when responding to stimuli perceived as threatening. Parents must learn to differentiate between their infants' aggressive assertiveness and their reactive aggressive responses to perceived threatening stimuli.

When confronted with threatening or distress-inducing stimuli (Lichtenberg 1989), infants' innate need to signal their distress is triggered. This in turn propels them to activate preprogrammed behaviors (e.g., crying, taste aversion, gaze aversion, auditory aversion, touch aversion) and thereby generate both *fight responses* (i.e., aggressive and antagonistic behaviors to ward off the source of perceived danger) and *flight responses* (i.e., withdrawing and avoiding behaviors). The fight responses generate the displeasurable feelings of crying distress, anger, and disgust, and the flight responses generate the displeasurable feelings of crying distress, fear, and, later, shame and low keyedness (Lichtenberg 1989).

Kagan (1989) noted that there could be a temperamental orientation toward exhibiting either fight or flight responses, citing innately shy and avoidant infants who manifested high withdrawal from new situations (i.e., exhibiting a tendency to initiate flight responses). Infants can also be either pharmacologically or genetically predisposed to a too early and abnormal development of their innate need to signal distress (Lichtenberg 1989). For example, infants who were exposed in utero to certain hormones (e.g., synthetic progestins, an androgen-based drug) can become more aggressive than those not so exposed. In addition, infants can be genetically predisposed toward being more aggressive. This group of infants can be broken down into labile genotypic infants, who will respond to emotionally positive nurturance, which in turn influences the degree to which the labile genetic input affects the eventual phenotypic expression, and relatively nonlabile genotypic infants.

In a study by Crockenberg (1987), mothers who had experienced rejection from their own mother treated their infant's signals of distress with physically rough, nonsoothing responses. Crockenberg found that, of those infants with rejecting mothers, those who were not easily soothed at age 3 months generally became more angry and noncompliant than those who possessed a temperament that enabled them to be more easily calmed. In time, an infant's innate need to signal distress can dominate his or her need to be assertive and engage in attachment transactions. In discussing these findings, Lichtenberg (1989) noted,

> When the baby enters the world highly inclined to aversive states and the mother is ill-prepared to meet any of her baby's needs, then the infant by the toddler stage (i.e., by 12 to 15 months of age) has aversive motivation that becomes a dominant system and little confidence in exploratory-assertive and attachment motives. (p. 192)

Parents can also influence the overactivation of their infant's need to signal distress by engaging in parental projective identification. For example, a mother complained that her son did not like her, based on her interpreting (in essence, misinterpreting) her infant son's signals of distress as indications of his dislike of her. It was later discovered that she stimulated her son's need to signal distress by poking him. In so doing, she was projecting her dislike of him onto him by antagonizing him and then identifying his fight response as a sign of his innate antagonism. Thus she was able to "confirm" her view of him as antagonistic.

Lichtenberg (1989) also identified certain social phenomena (what he called an *aversive motivational system*) that can trigger infants' innate need to signal distress:

1. *Noxious, frustrating stimuli* (e.g., ammonia brought close to the infant's nose).
2. *Frustration of infant expectations* (i.e., when the infant's pre-constructed contingencies are not reliable predictors of an event). For example, a 10-week-old infant girl sees her smiling mother approaching and eagerly responds in an attempt to activate her innate need to continue to attach to her mother. However, she hears the taped voice of another person instead of her mother's voice while seeing her mother. She becomes startled, her initial facial interest and joy turn to distress, and she uses gaze aversion to turn away from her mother. She is experiencing distress because she had already constructed some long-term implicit memories of contingencies involving herself, her mother's face, her mother's voice, and transactions between herself and her mother, and the current event did not match those contingencies.
3. *Experiences that generate displeasurable emotions.* Parens (1987) noted that some people are innately more vulnerable to emotional pain and irritability than others and some may become more vulnerable through their life experiences.

It is clearly difficult to assess the source of infants' aggressive responses, because both their innate need to be assertive and their innate need to signal distress are fulfilled through the use of aggression. Parens (1987) classified human aggression as being of two kinds:

- *Nondestructive aggression* is nonhostile aggression in the service of an infant's innate need to assertively pursue novel stimuli, generate plans, learn about contingencies, and assimilate

and accommodate to new stimuli. The result is the experience
of the emotion of competency pleasure. For example, a 1-year-
old infant boy who is trying to learn how to use a spoon assertively but quite aggressively grabs for it when his mother is
holding it. His empathically attuned mother senses that he is
not trying to hurt or disregard her but is simply enthusiastic
about acquiring new knowledge.

• *Destructive or hostile aggression* is a physically hurtful action
  or hurtful verbalization where the intent is to harm the other.

A rage or intense fight reaction can emerge in an infant when
his or her parents fail to respond or treat the infant's distress signals
with overt hostility or indifference. Through this type of reaction,
the infant attempts to hostilely attack the source of the highly displeasurable or threatening stimulation. Parens (1987) postulated that

> Hostile acts in children—those carried out under conditions of
> pleasure and/or premeditation—are preceded by an experience
> of excessive pain that has been recorded in the psyche [i.e.,
> stored as short- or long-term memories within the represen-
> tational world]. The hostility is acted upon later, under condi-
> tions that are easier for the child to deal with. (p. 14)

Hostile aggression is mobilized by the infant's being forced to
passively suffer displeasurable experiences, which make the infant
feel helpless. The infant wants to turn passive to active, or do to
others what others have done to him.

It is important to note that the feelings accompanying the innate
need to signal distress (e.g., crying, distress, anger, disgust) do not
normally become internal motivators for infants the way, for example, competency pleasure or joy would. Infants are preprogrammed to activate these feelings primarily as signals to their
parents. Initially, attuned selfobject parents must not institute
too long a delay in responding to their infant's distress signals.
Eventually they must respond more slowly to their infant's distress
calls. During the delay in responding, infants are given the opportunity to feel their own displeasurable emotions and begin to learn
self-soothing behaviors or how best to demonstrate a fight-or-flight
response.

In an earlier section I describe experiences of benign displeasure (e.g., separation anxiety) and how infants and children must learn what to do to alleviate their anxiety in such situations. However, when exposed to too many *malignant displeasurable experiences* (Parens 1987; these are what I have labeled as traumatic experiences), infants can react with an overactivation of their fight-flight responses. By living in a dangerous and nonprotective social world, these infants' need to signal distress can eventually achieve dominance over their other innate needs and can become an independently generated need in itself.

Chapter 4

Toddlerhood Phase of Mental Development
Age 18 Months to Age 3 Years

Major Developmental Tasks of Toddlerhood

During each phase of the life cycle, as a child accomplishes the major developmental tasks of that phase, he or she attains subcomponents of his or her overall identity. These subcomponents continue to be developed during each succeeding developmental phase.

Toddlers gradually attain by age 3 years the following major developmental changes, changes that are then stored as new representations and act as new psychological stimuli to motivate them:

1. Toddlers begin to construct an autonomous identity, in that they begin to believe that they are separate individuals who can be autonomous, despite their wish at times to be dependent on their parents or significant others. This awareness is achieved through their learning that their parents and others permit them to separate from them as they autonomously ex-

plore the world as a separate person, even though at times these separations lead to negative emotional experiences involving their parents and others.

2. Toddlers begin to construct a gender identity as they begin to attain the belief that they are boys or girls.

These identities are subcomponents—the first building blocks—of toddlers' continuously growing overall identity.

Functions of the Social Environment

■ Parental Functions

In nurturing their toddler as he or she begins to develop an autonomous and gender identity, parents must be particularly attuned to the following functions they must fulfill:

- Protect their toddler in his or her assertive explorations from experiencing too many episodes of distressful over- or under-stimulation
- Teach their toddler how to gratify each of his or her innate needs within the family and social environment while keeping within the limits and rules set by society
- Provide empathically attuned encouragement, support, and admiration for their toddler's growing autonomy, while at the same time teaching their toddler that his or her autonomy has limits and restrictions

In all these functions, the parents are faced with the issue of how to shape their toddler's growing sense of being an autonomous self. Inherent in their shaping efforts are each parent's view of what is a normal child.

■ Parental Concept of What Is a Normal Child

Throughout recorded history, children were not thought of as serious objects of study (Boswell 1988). Through the middle of the

19th century, few ancient philosophers or scientific thinkers in Western Europe or the United States pondered what constituted normality in children. Far too often, a normal child was simply thought of as a child who obeyed his or her parents, thought very little about life, and was not interested in his or her social world other than how this world gratified his or her needs.

Strongly influenced by Darwin's 1877 description of his son's "normal" development, Sigmund Freud, his contemporaries, and many developmentalists who followed him, pondered the issue of how humans develop. They all inevitably faced the issue of defining those infant and child behaviors, thoughts, feelings, and cognitive changes that would be considered normal in their respective societies. For example, in modern-day United States, parents prize instilling their children with a sense of autonomy and independence and a desire to be honest always about their wishes and feelings. Thus a 6-year-old boy who is angry at a playmate and does not express his anger for fear he would lose this friend's admiration and support would be viewed more often than not by his American parents as being too unduly dependent on his friend's approval; his behavior would be viewed as more abnormal than normal. Most American parents would encourage their children to be honest in telling their playmates when and why they feel angry. In so doing, children rely on their inner sense of attained self-reliance and a belief in their own sense of value without needing to be reassured of their value by their friends.

If, however, a 6-year-old Japanese boy displayed this normal, American behavior, he would most likely be considered abnormal in his society (Kagan 1984). In current Japanese society, parents more highly prize in their children a sense of interdependence, harmony in social relationships, and a willingness to hold back the truth—to foster the social white lie—in order to avoid injuring the feelings of another. This 6-year-old boy's parents would tell him that it is always wise to tell the minor social lie when it preserves social harmony.

Hence each society contributes to how parents define normality. Parents also seem to intuitively feel when the standards they are teaching their children are in keeping with those of their society. When they are not, parents feel stress.

Offer and Sabshin (1984) delineated four perspectives on how child normality is defined within any society:

1. *Simply being healthy (i.e., when there are no signs of any significant emotional or physical illness)*—What degree of emotional or physical illness would be considered abnormal is not addressed.
2. *Achieving an average standard on a bell-shaped curve*—An above-average child would possess those characteristics most highly prized by the society in which the child lived.
3. *Reaching one's optimal development*—This would be a universally defined achievement where the child would be competing with only himself or herself in trying to reach this goal.
4. *Engaging in interdependent transactions with one's parents and important others, with each member in those transactions progressing and developing in a healthy manner*—Some degree of developmentally enhancing transactions would be viewed as normal, wherein a developmentally enhancing transaction would be one in which the needs of the child and the needs and social taskings of the parents are both met to some degree. This view of normality is difficult to describe, break down into stagelike norms, or quantify behaviorally. However, it suggests that children's behaviors are the result of ongoing child-parent transactions and that a "normal" child is one who is engaged in a developmentally enhancing adaptation to both his or her needs and his or her parents' needs and developmental taskings. Such an adaptation is achieved by both children and parents in their constant attempt to achieve a goodness of fit, while the goal of socializing children is not lost sight of by the children or their parents.

This transactional adaptational view of normality (Sameroff 1975) recognizes that the goodness or poorness of fit the child is engaged in with the parents 1) is not static and 2) is a major determinant in whether the child is or is not adapting well to his or her environment. This adaptational fluidity is not allowed, for example, within the third view of normality noted above, in which parents may not take into account factors in their relationship with their child that prevent him or her from achieving optimal development. For example, a 5-year-old boy's parents might believe that their son should receive an "A" on the bell-shaped curve of normality. However, if this same child were to experience a major trauma 1 year later—such as lose his leg in an automobile accident—and, because of his amputation, begin to do poorly in school and become more emotionally dependent on his parents, then that boy might lose his father's support and admiration and therefore merit only a "C."

Psychologically attuned parents intuitively use the transactional adaptational view of normality as their overall definition of normality in assessing whether their child is developing normally. Parents are also flexible in using the first three definitions of normality noted above in their efforts to assess if their child is progressing normally. However, each parent's flexibility in using the first three definitions depends on his or her ability to observe and learn from the transactions that occur during the family's life cycle. Some parents rigidly hold to one definition of normal behavior, whereas other parents are much more flexible in being open to transactional processes. The majority of normal parents eventually learn through developing a transactional, goodness-of-fit attachment relationship with their child that one definition of normality is too simplistic and does not do justice to the complexity of human development— both their child's development and their own.

Development of the Ego in Relation to the Toddler's Developing Self

As I note in Chapter 3, the self exists unconsciously and therefore operates outside the toddler's conscious awareness. The self is different from the self-representation, which is consciously experienced. Whereas the self is present from birth, the self-representation is constructed at about age 18 months. The latter enables toddlers to be consciously aware of having all the personal characteristics that they will eventually come to know as their identity. They are able to say, "I am and my mom is."

All of the forerunners of toddlers' evolving self-representation are continuously developed during the first 18 months of life. These forerunners include infants' constructed representations of their innate needs, emotions, temperamental characteristics, body sensations, and transactions involving their parents. Infants' activity, as motivated by their innate need to be assertive, has been noted to be the most important trigger for the development of a sense of self (McDevitt 1987) in that, through activity, infants slowly become aware of themselves as agents who make things happen (Pine 1985).

The self-representation is the experiential or internal and external perceiving part of the self. The self is not consciously experienced because it is a theoretical construct that gives a label to the mind's ability to organize all of its component structures and processes and achieve certain goals. As the mind's main agent of organized activity, the self does not require conscious forethought. Further, the self is never experienced mentally. As Meissner (1986) expressed it,

> The self in its subjective experience [i.e., the self-representation] is something which can observe itself. The ego is free of this: the ego is something which functions, it does not observe itself. (p. 385)

Neither does the id or superego observe itself. The ego, as a metaphorical container of many of the mind's processing functions (e.g., perceiving, conceptualizing, memorizing, and remembering; temperamental characteristics, mental organizing principles) is never directly experienced by the child or the adult. Arlow (1988) described the ego as a theoretical abstraction that is found in books on psychoanalytic theory.

Aspects of the self-representation are conscious and unconscious, just as aspects of the ego and superego are conscious and unconscious. The determining factor for whether any aspect of each is relegated to the unconscious is the self's directing its ego to bar from consciousness those mental contents that are associated with a highly displeasurable emotional state.

Maturation and Development of Innate Needs

The Anal Phase

During toddlerhood, there are significant maturational changes in the toddler's innate need to 1) assertively explore for novel stimuli, 2) engage in emotionally pleasurable attachment transactions, 3) signal episodes of distress, and 4) seek pleasurable bodily sensory-sexual stimulation and gratification.

S. Freud (1923/1963) hypothesized a progression in body parts or *zones* through which infants and children seek sensual, and ultimately sexual, pleasure. In the infancy *oral phase,* sensual pleasure is experienced through the lips and oral mucosa. In the toddler phase—Freud's *anal and urethral phase*—the anal and urethral mucosa of the toddler become the erogenous zones. As Brenner (1965) remarked,

> The anus comes to be the most important site of sexual tensions [stimulations] and gratifications. Pleasurable and unpleasurable sensations are associated with the retention of feces and with their expulsion, and these bodily processes, as well as fecal odors, are the objects of the child's most intense interest. (p. 26)

Roiphe and Galenson (1981) and Galenson (1993) documented how, by age 18 months, toddlers are quite preoccupied with anal and urethral stimulation and with defecation and urination. Defecation now becomes an "event" for toddlers: at times they pull at their diaper; they may look pleasurably preoccupied when defecating and urinating in their diaper; they may want to keep their stool to explore and smell it; and they show a new interest in watching their parents and siblings go to the toilet and seeing their stools. Likewise, urination becomes an interesting event for toddlers. Galenson (1993) observed that at this age toddlers become aware of their urinary stream and play with it; become curious about their parents', siblings', and peers' urination; and engage in a great variety of derivative play behaviors that resemble urination (e.g., playing with faucets, watering hoses and cans, and squirting devices).

By age 2 years, toddlers know that they produce body products that create a response from their parents. They then begin to acquire new knowledge about what anal or urethral activities mean in their families and what it means to produce feces and urine. The next important development of this anal phase is to learn about the social behaviors involved in toilet training (see "Development of the Self and Object Relationships," below).

Maturation and Development of Physical Capabilities

Gross Motor, Visual-Motor, and Manual Dexterity Capabilities

During this period, toddlers display many signs of developing physical maturity; their newly found physical skills occur in the context of continuing social transactions. For example, parents begin to shape their toddler's manual dexterity by demonstrating their own use of eating utensils, thereby setting up transactions in which the toddler will attempt to imitate them; by age 3 years, the toddler learns to eat in a socially acceptable manner. (The major gross motor, visual-motor, and manual dexterity abilities and associated social behaviors that emerge between ages 18 months and 3 years are listed in Table 4–1.)

At age 18 months, toddlers engage in many behaviors that demonstrate their growing manual dexterity and hand-eye coordination. They walk fairly well, experiment with running, and learn more each day about how their hands can manipulate new objects and parts of their own body (e.g., they can pleasurably stimulate their genitals and are curious about exploring the genitals of opposite-gender individuals). Toddlers achieve particular competency pleasure in discovering actions that they can make recur. They revel in discovering contingencies between something they do and the results; thus they engage in throwing all sorts of items and having them be thrown back, opening and closing objects with lids, pouring liquids in and out of containers, and building objects and knocking them down (see Figure 4–1).

All of these walking and running activities are biological as well as social stimuli—biological in that they are stimulated by toddlers' maturing physical nature, and social in that they generate responses from their social environment. These stimuli in turn generate many developmental changes. For example, a 10-month-girl took her first steps when she stood up, using a toy with wheels designed to aid in walking as support. Her mother witnessed this first walking event and responded with an enthusiastic smile. In constructing an early representation of this new walking behavior, the infant girl was accomplishing a developmental change and, in further practicing this behavior, she engaged in learning how to walk without the assistance of a walker.

By definition, toddlers' maturing physical abilities become another aspect of their maturing developing ego, an ego that functions silently in generating sensations, perceptions, thoughts, feelings, memories, and actions. All these functional products of the ego come under the direction of a toddler's self as the organizer and initiator of the toddler's overall decision to initiate or not initiate behaviors.

Table 4–1. Major gross and fine motor skills that emerge between ages 18 months and 3 years

Age	Motor skill
1½ years	Can grasp, hold, and return objects Can walk unattended Attempts to feed self
2 years	Can walk quite steadily Begins to be successful in feeding self Can walk up and down stairs
3 years	Can run quite steadily Can put on some clothes Begins to feed self more consistently

Source. Adapted from Ames and Ilg 1976a.

Maturation and Development of Cognitive Capabilities

■ Emergence of Objective Self-Awareness

At age 18 months, toddlers can be objective and observe themselves as separate people in a world of others. At this point in time, their objective self is born and, with it, they possess the beginning understanding of the concepts I, you, and we. This objective self-awareness is in contrast to the infant's subjective, or entirely self-absorbed, self-awareness (Stechler 1982).

A toddler's conscious awareness of being a separate self is not possible without a concurrent awareness of the existence of others.

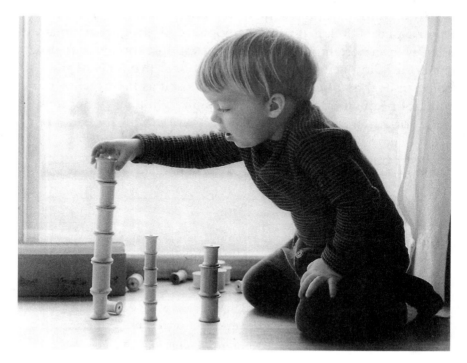

Figure 4–1. A toddler experimenting with stacking spools at different heights.
Source. Photograph by Florence Sharp; used with permission.

Interaction between the self and others provides meaning for both the self and others. M. Lewis and Brooks-Gunn (1979) described the toddler's progressive awareness of being a separate self in a world of others as a parallel process involving the toddler's concurrent acquisition of knowledge of self and others.

By ages 18–24 months, toddlers' fully developed schema of object permanence, coupled with the capacity for evocative memory, assists them in evoking mental images of themselves (i.e., a self-representation) and of others (i.e., objective representations of their parents, siblings, or other individuals who have been a predominant presence so far in their lives). They now use their ability to evoke object representations of important others to verify that people and inanimate things continue to exist even when they are not receiving sensory and perceptual input of that existence. These object representations include toddlers' sensations, perceptions, wishes, thoughts, and emotions as well as prior representations of each person. They exist within their inner world as representations of varying complexity—from the object representation of a neighbor with whom a toddler has only infrequently interacted (a representation that is most likely devoid of emotional content) to the object representation of a toddler's mother, which contains myriad emotions, thoughts, wishes, and so on.

Object representations are stored as long-term memories only when an object has achieved some degree of constancy in a toddler's life (McDevitt and Mahler 1989). For example, a 2-year-old boy will construct an object representation of a baby-sitter only if he has regular encounters with that baby-sitter, encounters that are colored by the toddler's wishes about and feelings toward the baby-sitter. These encounters will produce various images of the baby-sitter. Eventually, the boy will construct an object representation of the baby-sitter that is an amalgamation of all these different prior images. In storing this object representation as a long-term memory, the toddler will now possess an awareness of knowing the baby-sitter.

Toddlers' emerging objective self-awareness can be observed in their behaviors. Kagan (1981, 1989) described the following seven behaviors that emerge between ages 17 and 24 months (see Table 4–2). The emergence of these behaviors signifies the toddler's conscious beginning awareness of possessing a mind.

An appreciation of right and wrong, good and bad, valued and not valued. Through their growing capability to discriminate between good and bad behaviors and their ability to realize that parents attribute value to events, inanimate objects, and people, toddlers begin to recognize that they are individuals and that people are valued based on what they do. Toddlers learn that what is not valued is given up; thus, in their view, there is no danger to them unless they become judged worthless (Rochlin 1965).

Once toddlers begin to learn that some behaviors are thought of and admired by people as good and other behaviors as bad, they begin to monitor themselves as well as make inferences about others' behaviors. For example, if a toddler girl sees a broken dish, she may spontaneously say, "Broke, not me," and expect the parent to confirm her knowledge that someone else did the breaking (Kagan 1989). She is demonstrating to her parents that she has an intrinsic need to judge herself as valued and good.

Table 4–2. Toddlers' behaviors reflecting their developing self-awareness

- Ability to appreciate right from wrong, allowing them to choose between a right and a wrong behavior
- Ability to recognize that behavior A → event X and behavior B → event Y, allowing them to determine outcome based on their choice of behavior
- Ability to perceive another's emotional state
- Ability to assess the success or failure of a task and to experience anxiety based on their perceived failure at a new task
- Ability to begin placing value on behaviors and develop standards of behavior
- Ability to identify their own inner state, affects, ideas, and so on through language
- Ability to recognize themselves as separate individuals with a fixed identity

---

Source.   Adapted from Kagan 1989, pp. 221–242.

The recognition, through inferential thinking, that results have causes. After about age 18 months, toddlers begin to understand that events have causes (Greenspan 1979). Returning to the example of the broken dish, this self-aware toddler girl will understand that the dish was broken as a result of the action of a separate person who exists in her world. What now begins to occur is that toddlers become motivated to understand specific causes for many events. They will infer all sorts of ideas during this phase in their ongoing attempts to assimilate current perceptions into what they already know and accommodate to and therefore acquire knowledge about new and unexpected events. By about age 2½ years, toddlers begin to deluge their parents with "Why?" questions, and also begin to present their parents with many of their explanations or "theories" for why certain things happen. In their attempts to learn that events have causes, toddlers often become frustrated in the answers they receive to their questions because they are limited in their cognitive ability to understand many of the causes for observed events.

Using early forerunners of empathy to motivate and guide behaviors. By age 2 years, toddlers are able to infer the emotional state of another in their efforts to understand the effects of their behavior on that other person (Brothers 1989). This is a precursor to true empathy, which develops between ages 6 and 8 years. At this earlier stage, toddlers engage in the unconscious process of *projective identification*, through which they infer that someone else experiences the same feelings they would experience in the same situation; thus they project their own feelings onto others and then identify with the projected feeling. For example, a 3-year-old boy sees a little girl fall off a swing at a playground. The girl goes and sits on a bench and is not crying. However, the boy infers that he would feel pain if he had fallen off a swing, and he projects his own painful feeling onto the girl. He walks up to her, identifying this feeling in her, and says "It's okay. It hurts a lot, huh?" This boy's actions can be viewed as prosocial behaviors. *Prosocial behaviors,* which are often triggered by children's empathy, are "voluntary actions that are intended to help or benefit another individual or group of individuals" (Eisenberg and

Mussen 1989, p. 3). And in noting how empathy and prosocial behaviors appear to maturationally emerge in toddlers, Emde (1991) wrote, "The fact that empathy appears normatively in development suggests a biologically prepared, positive system for prosocial inclination" (p. 20).

In time, through empathy, toddlers become better able to assess correctly the emotional state they will generate in another if they execute a certain contemplated behavior (e.g., if they hit other children). This empathic awareness of being able to generate good and bad feelings in others is another way in which toddlers begin to attain more knowledge of themselves as independent agents whose actions can cause others to feel and behave in certain ways. As they learn the effects of their actions, toddlers are encouraged to adopt behaviors that are good and avoid those that are bad (see Figure 4–2). This process motivates them to identify with their parents' nonhurtful behaviors (i.e., parental behaviors that are more adaptive than maladaptive in helping the child gratify his or her innate needs). For example, Kagan (1984) described the following interaction between two 3½-year-old boys, one of whom was more dominant and the other, more passive: the passive boy seized and put on the only Batman costume there was. When the more dominant boy wanted the costume, the passive boy then "paraded around the room showing off his prize. And then, as if he understood the jealousy he was generating in the more aggressive boy, he said, 'You can hate me if you want'" (p. 127).

Toddlers' development of their capacity for empathy can be nurtured or extinguished by their parents' responses to their empathic overtures. Attuned parents communicate to their toddlers that empathy is a usable and valued way in which people interact with each other. On the other hand, when parents reject their toddler's empathic observations of the parents' feelings, the toddler eventually begins to try not to feel or perceive the feelings and associated wishes of parents and others. In effect, the toddler, to stay out of trouble with his or her unempathic parents, tries to become imperceptive to empathically sensing the emotional states within them.

For example, a 3-year-old boy sat at the breakfast table with his mother. He spontaneously said, "Here, Mom, I made you some cereal (he had mixed milk and dry cereal in a bowl) so you won't feel so sad." Even though the mother was feeling sad, she rejected her toddler's empathic perception of her emotional state by exclaiming, "What are you talking about? I feel just fine!" As time went by and the mother continued to reject her son's empathy, he began to avoid using his empathy to stay out of conflict with his mother.

The beginning construction of standards. After about age 18 months, toddlers become increasingly cognizant of the existence of standards that dictate whether a behavior is good or bad, and begin to construct two separate categories within their mind for these two types of behaviors. At this age, almost all behaviors are either good or bad. For example, take a toddler girl who has

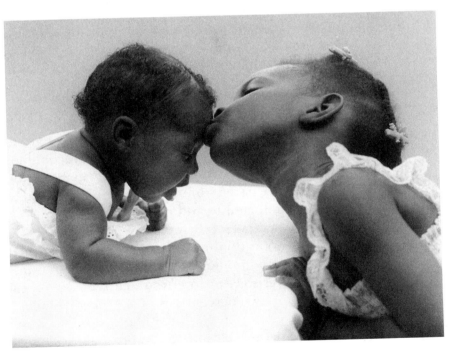

Figure 4–2. A toddler displaying affection and empathy toward a younger sibling as well as identifying with her parents' behaviors. *Source.* Photograph by Florence Sharp; used with permission.

just stacked a group of toy containers. Because all toddlers are basically performers and are in the process of discovering their separateness as an independent locus of actions and feelings, they desire to perform for themselves and achieve competency pleasure and mastery smiles as well as perform for their parents and receive mirroring smiles indicative of their valuing her. Thus this toddler girl regards stacking the toy containers as a good behavior because it causes her to feel competent and it pleases her parents, both of which enhance her self-esteem.

In the process of producing highly valued behaviors for their parents, toddlers are assisted in being biologically prepared to acquire standards (Kagan 1984, 1988). In essence, toddlers do not always need to learn through a direct assimilation or accommodation experience that a behavior is bad or harmful before they will inhibit that behavior. For example, 3-year-old toddlers will often experience jealousy and anger when a new baby sister or brother is brought home. However, despite the many opportunities available for the toddler to inflict bodily harm on his or her new sibling, most toddlers appear to maintain the standard that hitting a person much smaller than themselves is bad (see Figure 4–2).

The generation of anxiety when faced with possible failure in mastering a new experience. Toddlers who have finally begun to be aware of their mental and behavioral capabilities continue to be motivated to perform in assertively seeking stimuli, assimilate or accommodate to the stimuli, generate mastery smiles in response to acting competently, and receive admiring, mirroring feedback from their parents for their mastery of the new stimulating situation. Their motivation to perform arises from 1) their parents' use of operant conditioning (i.e., giving material rewards and positive mirroring responses) to encourage them to repeat valued behaviors, 2) their own perceptions of new developmental taskings given by their parents, and 3) their perception of a novel object or task that stimulates their innate need to assertively seek stimulation and master novel situations.

Kagan (1981) reported that 2-year-old toddlers will either observe an adult doing a new task or be shown a new task by an adult. They will then, either in the presence or in the absence of the adult, try to imitate the new task until they succeed. When they fail at accommodation, they begin to express their distress through crying, fretting, protesting, and other similar behaviors. These behaviors likely reflect the fact that they experienced an obligation to duplicate the adult's actions but recognized that they were unable to do so. They would not become distressed unless they were dimly aware of a deficit in their ability. In this case, toddlers show that they are capable of experiencing anxiety when they believe they cannot meet a self-imposed standard (Kagan 1981). On the other hand, when toddlers are able to master a new task, they first generate a private mastery smile and then seek a mirroring smile from their parents.

The use of verbal language to identify actions. By age 2 years, toddlers begin to discover that they have a mind that senses, perceives, feels, thinks, and remembers (Leslie 1987). They also become more aware of their gender identity, of possessing a name, of being able to choose behaviors that bring praise from their parents, and, as perhaps the most remarkable capability possessed by humans, of being able to speak and use words to identify and differentiate their characteristics from the characteristics and behaviors of others. The use of the words such as I, me, Mom, and Dad becomes quite dominant at about age 18 months, when toddlers begin to use memories to evoke images of themselves, their parents, and other important family members. As P. Tyson and Tyson (1991) expressed it,

> The use of words helps the toddler begin to perceive his own inner state, his own affects, differences between a wished-for state and his actual state, and differences between his wishes and his mother's. (p. 179)

The ability to visually recognize one's separateness as a person. M. Lewis and Brooks-Gunn (1979) documented how, at about age 18 months, toddlers will look in a mirror after their face has been altered by a spot of rouge on their nose and be able to touch the spot, an ability they did not possess earlier. Because they recognize that something in the reflection is not "just right," it is thought that they are able to recognize that the reflection in the mirror is not exactly their own. By age 3 years, however, those same children will immediately know that their face has been altered and that the altering hides in some way their true facial image. Most children at this age will touch the spot, laugh, and immediately assume that someone wants them to pretend to be a clown, hide their identity, and so on.

■ Continued Development of Conceptual Thinking

Toddlers ages 18–24 months have already constructed an object representation of their mother. For example, they know that their mother is the person whom they trust to protect and nurture them. This trust is much more than a perception of their mother; it is a thought with personal understanding (i.e., a conception of what a mother means to them). Beginning at about age 18 months, toddlers' conceptions become a new part of their developing identity as a separate individual.

Ability to symbolize. One cognitive advance that emerges with toddlers' maturation of conceptual thinking is the ability to symbolize (Klein 1930/1975; Werner and Kaplan 1963). With this new ability, toddlers begin to form symbolic representations, or symbols for short. They construct symbols about their experiences with inanimate objects (Galenson 1984; Galenson et al. 1976). For example, a toddler takes much pleasure in imbuing a stuffed teddy bear with the qualities of affection and trust. As one 2½-year-old girl said, "My teddy bear loves me and never goes away."

One characteristic of toddlers' symbolizing is that they cannot distinguish between the symbol and what it symbolizes. For example, a toddler boy and his mother are playing with puppets, one of which is a puppet of a dog. The toddler attributes a symbolic meaning to the dog puppet, imbuing it with the quality of being alive (this is called *animism*). Thus he smiles if his mother, in talking for the dog, talks in a friendly manner, and becomes frightened if his mother verbalizes a menacing growl for the dog puppet. Toddlers also imbue parts of their body with the quality of being alive (e.g., a toddler might say, "My tummy is being bad today"). It is as if the objectively aware toddler has become aware of his or her own aliveness and goes around assuming everything else in the world has this quality too.

A toddler's attributions of life to nonliving things are particularly involved when the inanimate object symbolizes a real person or the toddler himself or herself. For example, a 3-year-old girl saw a puppet in my interview playroom and said with joyful interest, "Oh, the cookie monster is here." When I put the cookie monster on my hand and made a slight "grrr" sound to imitate a growl, she became very frightened, stating, "Take him away! He's scary! He'll bite me!" She could not distinguish the cookie monster puppet from what it symbolized, which was her own angry feeling projected onto the cookie monster in an attempt to solve her own internal conflict. This conflict involved her wanting on that day to eat as much junk food as she wanted (the way a cookie monster can eat unlimited amounts of cookies) and her knowing that her mother had restricted this food intake before the interview.

DeLoache (1987) demonstrated the inability of toddlers to recognize that a symbolic object stands for something else until about age 3 years. In that study, children ages 2–3 years were shown a model of a room and were told that the model stood for, or was a picture of, the real room they were in at the time. The toddlers were then allowed to watch as a researcher hid a tiny stuffed dog in a certain place in the symbolic model room. Each toddler was then asked to go find a larger stuffed dog in the real room. The 3-year-old children usually looked for and found the larger stuffed dog in the same place in the real room in which the tiny stuffed dog was hidden in the symbolic model room. However, the 2½-year-old toddlers could not find the larger stuffed dog because they could not understand that the model room was a symbol for the real room.

Toddlers also do not realize the transparency of their symbols; that is, they are unable to recognize how they use a symbol. For example, the 3-year-old girl noted above was entirely unaware that the cookie monster puppet stood for an aspect of herself: her wish to have no limits placed on her eating junk food by her mother. Parents, however, know that their toddlers' symbols often stand for their wishes or feelings; parents take pleasure, to a point, in supporting their toddlers' belief that symbols are real. Thus, if a toddler girl falls and says, "The stick made me fall!" and really means it, her mother might say "Bad stick! Don't you ever do that to my little girl again!"

For example, I interviewed a 2¾-year-old boy after his parents had reported that he was having frequent temper tantrums. The boy had a 1-year-old sister whom the parents described as difficult to soothe and who required a lot of their attention. In the interview playroom, when I asked the boy about his sister, he picked up a toy doll and called it "my sister." He then took play dough and smeared it in the doll's face and into her eyes. With much enjoyment he stated, "My sister has poops on her face and her eyes. Mom will hit her now!" He did not realize the transparency of what his symbolic object doll stood for: his recently intense aggressive outbursts toward his sister to which his parents were responding by spanking him often and, sometimes, I later learned, quite excessively.

Ability to understand concepts expressed in verbal language. Not coincidentally, the period from age 18 months to 2 years is the time when the ability to comprehend and express a verbal language begins to emerge because, to acquire verbal language, which is a system of word symbols, a toddler must have the cognitive ability to symbolize.

After age 18 months, toddlers' ability to form symbolic conceptions and learn words enables them to begin to store explicit memories—information stored either in verbal form; in visual, auditory, tactile, and olfactory perceptions and conceptions; or in a combination of these forms. Explicit memories are usually stored within their preconscious mental domain, which make them accessible to the conscious domain through their recall abilities. However, as I note in Chapter 1, an explicit memory can be automatically relegated to a toddler's unconscious mental domain through repression.

Toddlers' construction of all conceptions is driven by their innate need to recognize and assimilate the familiar, recognize and accommodate to truly novel stimuli, and acquire new knowledge—the process I conceptualize here as *developmental change*. Inherent in this innate need is their need to generate predictive expectancies about their future.

Ability to form object relations units.   As toddlers continue to use their symbolizing and verbal language abilities, they begin to form another type of complex representation: the object (or person) relations unit (see Figure 4–3) (Hamilton 1988). This type of complex representation comprises three mental representations, two of which may be the following: two aspects of the toddler's self-representation (Example 1 in Figure 4–4); an aspect of the toddler's self-representation and an aspect of one of the toddler's object representations (Example 2 in Figure 4–4); two aspects of the toddler's object representations (Example 3 in Figure 4–4); or two aspects of the toddler's categories. The third representational component is a representation that establishes a relationship between the first two representations. This relational structure can be a fantasy (Example 1 in Figure 4–4), a belief (Example 2 in Figure 4–4), or an emotion (Example 3 in Figure 4–4).

Fantasies.   Fantasies are constructed from the same ingredients as beliefs: current sensations, perceptions, thoughts, emotions,

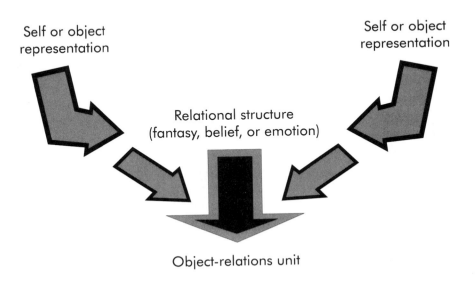

Figure 4–3. Components of object relations unit.
Source. Adapted from Hamilton 1988.

and wishes, and the memories of any or all of these, including earlier fantasies and beliefs that are associated with the current experience. However, the fantasy is primarily a wishful conception, in that the person's wishes are the motivating force for constructing the fantasy. Person (1995) described fantasy as "an imaginary story or internal dialogue that generally serves a more or less transparent wish-fulfilling function" (p. 7). A fantasy conceptualizes what and how a person wishes his or her world could be and incorporates the way that person would change things and people so that his or her wishes would come true.

Fantasies help toddlers learn how to cope with parental developmental taskings (see "Development of Play," below). In the toddler phase of development, all fantasies are toddlers' attempt to deny aspects of reality that they would prefer to ignore. Toddlers who have come to trust in their parents' ability to protect them

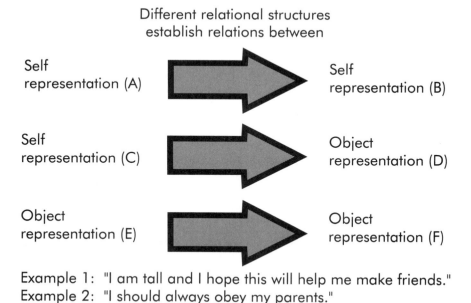

Example 1: "I am tall and I hope this will help me make friends."
Example 2: "I should always obey my parents."
Example 3: "Fathers and mothers love each other."

Figure 4–4.   Relational structures for object relations units.

from danger will eventually use experiences with their parents, siblings, peers, and other adults, as well as their emerging new cognitive capacities, to reconstruct their fantasies into reality-based beliefs.

A fantasy can be transformed into a belief about reality when a toddler's reality is so abnormal that it becomes emotionally intolerable for him or her. Consequently, the highly displeasurable emotions associated with the intolerable reality may be repressed into the toddler's dynamic unconscious while he or she constructs a fantasy that he or she chooses to believe as being a more tolerable reality. A toddler in this situation can border on the brink of abandoning all attempts to deal with reality, instead making his or her fantasies the only reality. At the extreme, such a child might develop a delusional belief that a fantasy is true, despite irrefutable evidence to the contrary.

Beliefs.   A *belief* is a conception that establishes the relationship between two or more inanimate objects, aspects of nature's laws, or people. A belief's truthfulness can be judged on a spectrum from being highly truthful to being completely false (Meissner 1992). Two pieces of knowledge become related within the toddler's mind through a belief. The belief allows the toddler to make declarative statements about his or her social and inanimate world. The declarative statement then becomes the substance of a declarative (or explicit) memory. The declarative statement may have only a subject and a verb, or it may contain a subject, verb, and object. Thus a belief of a 3-year-old child might be, "The earth moves," or "The sun makes the earth warm." In the belief, the toddler can be stating just a fact or two or more factual phenomena.

Beliefs, as with all representations constructed by the child, will be modified during the normal development process. In their daily discoveries, toddlers continually not only construct but reconstruct beliefs, particularly earlier beliefs and fantasies that in some way become contradicted by a current experience. Many of toddlers' beliefs replicate the edicts, standards, and moral values of their parents and their parents' aspirations for them. Therefore, the declarative statements of people whom toddlers view as authorities will contribute to their beliefs (Kagan 1984).

Categories. A *category* can be defined as "the symbolic representation of the qualities shared by a set of events" (Kagan 1989, p. 230). Toddlers automatically construct categories as another function of their maturing cognitive abilities. Kagan (1989) noted that, although children appear to be biologically prepared to detect physical and functional qualities shared by events, it is not clear why they sort objects into categories based on their similarities. For example, toddlers construct object representations of their mother, female baby-sitters, grandmother, and other women. Eventually, and quite automatically, they then construct the category of "woman," noting that one of the common features among people in that category is that they care for babies. Then, when toddlers perceive a young boy, they know that this boy is not a woman. A category such as this, according to Kagan (1989), becomes a "stabilizing force permitting the person to talk about the whole class of previously encountered women" (p. 232).

Although parents can, and often do, directly teach their toddlers to put people and things into categories, most of toddlers' categories arise through their automatic categorical constructions. Thus, as is depicted in Figure 4–5, the girl recognizes that the figure in the bed is not her grandmother, nor does the figure occupy any category such as woman, friend, or teacher. The girl then scans her file of categories and realizes that this figure is an animal and something, she has already learned, of which she should be wary. She is able to make this judgment without having any prior direct experience with a wolf dressed in human clothing.

The content of toddlers' growing categories is based on whether people, animals, or objects share common features; toddlers sort these features using the following abilities (Kagan 1984):

- *Perceptual commonality* (e.g., thunder, explosions, and talking loud all share the quality of loudness).
- *Functional commonality* (e.g., chairs and benches share the quality of being something to sit on).
- *Emotional commonality* (e.g., a dog, a person, or an inanimate object perceived as threatening all share the feature of generating anxiety).

- *Conceptual commonality* (e.g., checkers, tennis, and stamp collecting all share the conceptual construct of being a game or hobby). This is considered to be an internal, not an external, perceptual quality, in that a toddler recognizes not these items' external similarities but instead his or her common attitude toward them.
- *Word label commonality.* As explained by Kagan (1984), "The fact that flies and roses are called 'alive,' and Zeus and Athena are called 'gods,' can be a sufficient basis for a child to treat both pairs as members of separate categories, even if the child does not know the biological qualities of life or the function of gods" (p. 212).

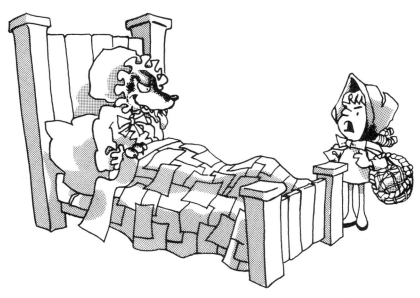

"My gran'ma, eh? Let's see some I.D."

Figure 4–5. A toddler girl uses her previously constructed category of "woman" to confirm that a wolf dressed like a woman is nonetheless not a woman.
Source. Copyright 1987; reprinted courtesy of Bill Hoest and *Parade Magazine.*

- *Belief and fantasy commonality* (e.g., the characters Super-man, Spiderman, and Batman all share the quality of possessing unlimited strength and power).

Self-reflection. Concurrently with their development of the above complex conceptual structures, toddlers develop the ability to revise old complex conceptions through the process called *self-reflection*. Piaget (1967) referred to this process as one in which the toddler reshapes previous thoughts into new or revised ones. In Chapter 2, I discuss how pre-self-aware infants use the accommodation-transformation process to accommodate new biopsychosocial stimuli and thereby transform old representations. Objectively aware toddlers continue to use this process, but now can also use their new ability for self-reflection to think about prior beliefs and fantasies about themselves, their parents, and objects and transform them. In addition, through self-reflection, toddlers slowly begin to prioritize their wishes, beliefs, and fantasies in accordance with the hierarchical restructuring principle (also discussed in Chapter 2). These self-reflective processes enable toddlers to prioritize their representations in ever-changing hierarchies related to their importance, their complexity, and other features.

For example, a 2¾-year-old boy constructs the following conceptual representation of a hat: I like hats because they have funny things on them. By age 4, his concept of a hat is more complex: I like baseball hats best of all because my dad and big brother wear them. By age 8, more complexity is added to his hat schema: Sometimes I like to wear baseball hats so I don't have to comb my hair, but usually I like them because I like to play baseball. This boy's priorities in reference to hats will change over the years as the importance of hats in his life changes; eventually, he might say: Hats are no big deal for me.

Kagan (1989) also noted that toddlers begin to transform their beliefs, wishes, and fantasies based on their new cognitive ability to use intuition and logic. They revel in being able to use their new intuition not only in responding to new stimuli but also in making inferences and generating new thoughts. Toddlers are quite limited, however, in their ability to intuit explanations and use logical thinking in comprehending many of life's events and physical phenomena. For example, the following exchange took place between a 3-year-old boy and his mother:

Son: Mommy, how do you make babies?
Mother: You plant a seed and it grows in the mommy's belly.
Son: It's good you didn't plant it in the yard, because it would grow up looking like a tomato.

Use of primary and secondary process thinking. The further development and differentiation of toddlers' primary process thinking from their secondary process thinking is enhanced by the development of their ability to 1) use self-reflective, intuitive, and logical thinking, 2) use verbal language, and 3) create and use symbols. Symbolic representations assist toddlers in developing a verbal language, which in turn helps them develop their secondary process, reality-based form of thinking. However, symbolic representations can also help them develop their primary process, magically oriented form of thinking. When a toddler forms a symbolic representation of, for example, a stuffed teddy bear and endows the teddy bear with comforting and protective qualities, the toddler is developing his or her ability to use primary process thinking in an adaptive way. In constructing symbols, toddlers are able to use magical thinking at the same time as they are developing and using their secondary process thinking.

As they develop, toddlers confront many facts of life that are difficult to accept all at once. Primary process symbolic representation allows toddlers and children up to about age 6 or 7 years to use magical thinking to deal with displeasurable life events. Parents allow this, knowing that their child's belief in a magical teddy bear that protects him or her from all loneliness and danger—something on which the child relies when experiencing separation anxiety during his or her parents' absence—will give way to new, reality-oriented behaviors that help their child tolerate and master his or her separation anxiety. This use of a teddy bear is an example of the child's creation of a transitional object (Winnicott 1953/1971, 1959/1989). A *transitional object* is so called because it allows toddlers to make the transition from the infancy phase—in which they developed basic trust and a sense of separateness and value—to the toddler phase—during which they must begin to exercise their separateness and value in acting autonomously without excessive doubt and separation anxiety (Erikson 1959). The transitional object is not just a substitute for the mother or father, but a magical creation by the toddler. It is a symbolic representation of the mother and is imbued with magical powers to soothe, protect, and empower the toddler to continue to explore the world. Transitional objects are created by toddlers most often between ages 15 months and 2 years. They can then persist in the child's life up to ages 4–5 years.

Deferred imitation. Toddlers' use of transitional objects involves their use of thought as a "trial action" within their mind—that is, as a tactic to delay initiating a surface behavior. This is in keeping with Piaget's labeling the second phase of cognitive development (ages 18 months to 6 years) as the *preoperational phase.*

One of the hallmarks of the toddler phase of cognitive development is when toddlers demonstrate what Piaget (1954b/1981) called "deferred imitation." Through this process, toddlers can develop thoughts other than those linked to direct sensorimotor experiences. In deferred imitation, instead of having to imitate an observed behavior immediately (as in the sensorimotor cognitive stage of infancy, where sensory manipulation of objects is paramount), toddlers may spontaneously attempt to imitate and repeat the behavior at a later time, often hours and sometimes days later. Deferred imitation helps toddlers learn by imitating a behavior and discovering some new behavior or fact about their body or social world. For example, a 2-year-old girl sees her mother bathe her baby brother and asks her mother if she could help. The mother agrees. One day, the mother leaves her daughter with a baby-sitter. After the mother leaves with the baby brother, the 2-year-old girl goes to the sink and gives her doll baby a bath, imitating what she remembers of how her mother bathed her baby brother. In this way the girl is acquiring new knowledge (a developmental change) and applying this knowledge in learning by deferred imitation.

Ability to delay action. Another aspect of cognition that emerges at about age 18 months is toddlers' ability to delay action in response to a novel object, person, or event. Before age 18 months, when they see a new object or behavior, infants invariably act to perform an "experiment" on it, immediately trying to assimilate the new object or behavior into one or more of their existing representations. If they are unsuccessful, they then attempt to accommodate to the new perception and, in the process, construct a new representation. However, beginning at age 18 months, toddlers do not always immediately act but sometimes delay their action. During this delay, they are thinking: they are comparing the newly perceived object or behavior with their internal representations. They may 1) recognize that this new object or behavior is similar to another object or behavior of which they have knowledge and, hence, delay their imitation of the behavior or exploration of the object for another time, or 2) become joyfully excited by recognizing their ability to internally think about a perception without having to act. This delay in action to allow thinking is a cognitive processing capability that assists toddlers in their concurrent learning of a verbal language (see below). As they delay, toddlers have time to listen to their parents' verbalized directions about whether or not it is okay for them to act in a particular way.

Inability to understand conservation.   During toddlerhood, toddlers' are unable to understand the concepts of conservation of mass and number. For example, a 2-year-old boy is shown two same-size circular apple pies, one cut into four pieces and the other cut into eight pieces. If asked which pie he wants, he will choose the eight-piece pie. His current cognitive capabilities cause him to believe that an object containing more parts contains more of the object. He is cognitively unable to integrate his perceptions of both pies and comprehend that matter stays constant or is conserved regardless of a change in its overall physical appearance.

Toddlers also are unable to understand the concept of conservation of number—that is, that the number of objects stays the same regardless of the change in their dimensions. For example, a 3-year-old girl is shown two rows of checkers, equal in number. The adult then says, "One pile is mine and one pile is yours" (Gleitman 1987). The adult spreads both checkers in rows that are the same length. The adult asks, "Do we both have the same?" The child nods yes. The adult then rearranges the rows so that his row is spread out in a longer row. The child now says, "Your row has more."

Egocentrism. The inability to understand conservation of both mass and number points to a more general cognitive inability in toddlers: the inability to perceive two physical dimensions of an object and understand that both dimensions are properties of the same object. This inability to take in two simultaneously perceived dimensions leads them to manifest egocentrism or an egocentric view of the world. *Egocentrism* is the belief that one's point of view or perception of an event is the only point of view that can exist for that event. Because of their egocentric view of the world, toddlers have difficulties in completely understanding that their parents and other individuals each have a self and mind separate from their own.

Gleitman (1987) described an experiment conducted by Piaget and Inhelder (1956) in which they demonstrated egocentrism:

> If two adults stand at opposite corners of a building, each knows that the other sees a different wall. But according to Piaget, pre-operational children don't understand this. In a study, children were shown a three-dimensional model of a mountain scene. While the children viewed the scene from one position, a small doll was placed at various other locations around the model. The child's job was to decide what the doll saw from *its* vantage point. To answer, the child has to choose one of several drawings that depict different views of the mountain scene. Up to four years of age, the children didn't even understand the question. From four to seven years old, this response was fairly constant— they chose the drawing that showed what they saw, regardless of where the doll was placed. (p. 378; italics in the original)

Toddlers' egocentric view of the world at times makes them tell the toddlers' parents that their perception is the only perception of an event. At other times, toddlers, in their wish to see their parents as all-powerful protectors, project their egocentrism onto their parents as an omnipotent idealization of the parents. This idealizing view of the parent does not become truly prominent until after toddlerhood (i.e., after about age 3 years). For example, a 2½-year-old girl saw a sunset with her father. The next morning, she implored her father, "Dad, do it again!" (M. L. Lewis 1978). However, this omnipotent and egocentric view of herself and her father slowly changes as she begins to realize that things happen that are not controlled by herself or her parents. By age 3½ years, she would still be overly preoccupied by her own perceptual experiences, but less egocentrically so. At this age, she asks her dad, "How does the sun go down like that? How does that happen? What is a sun?"

Play. In toddlerhood, the quality and meaning of toddlers' play changes greatly (Waelder 1976a, 1976b). Play may be thought of as the primary means by which toddlers and children up to age 6 years teach themselves. Even when formal grade school begins at about age 6 or 7 years, play is still crucial in helping children learn and adapt to their social world. Toddlers do not necessarily view their play activities as play. For them, play is a natural aspect of their life. Or, as one 3-year-old answered when asked why he liked to play, "I don't play. This is what I do!"

The function of play for toddlers is threefold:

1. To act out, in playful fantasy, a pleasurable life experience using toys, other adults, and children as symbols for the real experience, acquiring new knowledge in the process. Acting out a fantasy in play is one of the ways that toddlers manifest their ability to evocatively remember, defer imitation, and re-create an aspect of their world in a play "drama." In this drama, toddlers assign various roles to their symbolic objects, which represent their self and object representations. Children's stories, both modern and classic fairy tales (Bettleheim 1985), appeal to toddlers and older children mainly because they symbolically express toddlers' common wishes, fears, and conflicts. Bettleheim noted that classic fairy tales assist toddlers in developing playful fantasy by often expressing the theme that, despite life's conflicts, toddlers' assertion and good deeds overcome their bad behaviors or the malevolent motives of bad people.

Stern (1985) noted that, through their new capacity for objectifying the self and coordinating different mental and actional schemata, toddlers can share their representational world, knowledge, and experiences as well as work on their world in imagination or reality. For example, a 2¾-year-old girl expresses much joy in continually making a teddy bear appear from and disappear within a box by pushing a button that controls the opening and closing of a lid. This play mimics similarly joyful play in which she had appeared to her father earlier in the day, went off to another room to hide, then reappeared and laughed when her father acted surprised. This behavior with her father had continued for several minutes. When the father returns and sees his daughter playing this appearing-disappearing game with her teddy bear, he asks her, "Is that teddy bear me?" She replies, "No, I'm just making believe." Her belief that her play is pretend enables her to enjoy the play activity. Pretending does not detract from the immense enjoyment she receives in her play.

Toddlers' enjoyable play functions as a substitute for the original situation that the play symbolizes. By the time a child reaches ages 6–7 years, play will not work as well in being a substitute for receiving real gratification of his or her wishes and needs. But this remarkable aspect of play in early life assists toddlers in being socialized in that it gives them a way to make themselves happy. Without this ability of play to give substitute enjoyment for the "real thing," toddlers might "tell" their mother, "Don't give me toys when I want you to drop everything and play with me right now!" On the contrary, during periods when toddlers must occupy and stimulate themselves, they act out a script based on real life experiences. In the process, they are also stimulating their own acquisition of new knowledge. Thus, while playing with the teddy bear, the girl in the above example is accommodating the perception of the new box and adding to her knowledge of boxes by learning that some boxes open and close by pushing a button. Also in her play, she is making intuitive guesses about what she experiences; these intuitive thoughts will lead to new behaviors that ultimately lead to new representations. For example, she intuits that if a button can open a box, then maybe the button on the other objects will open them or produce some other result. In thinking about such actions, toddlers are able to use self-reflection in order to reconstruct preexisting representations by constructing new beliefs and fantasies.

2. *To practice delaying the behavioral or verbal expression of wishes and feelings that are causing developmental conflicts with parents.* Toddlers use play to deal with situations of developmental conflict. A *developmental conflict* is a disparity between a toddler's current wish and the wishes of his or her parents that are connected to the socialization of the toddler (Brenner 1979). These conflicts are called developmental because they normally occur in the process of toddlers' becoming socialized members of their family and society. Many times each day, toddlers are faced with developmental conflicts (e.g., when their parents prohibit their wishes, when their parents make it clear that gratification of their wishes must be delayed). In these situations, toddlers experience a benignly displeasurable level of anxiety caused by their fear of losing their parents' positive mirroring and attributions of value and love if they were to suddenly express in behavior or speech their restricted wishes. For example, no matter how much a toddler boy may wish that his parents would never leave him, he must deal with this (hopefully) benignly displeasurable fact of life, albeit initially with much separation anxiety. He must learn ways of tolerating and dealing with his separation anxiety as one of the emotions that go along with having a relationship with his parents. Through play, toddlers are able to symbolically repeat situations of conflict and arrive at creative solutions to the developmental conflict facing them.

S. Freud (1917/1963) delineated a series of potential "normal developmental calamities" of life that a child would experience as traumatic, the first of which was abandonment by his or her parents. Separation anxiety triggered by parents' actually leaving their child can eventually be ameliorated by the parents' demonstrating their trustworthiness by returning time and time again. A different type of anxiety is called *signal anxiety,* in which children use anxiety to signal to themselves that the behavior they are considering might bring on their parent's disapproval and a potential developmental calamity.

One time of day during which toddlers often experience separation anxiety is at bedtime, particularly on a day when they have done something to displease their parents. When left in bed, toddlers must comfort themselves—sometimes through symbolic play with a transitional object—and reassure themselves that their parents will be there if they need them and also when they awaken. For example, Piaget (1952) described the play of his 2-year-old daughter in which she invented a game where she lay in bed and opened and closed her eyes. Eventually she restructured the game into one in which she would pretend she was lying in bed by putting her head down (e.g., at a table) and closing her eyes. She would then open her eyes and smile. Although she did not use a transitional object, her pretending to be in bed when in reality she was not was interpreted by Piaget as her constructing symbolic play. This play helped her practice tolerating her separation anxiety associated with going to sleep at night alone in her bed. Thus, while pretending to go to sleep and then waking up, Piaget's daughter was convincing herself that, although she must go to sleep, she could also wake herself up and find that everything was fine.

Freud also labeled as separation anxiety the benignly displeasurable emotion that is generated within toddlers when they perceive they have acted poorly. This form of separation anxiety—the fear of being separated from their parents' love and admiration—is particularly painful for toddlers because of their continuing need for admiring, mirroring responses from their parents to develop self-esteem. (Kohut [1977] used the term *disintegration anxiety* to describe toddlers' internal response to their parents' threat of the withdrawal of their loving functions, an anxiety that has also been described as *psychological death* [Baker and Baker 1987].) Thus separation anxiety can refer to the threatened loss of parents' physical presence or the threatened loss of parents' admiration, support, and love both as selfobjects that develop toddlers' self-esteem and as whole objects that fulfill the other functions of the social environment.

Thus, in the normal family, situations of developmental conflict create separation anxiety (A. Freud 1951, 1965). Toddlers' play becomes a vehicle for their periodic need to temporarily deny their separation anxiety. This *denial in fantasy* functions as an adaptive defense mechanism: it assists toddlers in attaining a sense of mastery over their inevitable episodes of separation anxiety, while momentarily barring from their consciousness the displeasurable emotion of separation anxiety. Playing out a fantasy as an adaptive defense should either 1) enable toddlers to figure out a solution to the developmental conflict, or 2) enable toddlers to alleviate their separation anxiety and other displeasurable feelings generated by the developmental conflict (e.g., the toddler's anger at being left with a baby-sitter) for the moment, and then verbalize their conflict to their parents and invite their assistance in solving it at a later time (the latter is possible only when the toddler can speak). In one sense, then, many adaptive defenses toddlers begin to use will fuel the development of their forming identifications with their parents (McDevitt 1979). They begin to solve some of their developmental conflicts by identifying with the behaviors their parents offer them as ways of solving those conflicts.

Play also helps toddlers to learn self-confidence in facing events that generate separation anxiety. As a result, toddlers learn to be less fearful that these events will become developmental calamities.

Many examples can be observed of how toddlers are busily playing away at dealing with situations of developmental conflict. The following is one example:

> A 2¾-year-old girl is told repeatedly by her mother not to touch her good dishes in the cabinet, the very same cabinet that, to the toddler, looks so interesting, novel, and mysterious. Consequently, the toddler busies herself in playing with a set of toy dishes, putting them in neat stacks as she identifies with what she has seen her mother do on many occasions. In this play, however, she periodically messes up her neat pile and enjoys the symbolic and vicarious gratification of her original wish to explore and mess up her mother's prized dishes. In achieving vicarious pleasure, she also, in a repetition process that mediates learning, learns how to stack dishes. This accomplishment causes her to achieve competency pleasure and she gives herself a mastery smile. Her mother notices her toddler's ability to stack her toy dishes and gives her a mirroring smile to reinforce her feeling of mastery as a dish stacker. What was originally the toddler's perception of her mother's stacking dishes in a neat pile has now become, through playing out an identification with her mother, a part of the toddler's self-representation: I can stack dishes myself! Thus, what began as a developmental conflict between this girl's wish to explore the fragile dishes in the cabinet and her mother's prohibition of her wish emerged into a further advance

in the toddler's self-representation in viewing herself as more autonomous from her mother.

Identifications, therefore, become one of the major ways in which toddlers develop their autonomous identity as contained within their self-representation.

In the process of discovering that they have developmental external conflicts between their internal wishes and the external prohibitions of their parents, toddlers begin to learn that sometimes they possess one internal wish that goes counter to another internal wish. In this way, toddlers become aware of possessing developmental internal conflicts within their representational world (Shapiro 1981). These internal conflicts give them a sense of how their representational world is becoming increasingly structured (at a time that still predates their construction of a superego or conscience) and also provides them with their first experience of possessing ambivalent feelings. For example, say that at a later date the 3-year-old girl mentioned above discovers as she plays in the backyard that the sun casts reflections off shiny objects. This new perception of the sun motivates her to want to conduct a few experiments in letting the sun shine on objects. She then enters the dining room and sees her mother's shiny good dishes. At that moment she becomes aware of two wishes: to play with the dishes by unstacking them and to leave the dishes in a neat stack and let the sun shine on them.

These situations of ambivalence create situations of choice. They enable toddlers to gain a developing awareness of being able to choose the good over the bad or the right over the wrong, and, based on their choice, become either a good or a bad child. As noted earlier, once toddlers achieve objective self-awareness and can evoke an image of themselves (as contained within their growing self-representation), they begin to become cognizant of the fact that their parents are forever observing their behaviors and evaluating them.

Toddlers' using play to learn standards of behavior as they solve external and internal conflicts, often by forming identifications with their parents' behaviors, are the early seeds of the development of their conscience or superego (Buchsbaum and Emde 1990). (This is discussed further in "Development of the Superego," below).

3. *To act out a compensatory fantasy developed in an attempt to reconstruct a conception, resulting from a traumatic experience, into a new conception.* Toddlers who have experienced a traumatic event eventually construct a conception of the event that is usually repressed and relegated to their dynamic unconscious to keep them from remembering the highly displeasurable emotions (i.e., the feelings of intense separation anxiety and rage and the sense of helplessness) associated with the trauma. These toddlers will become unconsciously motivated during toddlerhood to re-create the traumatic event symbolically, and then "write" a play drama in which they are a victor and thus are in control of the original traumatic event. The result is their attaining a sense of mastery over the original trauma in which they experienced themselves as being a helpless, passive victim. Through this process, another organizing principle of mental functioning is in operation: the repetition principle.

In essence, the *repetition principle* states that the human mind will be unconsciously motivated to attempt to re-create an event in the present that is similar to a past traumatic event. The goal is to experience in the re-created event more of a sense of control and a feeling of competency pleasure in being the victor as opposed to the rage, panic, and sense of incompetence and helplessness associated with being the victim in the original trauma. The repetition principle is enacted when toddlers are exposed to an experience that is in some way related to their repressed traumatic memory. As they try to re-create a facsimile of the trauma, they remain unaware of how their unconscious traumatic memory is dictating their re-creation. Toddlers are aware only of being motivated to create what they believe is a new scene (Terr 1994). This principle is played out in the following scenario:

> A 2¾-year-old boy is playing in the backyard of his house when a large German shepherd jumps over his fence and knocks the boy down. In a panic, he screams once and then becomes passive and suffers a silent panic as the dog walks around the yard for several minutes. The dog then rejumps the fence and leaves. The screaming boy then runs to his mother. It takes her several minutes to calm him down. For the next few days, the toddler will not play in his yard unless his mother is with him. But after a week he is

able once again to play alone in his backyard. A week later he sees a small stuffed dog in a toy store and asks his mother to buy it for him. He then plays with the toy dog without being aware of his attempt to re-create something of his trauma with the German shepherd. He engages in fantasy play in which he is more powerful than, and in complete control of, the stuffed toy dog. Through this play, he begins to replace his traumatic memories of feeling frightened by the real dog with new memories of feeling enjoyment in controlling his toy dog.

In the process of his playing, this toddler eventually reconstructed a traumatic memory in which he had experienced himself as a helpless victim in the face of an overpowering dog into a playful fantasy in which he was the active and assertive victor, thus fantasizing that he was no longer afraid of dogs. Gradually, he might play with a real dog, provided the dog is a puppy. Finally, he might be able to play with the same-size dog that had originally frightened him. Consequently, his frightening feeling associated with dogs might gradually become replaced with more pleasurable feelings. All of these new pleasurable experiences with toy and real dogs will help him to restructure his original traumatic memory so that it no longer causes him to avoid large dogs.

Although this boy's posttraumatic play helped him restructure his traumatic memory, more often than not a young toddler's posttraumatic play is not sufficient in itself to undo the effects of the original trauma. Posttraumatic play tends to be effective when the trauma is a single one, instead of multiple traumas, and when it takes place in toddlers engaged in good attachment relationships with their parents (Kahn 1963; Terr 1994). However, if a toddler boy who was periodically abused by his father experienced the above-described trauma with the dog, that event would only compound the chronic emotional and physical trauma he constantly experienced at the hands of his father. In such an acutely and chronically traumatized child, his posttraumatic play might be "grim, long-lasting, and a particularly contagious form of childhood repetitive behavior" (Terr 1991, p. 12).

If a toddler's posttraumatic play either is grim and repetitive or contains a fantasy in which the toddler is attempting to deal with an intolerable, constantly traumatic reality (e.g., in fantasy he tries to change his abusive alcoholic father into a good king), then the assistance of a mental health professional is necessary. For example, Stern (1985) described a case reported by Herzog (1980) that involved a toddler experiencing a trauma when his father moved out of the family home. In the description of this toddler's posttraumatic play (which follows, below), it is clear how the toddler's fantasy of bringing his father back is temporarily soothing, but how his use of play as denial in fantasy will not suffice in helping him deal with his strong wish to bring his father back home.

> An 18-month-old boy is miserable because his father had just moved out of the home. During a play session with dolls, the boy doll was sleeping in the same bed room as the mother doll. [The mother did, in fact, have the boy sleep in her bed after the father left.] The child got very upset at the dolls' sleeping arrangement. Herzog tried to calm the boy by having the mother doll comfort the boy doll. This did not work. Herzog then brought the daddy doll in bed next to the boy. But this solution did not satisfy the child. The child then made the daddy doll put the boy doll in a separate bed and then get into bed with the mother doll [construction of a compensatory fantasy]. The child then said, "All better now." [In Stern's view] the child had to be juggling three versions of family reality: what he knew to be true at home, what he wished and remembered was once true at home, and what he saw as being enacted in the doll family. Using these three representations, he manipulated the signifying representation [the dolls] to realize the wished-for representations of family life and to repair the actual [traumatic] situation. (pp. 166–167)

Maturation and Development of Temperamental Characteristics

Development of Toddlers' Optimal Stimulation Range

In Chapter 3, I define an infant's temperament as his or her innate style of expressing activity, reactivity, emotionality, and sociability.

I also note how an infant's attachment relationship can bring about changes in or maintain some of the infant's temperamental characteristics. Infants and toddlers also undergo changes in temperament because of the maturation of their temperamental characteristics. One such maturational change in toddlers involves modifications in their optimal stimulation range and the point at which they signal their distress as a result of being over- or understimulated. This maturation enables toddlers to habituate to more stimulating experiences with their parents, siblings, and others. J. D. Baldwin and Baldwin (1978) observed the following with regard to temperamental changes:

> After repeated experience while exploring, the infant habituates a step at a time to higher levels of stimulus input. . . . As it familiarizes itself with broader ranges of novel, unpredictable stimuli and habituates to higher levels of stimulus quantity and intensity, the infant is reinforced for leaving the mother's side and venturing into ever more stimulating activities. Thus, in many environments, one sees infants progress through a series of overlapping stages from early maternal contact, to exploration of the non-social environment, to social exploration, then to social play. Within the realm of social play there is often a sequence from gentle wrestling play, to chasing and noncontact play, to play fights. The rate at which these stages appear is constrained to some degree by biological factors (i.e., the maturation of the child's psychological nature, in this case the child's temperamental characteristics). (p. 182)

It is quite difficult to predict the sequences of changes in toddlers' optimal stimulation level (J. D. Baldwin and Baldwin 1978). This is because how each toddler processes transactions between his or her biological advances (e.g., muscle coordination, manual dexterity, locomotion), psychological advances (specifically, the maturational expansion of their optimal stimulation range), and social advances (i.e., the goodness of fit between their capability to remain within their optimal stimulation range and their parents' ability to assist them in this goal) is unpredictable.

Most parents notice how their toddler is exploring more and signaling his or her distress less. They also intuitively provide new and more challenging stimuli to help in the expansion of their toddler's optimal stimulation range; they sense how much to push. As one mother told me,

> Our first son Tom had such a spunky temperament. He seemed like he was always getting bored if we didn't let him explore a lot with all sorts of new things. Our second son David seemed to need us to be there more for him. When he was 3 the same kind of situations Tom handled quite easily when he was 3 would get David overwhelmed. So we had to go slower with Tom and let him develop his independence at his own pace.

Maturation and Development of Emotions

Emergence of Social Emotions

Toddlers' growing awareness of their own emotional life changes into a more complex awareness as 1) their conceptual thinking ability develops (Izard 1971, 1972); 2) their parents continue to use their empathy for them in correctly identifying, admiring, and providing the right word labels for their emotions; and 3) their parents communicate to them that verbalizing their emotions can provide useful information for their parents to help them better understand their inner world.

When a toddler achieves self-awareness and begins to recognize himself or herself as 1) a separate agent of assertive behaviors who expresses innate needs and interests in the environment, 2) a constructor of memories, 3) a possessor of an intact and whole body, and 4) a possessor of emotions in response to sensations and perceptions, the toddler begins to construct emotional conceptions about his or her emotionally tinged experiences with the environment.

Self-aware toddlers' ability to cognitively appraise their interactions with others enables them to generate a new set of emotions: these are the emotions of shame and shyness, followed later by the emotions of guilt, contempt, and hatred (Demos 1981; Emde 1984; Harris et al. 1986; Henry 1973; Hoffman 1983; Zajonic 1980). These emotions are not thought to be experienced in the pre-self-aware stage (up to age 18 months) because they require that the one experiencing them be objectively aware of himself or herself with regard to others. For this reason, the above five emotions are called *social emotions.* The child generating these emotions must first be able to cognitively appraise what behaviors are expected of him or her (Emde et al. 1991). Take the emotion of shame. This emotion is the feeling generated when toddlers are observed by a parent when they are behaving in a way their parents do not approve. For example, a 2½-year-old boy feels shame when he is writing on the kitchen wall, which his mother recently told him not to do; he then looks up and sees her staring disapprovingly at him.

As they develop an autonomous identity concurrently with developing standards of right and wrong behavior, toddlers must contend with these new "social" feelings. They need their parents to help them label them and assist them in verbalizing them so they can better understand them. How much or how little permission is given by their parents to express these social emotions as well as the emotions that emerged during infancy (i.e., joyful interest, surprise, sadness, anger, disgust, fear, and anxiety) will influence the degree to which toddlers will be "in touch" with the emotional aspects of their representational world. Thus a toddler girl whose emotions are empathically sensed and positively mirrored by her attuned parents will enjoy using her maturing cognitive capabilities to discover the emotional part of herself and to construct representations of her emotional experiences that will enhance the development of her self-representation. She will internally perceive her emotional states as aspects of herself that can be communicated and shared with her parents. This sharing will generate, for the most part, a sense of mastery and competence within her. Consequently, she will not have to externally flee from perceiving emotions in others or internally flee from perceiving emotions within herself (e.g., by activating defense mechanisms to bar from her consciousness the awareness of her emotional life). Her emotions will function for the most part as motivators for future actions (Tomkins 1970).

Maturation and Development of Verbal Language Abilities

■ Development of Verbal Language

Toddlers' development of verbal language, like most of the important capabilities that can be conceptualized as being contained in the toddler's developing metaphorical ego, results from the interaction of maturational advances within a socializing human environment.

Chomsky (1957) postulated that an innate preparedness for language exists. In this view, infants possess preexisting mental informational structures that enable them to begin to become attuned to the sounds of human speech, as well as enable them (beginning at about age 10 months) to begin to detect subtle differences in human spoken sounds. For example, within the first months of life, infants are innately capable of detecting the subtle differences between the spoken sounds of "ba" and "da." This sound discrimination ability manifests itself without prior training and leads infants to manifest a remarkable new ability: to hear discrete bursts of sounds while looking at, feeling, or smelling an object and, through inference, associate the two as related (Kagan 1984). For example, as a toddler girl begins to eat with a fork, she hears the word "fork" and at the same time sees her father's smiling face and senses his admiration. In time, she will reach for a fork or spoon, smile at her father, and say "Fork?" Thus much speech is learned in the context of playful interaction in which toddlers' behaviors are evaluated and labeled by the parents.

The emergence of actual spoken speech, at about age 18 months, coincides with toddlers' maturationally emerging abilities to discriminate between sounds (e.g., "da-da" versus "ma-ma") and to symbolize. The result is the emergence of the ability to form distinct words as symbols for people and things and to store them in long-term memory as the representations called symbols. Another maturational change that occurs at about this time is the increased ability to use evocative memory. Therefore, at about age

18 months, toddlers begin to evoke, through memory, words that were stored within their representational world. This evocative aspect of speech production becomes another, if not the most significant, competence that allows toddlers to generate thoughts and feelings without antecedent sensory stimuli—that is, to activate delayed imitation.

A toddler's ability to discriminate among the sounds that comprise human speech requires that the toddler be nurtured in an environment in which human language is spoken and heard. When no human language is heard by an infant, that infant does not develop human language (Bruner 1983). However, it is also known that the chronology or timetable for the maturational readiness for and the development of language cannot be significantly altered by social influences. No matter how much infants are exposed to a rich speech environment during their first year of life, they will not speak intelligible words until between ages 10 and 20 months (Gleitman 1987; Slobin 1973). Developmental research has also shown that there is no clear correlation between verbal stimulation before age 1 year and the later cognitive development of the child. However, there is a positive correlation between a child's having been exposed to a stimulating verbal environment between ages 1 year and 3 years and that child's cognitive competence at age 4 years.

Speaking a language becomes another characteristic that toddlers discover about themselves as they begin to attain objective self-awareness (beginning at about age 18 months). Pre-self-aware infants, however, have given evidence of selectively responding to the sound of a human voice and being able to learn to be discriminate in these responses. Mothers and fathers quickly notice and expect that their infants will react to the sounds of their voices. From the moment their infant is breathing, seeing, feeling, and learning, they talk to their baby without really expecting their baby to understand the content or message in their words. They talk more to communicate to their infant their emotional attunement and attributions of value.

Two components of toddlers' earliest language are *syntax* (the structure and rules of language) and *semantics* (the meaning of language). In toddlers' maturation and development of verbal language, comprehension of the verbal message precedes the expression of the words and the understanding of the rules of verbal language. Thus throughout toddlers' emerging ability to understand and speak a language, they will know what they mean to say before they know how to say it. Stated in terms of representational structures, conceptual mental structures precede linguistic mental structures. Thus toddlers will learn the meaning of the word repetition "bye-bye" and deposit that meaning within their representational world as a symbol before they acquire the voluntary motor speaking ability to say "bye-bye."

In general, speech-language milestones for the normally developing child are as follows:

- *Age 18 months*—Can comprehend two-word commands, point to one body part, use five words
- *Age 2 years*—Can use two-word structures, point to four body parts, and use about 50 words
- *Age 3 years*—Can use "short sentences to announce current, completed, or intended activity. . . . Words confirm and support whatever the child is doing" (Ames and Ilg 1976a, p. 54)
- *Age 3½ years*—Can use language to predict future events and to express beliefs
- *Ages 4–5 years*—Has a 2,000-word vocabulary
- *Age 5 years*—Has mostly internalized rules of language

Evidenced by the fact that, by age 4 or 5 years, children have a 2,000-word vocabulary, it would seem that children from ages 2 to 5 years have a "word hunger." The 2- to 3-year-old toddler also quickly learns that producing the name for something generates a mastery smile of competency pleasure and usually a reciprocal, mirroring smile from his or her proud parents.

Speech development tends to be optimal in families in which parents use both simplified syntax and slower and simpler speech, as well as speak to their toddler in a repetitive fashion (L. Nelson 1982; Snow 1972). Attuned parents sense when the content of their speech is understandable to their toddler and when it is not. They then begin to focus more on their speech content while monitoring how different ways of saying the same thing will be responded to by their toddler. This is one of the reasons a well-meaning adult other than a toddler's parent may fail to verbally communicate something to a toddler when the toddler's mother or father is able to communicate the same thing by using the syntax and vocabulary they know their toddler can comprehend. Speech becomes another opportunity for parents to become attuned to their toddler's language-learning capabilities and attempt to achieve a goodness of fit between what they expect of their toddler and what their toddler can achieve.

■ Speech as a Facilitator of an Autonomous Identity

The ability to use speech as a language to communicate one's wishes, feelings, and conceptions of oneself and others facilitates toddlers' development of their self-representation, specifically by facilitating their development of an autonomous identity. This is accomplished by the effect of speech development on the following aspects of toddlers' developing autonomous identity.

Self-esteem.   A parent's image of his or her toddler is mirrored in how that parent speaks to the toddler. In time, toddlers learn that speech is one of the principal socially accepted ways of receiving feedback about their uniqueness and performances and of exhibiting their newly developing sense of possessing an autonomous identity. They learn that their words are valued and responded to by their parents with love and support. H. Ross (personal communication, November 1975) expressed this in the following manner: "In the loved and responded to child, verbal communication and love begin to become synonymous."

In each society that values speech, it is impossible for toddlers to develop a sense of self-value without receiving admiring feedback about their speech productions. Hence, speech is one of the most important possessions that self-aware toddlers desire to exhibit. Toddlers also expect their parents to mirror their own smiles of mastery as they demonstrate their speaking abilities. The result is a correlation between toddlers' self-esteem and their speech competence.

Self-assertion and autonomy. Speech emerges at the same time as when toddlers are furthering their locomotive skills, their ability to defer imitation, and their ability to symbolize as well as discovering that they are separate people in a world of others. In the midst of these advances, as toddlers begin to become aware of their increasing autonomy from their parents, they begin to use their first words. Toddlers particularly revel in the ability to assert their autonomy in being able to say and understand the meaning of the word "no." This word, as well as others that begin to communicate toddlers' wishes to explore independently the world away from their parents, must receive support from the parents lest toddlers begin to learn, through operant conditioning, that the assertive verbalization of independent wishes is responded to by parental withdrawal of admiration, nurturance, or both. Indeed, I have worked with families in which a toddler's development of the emotionally painful symptom of stuttering was attributable, in part, to one or both parents' mislabeling their 2-year-old child's normal assertive expression of autonomy as a refusal to obey and an aggressive wish to hurt and attack them (Gemelli 1982a, 1982b, 1985). By age 3 years, these stuttering toddlers gave evidence of possessing a conception that their own autonomous wishes were bad and would bring parental rejection or punishment.

Empathically aware parents are attuned to their toddlers' struggle to achieve self-autonomy and assertion. They also understand how their toddlers can experience stranger or separation anxiety when their assertive expression of independence brings them face-to-face with things, people, or situations perceived as threatening, or how they can experience anger when their autonomous excursions are limited by their parents. Because of these displeasurable feelings their search for autonomy can generate, toddlers' parents must also develop empathy for how their toddlers can be ambivalent about their autonomy: one moment a toddler wants autonomy, but the next moment he or she may want to give up all assertive explorations and become reattached to his or her parent's "apron strings." Noshpitz and King (1991) articulated this dilemma as follows:

To distinguish himself as a person, the child must define a difference, indicate a boundary, draw a line. The easiest way to assert non-dependence is to be noncompliant, to do the opposite of what someone else expects. Hence, whatever the mother may ask of the child, he says: "No!" In negativism there is a declaration of selfhood, which is what the child seeks with his defiance. It is the easiest way for the child to declare his separateness and assert a modicum of independence. (p. 232)

Parents also use their empathy in this rapprochement aspect of their child's separation-individuation process (see "Development of the Self and Object Relationships," below) by trying to sense what their toddler's emotional state may be as expressed through his or her nonverbal behavior. They then provide words for the toddler's inner feelings, which helps the toddler begin to use speech to achieve emotional self-regulation and delay of action, as in the following example:

A mother is confronted by her almost 3-year-old daughter, who comes into the house after being in their backyard. The mother had just observed, in looking out the backyard window, that her daughter became frightened by the neighbor's dog, who barked at her from across the fence. The mother now notices that her daughter is tense. The girl tells her mother, "I won't play in the yard," and then throws a cookie on the floor. The mother then tells her, "You are angry with Mommy, because I wasn't there when the dog barked at you. It scared you, and you can tell me that you are angry and afraid. You don't have to throw things to tell me. If you talk, then these feelings won't be so scary. Next time, if you see the dog and you get afraid, you can come and tell me, and even if the dog barks at you, you won't get so afraid."

In this communication, the mother is in effect telling her daughter that 1) she can identify with her mother in using speech to verbalize the signal anxiety she experiences when her exploration of the environment makes her feel afraid, 2) speech is a valued way to master fears and anxieties, and 3) when she is afraid and angry, sharing those feelings with another person whom she trusts lessens the unpleasant emotions associated with the fearful experience.

Through such interactions, toddlers begin to have emotional experiences in which they construct object relations units that define the internal rules they will follow in verbalizing their wishes, feelings, beliefs, and so on to their parents, siblings, and other important people in their social world. For example, the almost 3-year-old girl might construct the object relations unit, "I get angry at Mommy when she is not there, and I get afraid, but it is okay to tell her when I get afraid and when I am angry at her. She loves me better if I tell her instead of throwing and hitting things." Such an object relations unit contains the following *emotional display rule:* The verbalization of anger and anxiety is permitted. In contrast, the father of a very anxious and troubled 2¾-year-old boy told me, "In our family anger is not allowed. Talking angrily is a waste of energy. My son has been taught that when he is angry he is to leave the room and only come back when he's gotten rid of it." Thus the emotional display rule in this family was: The verbalization of anger or anxiety is not permitted. Both the toddler girl and boy (above) will eventually make their separate emotional display rules part of their future consciences. The boy's conscience will threaten guilt if he thinks of verbalizing his angry feelings to his father; the more normally reared girl's conscience will give her internal approval when she verbalizes her angry feelings.

Self and object (other) interdependence. In acquiring speech, toddlers discover that they can share so much more of what they perceive externally and internally. As Stern (1985) expressed it,

> With each word, children solidify their mental commonality with the parent and later with other members of the language culture, when they discover that their personal experiential knowledge is part of a larger experience of knowledge, that they are unified with others in a common culture base. . . . Language, then, provides a new way of being related to others by sharing personal knowledge with them, coming together in the domain of verbal relatedness. (pp. 172–173)

Once toddlers begin to experience the joy, mutual admiration, and other pleasurable feelings associated with both speaking to their parents and being spoken to by them, they will experience displeasurable feelings when this language "bridge" of emotional intimacy is temporarily broken. Toddlers quickly learn that they can "punish" their parents by withholding their speech from them, as parents can "punish" them by either not speaking to them or ignoring their spoken words. The withholding of speech, both by toddlers and by parents, is much more than withholding words; it entails the withholding of emotional involvement.

Self-regulation and control. Speech assists toddlers in attaining emotional self-regulation in that speech can be used to verbally signal their emotional reactions in relation to the amount of stimulation they are experiencing. Their use of speech to communicate signal anxiety will also be influenced by their temperamental characteristics. As such, toddlers will differ as to when they begin to use speech to signal their distress.

In time, toddlers begin to use speech in the same manner as a trial action: 1) to delay their intended immediate action, 2) to verbalize their thoughts out loud, 3) to say what they want or do not want to do, and 4) to say how they feel but not immediately act on those feelings. Toddlers learn how to handle their feelings toward others in a socially acceptable manner only by delaying action and speaking instead (Inge et al. 1986). This gives them more time to think and remember behaviors they used in the past that helped them gratify their needs in a socially acceptable manner.

In learning to trust their use of speech to effectively attain self-regulation and maintain a developmentally enhancing relationship with their parents, toddlers progress through three stages:

1. *Action dominance (infancy and toddlerhood)*—Infants and toddlers for the most part are not expected to verbalize their wishes, fears, or feelings. Parents expect their infants to communicate through actions (e.g., visual gaze, social smile, emotional refueling, reaching, walking). They attempt to teach them specific actions or surface behaviors in lieu of others (e.g., a mother is pleased when her 1-year-old infant hands her

a cup when he wants more milk instead of throwing the cup on the floor). Once infants reach toddlerhood, at which time their parents work toward socializing their behavior, parents develop greater expectations of them. When speech emerges at about age 18 months, parents slowly introduce the concept of using speech in lieu of action. By age 3 years, toddlers generally enter the next stage in their communicating to their parents and others.

2. *Speech dominance (ages 3–6 years)*—Once toddlers reach early childhood, their parents are well into changing their message from one of "actions speak louder than words" to one of "words are usually better than actions." Psychologically aware parents, in all their interactions with their children, communicate their wish that their children begin to use their emerging speech ability to express their wishes, feelings, beliefs, and fantasies. Quite often during this era of the child's life, parents are heard telling their child, "You can talk about what you want and how you feel, but you can't just do what you want." As children begin to accept this "invitation," parents permit them to say things in ways that they tolerate but then gradually begin to modify and shape more along socially acceptable ways of speaking. For example, a 4-year-old boy was being excessively teased by a female cousin. He went to find his father and told him, "I wish she was taken away by a witch. I hate her!" His father permitted such a statement, putting less emphasis on his son's specific words and more on his son's use of speech to express his anger toward his cousin.

The following developmental axiom that emerges in the above example is applicable to all of children's emerging capabilities: when a new capability first manifests itself, parents must not place too much or too early a restriction on it or expect their child to perform the new ability too well lest their child begin to restrict its functioning prior to its full emergence. When parents too quickly attempt to excessively shape and overly socialize a new behavioral competence in their child or expect their child to perform perfectly, they can cause the child to give up the new behavior entirely or regress by manifesting a developmentally earlier ability or competence.

3. *Thought dominance (late childhood: ages 7–11 years)*—By age 7 years, children begin to be increasingly told by their parents to stop and think before they speak. This parental message is often given in situations in which children possess feelings and wishes about which they have conflictual feelings or which are in conflict with the feelings and wishes of another. When children begin to delay both acting and speaking, they are functioning more in accordance with thought dominance in deciding how to communicate with others. In interpersonal interactions, they now possess the conceptual belief that it is often best to engage in thinking before speaking. This belief assists them in becoming more socialized and learning more about complicated interpersonal issues such as compromise, negotiation, and placing one's needs secondary to the needs of a family member or a friend. Thought dominance basically means that a child has learned that thinking should direct one's speech and actions if speech is to be used to communicate as well as assist in relating to others.

Self-inhibition and mechanisms of defense. Shortly after speech acquisition begins to increase (i.e., around age 2½ years), toddlers are observed to generate inner speech (i.e., speech not spoken before an audience) (Berk 1994). Toddlers typically repeat aloud the shoulds and should nots they either have been taught by their parents or have arrived at through their own empathic and inferential thinking. Through inner speech, toddlers work on interpersonal conflict situations as well as on consolidating the emotional display rules they have been learning. For example, a 3-year-old girl playing with a dollhouse and two figures was overheard to say, "Now Sis, don't hit Brother. Brother don't be mean to Sis. Mom's happy when you don't fight."

Speech also enables toddlers to put defense mechanisms into operation. For example, verbalized denial can be useful as an adaptive mechanism (operating as a defense mechanism) in dealing with others, as in the following example:

> A 3-year-old boy did not receive a new bicycle but his sister did.
> He is extremely angry at his sister, but when his mother questions

him about whether he is upset he responds that he is not angry, upset, or envious of his sister. After denying his feelings to his mother, he goes to his room and decides to "express" his anger by engaging in symbolic play with his toy puppets where he meanly treats his sister. By verbalizing his denial to his mother, this boy refocused his thoughts from his own anger and envy onto something else until he was more in control of these emotions. His denial gave him time to delay and think about what to do, while he temporarily avoided the situation with his sister.

Many of the defense mechanisms toddlers use are the ones they see and hear their parents use. In an automatic—and thereby un-conscious—process of identification, they begin to use the same defenses as their parents in order to avoid the same displeasurable emotional state stimulated by a similarly interpersonal situation, as in the following example:

A mother frequently projects her own sad feelings onto her daughter, telling her that she [the daughter] is sad. The mother's projection of her own sadness is related to her being frequently physically abused by her husband when she tells him that she is sad. Her daughter senses her mother's denied and projected sad-ness and in time begins "seeing" sadness in others but denies its presence in herself. She needs to deny and protect her own sad-ness because, in identifying with her mother, she is convinced that she would also be hit by her father if she ever told him that she was sad.

In referring to the concealing and defensive use of speech, Stern (1985) wrote,

With the advent of language and symbolic thinking, children now have the tools to distort and transcend reality. They can create expectations contrary to past experience. They can elabo-rate a wish contrary to present fact. . . . Prior to this linguistic ability, infants (and toddlers) are confined to reflect the im-press of reality. They can now transcend that, for good or ill. (p. 182)

Continuing Influences of Preexisting Representational World

Development of Semantic and Episodic Memory Capabilities

By the time they reach toddlerhood, infants have already constructed a varied and complex representational world. This increasingly complex memory "database"—involving preconscious explicit memories, unconscious implicit memories, and unconscious repressed explicit traumatic memories—is viewed as another part of their developing ego (Rothstein 1988). As such, the memory parts of the toddler's representational world—as psychological stimuli—influence how he or she perceives and processes new biopsychosocial stimuli.

Once mental development begins at age 18 months, the developing mind, in storing a record of toddlers' experienced past, makes its own contributions to its continued mental development. As toddlers begin to construct, store, and retrieve explicit memories, they begin to differentiate these explicit memories into two types: semantic memories and episodic memories (K. Nelson 1990). *Semantic memories* store information about abstract concepts or events in time (Seigal 1993). An example of an abstract concept would be a 3-year-old girl's retention of the fact that crayons produce color on certain surfaces; an example of an event in time would be a 5-year-old boy's retention of the fact that Christmas comes every year in December. *Episodic memories* involve the retention of information about a child's life experiences. It refers to something that happened at a specific time and in a specific place (K. Nelson 1993a, 1993b). Many toddlers' episodic memories are not retained as long-term explicit memories because 1) these memories have no particular significance in the child's life (e.g., a 2½-year-old boy will remember only for an hour or so that his mother made him pancakes for breakfast, unless this pancake experience had some particular significance for him) or 2) parents do not reinforce these memories (e.g., parents do not feel it important to ask their 2½-year-old boy if he remembered what he ate for breakfast).

Beginning when toddlers reach age 2½ years, their parents affect what episodic memories they retain as part of their autobiographical memories. These are long-term explicit memories that become the memorial part of toddlers' ever-growing self-representation. Parents develop the growth of these memories when they engage in *memory talk,* through which they help toddlers organize their memory fragments of a particular event into narratives they can understand (K. Nelson 1993a, 1993b). In composing these narratives, parents assist their toddlers in their retrieval mechanisms and give a sense of meaning and importance to the memory of the event. For example, the mother of a 2¾-year-old girl told her daughter that they would visit Grandma's house the next day. In engaging in memory talk, the mother then reminded the toddler about certain events that had occurred during their last visit to Grandma's. When the toddler recalled, "Grandma and I went on the swings at the park," the mother enthusiastically supported her daughter's remembering and encouraged her to say more.

When toddlers are encouraged to engage in memory talk with their parents and others, they develop the belief that telling stories about oneself and one's life and interests will bring attention, mirroring smiles, and admiration. In one study, S. Engel (1986) compared two groups of mothers who approached memory talk differently. The first group talked with their 2-year-old toddlers about current and past events using narratives that emphasized details (e.g., what happened and when, where, and with whom); these mothers also viewed memories not only as a source of their toddlers' learning about how to behave but also as a means of their revealing themselves and how their mind worked. To them, memories comprised an emotionally rich aspect of parent-child interaction. The second group of mothers had a pragmatic view of their toddler's memories, tending to view them as a means of retrieving past information in a rather uninteresting and unimaginative manner. Engel found that, at age 4 years, toddlers of the first group gave more information in their memory talk than those of the second group.

Some toddlers' autobiographical memories are partly based in reality and partly based in fantasy (Tessler 1986, 1991). As toddlers age, their parents help them to sort through these memories and separate out the fact from the fiction, as in the following example (Deborah Belaga, personal communication, July 1995):

> The mother of a 3-year-old boy was recounting to an adult friend an incident in which her husband had come to the assistance of a woman who was being harassed by a man while in a gift shop. The mother was telling her friend about how the man in the shop was frightening a woman and how her husband forcibly led the man out of the gift shop. Suddenly, her son, who had been overhearing her conversation while playing with blocks, walked up to his mother and said, "When Daddy and me were in the woods there was a ghost, but I wasn't afraid. Dad chased the ghost away."
>
> His mother listened intently and then smiled and said, "That is an interesting story. Dad and I will never let ghosts hurt you." The mother took pleasure in her son's wanting to contribute his story to her own. She knew he was mixing fantasy and reality as he was extrapolating elements of his mother's narrative into his own narrative about his fear of ghosts and his need for a protective father. In the process he was developing his use of autobiographical memories. In time this mother helped her son separate the fantasy from the reality in his memories of his life experiences.

K. Nelson (1993b) listed the functions of autobiographical memories for children ages 2½–3 years as follows:

1. To share memories with others as a socially accepted way of sharing one's accumulated knowledge in relating with others.
2. To guide present verbal and other behaviors.
3. To predict the future by creating expectancies (e.g., positive and negative transference reactions to others).
4. To define oneself both socially and privately. The established autobiographical memory system takes on a personal as well as social value in defining the self.

Development of the Self and Object Relationships
Development of Autonomous and Gender Identity

Identity is developed through all phases of the life cycle. In the Lego-style, continuous view of developmental process (see Chapter 2), children must add new interlocking blocks at each phase in the life cycle that become new parts of their overall identity. After interconnecting these new blocks with the preexisting blocks, children continue to develop their emerging composite identity in order to possess an emancipated identity by the end of adolescence (see Chapter 7). The parts of that identity are their autonomous identity, gender identity, sexual identity, peer identity, and social identity. In this section, I more fully describe toddlers' construction and further development of an autonomous identity and gender identity. Although both of these identities develop concurrently for the most part, a gender identity is constructed before an autonomous identity.

■ Formation of a Gender Identity

Somewhere between ages 18 months and 2 years, after toddlers have attained self-awareness, they construct a gender identity (Emde 1983; M. Lewis and Brooks-Gunn 1979). According to J. Meyer (1982), *gender identity* can be defined as

> a psychological construct [or conceptual belief] which refers to a basic sense of maleness or femaleness or a conviction that one is male or female. (p. 382)

A toddler's gender identity becomes a new structural addition to his or her self-representation and establishes the toddler's early belief in his or her basic maleness or femaleness. As noted in Chapter 3, the four forerunners of a toddler's gender identity that are seen during infancy are 1) the infant's observable biologically generated sex, 2) the parents' proper gender assignment at birth in labeling their infant as male or female, 3) parental attitudes and beliefs about the infant's gender, and 4) the infant's experiences with his or her own body. I now focus on this last element.

During the first 18 months of life, infants learn about their genitals as part of body boundary exploration (R. Tyson 1986). Manual genital self-stimulation begins between ages 15 and 19 months (Galenson 1993). For example, some toddlers will stimulate their genitals when their parents are changing their diaper or bathing them (Galenson 1993). Galenson noted that, in both boys and girls, their self-stimulation

> is intentional and is accompanied by behavioral evidence of erotic arousal, including facial flushing, rapid respiration and diaphoresis, and penile erection in boys. (p. 387)

Boys will exhibit more vigorous and more frequent genital stimulation than is seen in girls of the same age. Boys focus their stimulation on their penis, which is more visible and accessible than a girl's clitoris. Girls are less vigorous and less focused in their self-stimulation than boys. By age 18 months, both girls and boys touch their genitals while concurrently lowering their gaze and withdrawing their attention to the external world, including decreasing their interaction with their parents. Galenson (1993), in addressing this decreased interaction between toddlers and their parents, noted,

> At the onset (i.e., beginning at 15 months), infants tend to embrace the caretaking adults as the genital stimulation continues. Because most caretakers discourage these embraces by various inhibitory behaviors of which they are quite often unaware, however, these object-directed overtures are soon replaced by the familiar inward gaze during the genital self-stimulation—an inhibition of action, which promotes the elaboration of fantasy. (p. 387)

Somewhere around age 18 months, both boys and girls begin to show curiosity about anatomical differences between adults, children, and animals. Genital play behavior between children begins somewhere around age 22 months. This genital play involves viewing each other's genitals with much questioning and, at times, excessive curiosity (Martinson 1976). This curiosity needs to be limited for toddlers to begin to acquire knowledge about body privacy. For example, it is a common practice in nursery schools that care for children ages 2–4 years to closely monitor the use of the toilets. Rules allowing only one child in a unisex bathroom at a time or the use of separate toilets for boys and girls communicate to toddlers that their normal developmental curiosity about anatomical differences must be restricted. However, boys' and girls' curiosity propels them to try to circumvent the rules. I remember observing a class of 3-year-old children in a preschool. One boy, in thinking no one was watching him, followed a girl after she told him she was going to the toilet. Their teacher was preoccupied so she did not see both of them enter the unisex toilet (the rule was that only one child was allowed in the toilet at a time). After both toddlers had left the toilet, I engaged the boy in some play (without mentioning the toilet scene). Spontaneously he began to play in the sandbox with oblong squirt bottles. As he squirted water into the sand, another girl came up to the sandbox. He then said quite spontaneously, "Boys can squirt with their things and girls don't even have one!"

In being aware of being a separate person who possesses a particular gender, toddlers, by age 2 years, are engaged in a process of *gender categorization,* forming early categories of what it means to be a boy or a girl (J.–K. Meyer 1980). Toddlers are propelled to identify with their same-gender parent; boys wonder about being a man like their father and girls wonder about being a woman like their mother (Erikson 1963).

This process of identifying with the same-gender parent helps toddlers begin to consolidate their early gender identity. Kagan (1984) described the process of identification as one in which toddlers, in possessing the conscious awareness of being a separate self, begin at times consciously and at other times unconsciously to infer that if they share some qualities with a parent then they must automatically share other qualities with the parent as well. In essence, *identification* is a mental process whereby toddlers assimilate an aspect, property, or attribute of another person, at which time they are transformed—wholly or partially—according to the model the other person provides. It is this apparent "absorption" of the other person's (usually the parent's) qualities without specific training, either by reward or by punishment, that leads to the hypothesis that identification circumvents the direct training process. It is as if toddlers learn a general principle "to be like my father and mother." They then unconsciously incorporate many of their parents' characteristic behaviors into their own repertoire of behaviors without, in each instance, appearing to receive overt rewards for doing so. For example, a boy and his father share the same hair color. This son perceives this similarity and adds to his belief—which supports his gender identity as a male—that he and his father are the same in many ways. Then, when the son sees his father hit a baseball well, he feels proud, and at that moment makes the inference that he also will be able to hit a baseball well.

Often toddlers will identify more with their parents when their parents begin to expect them to start doing things for themselves that were originally done by the parents. If the demands exceed their capabilities, toddlers will find it difficult to identify with their parents' behavior.

Identification can be detrimental if parents force their toddler to become more like themselves (Fraiberg 1982; Fraiberg et al. 1975). Some parents threaten withdrawal of love if their toddler does not behave like them. These parents will often foster identifications in their toddlers that are based in fear, not love. This kind of toddler will often identify with behaviors in the parents that caused him or her to experience excessive anxiety and reactive rage. A. Freud (1936/1966) labeled this as *identification with the aggressor* (see "Types of Defense Mechanisms," below). One type of family scenario that is particularly detrimental to a toddler's developing gender identity is when the same-gender parent is demanding and hostile and the opposite-gender parent is more accepting and kind. The toddler may, as early as age 18 months, begin to be in conflict with identifying with the hostile and demanding same-gender parent and thus begin to identify much more with the more nurturant and loving, opposite-gender parent. If the toddler's identification with his or her opposite-gender parent continues to be more prominent than his or her identification with the same-gender parent, the toddler's gender identity will inevitably become confusing for him or her.

In toddlers being raised by psychologically aware and loving parents, a healthy gender identity is constructed, leading to gender-appropriate behaviors. These gender-linked identifications also foster the development of qualities and standards of conduct and behavior that become the building blocks of the early conscience in toddlers (see "Development of the Superego," below).

■ Formation of Autonomous Identity

From birth through age 18 months, infants must accomplish the major developmental task of attaining a sense of separateness and value and a basic trust in others. Once this task is accomplished and they emerge into toddlerhood, they are able to construct their first objective view of themselves as having a separate and valued sense of self (Tolpin 1971). Toddlers are now interested in assertively activating their own wishes to explore the world. Accordingly, they can begin to take the initiative in being curious about the world and not be inhibited by the inevitable episodes of stranger and separation anxiety. Toddlers who have achieved some measure of basic trust and have established a good selective attachment relationship with their parents (enabling them to tolerate the separation anxiety that is associated with excursions away from the parents) are most successful at this task (McDevitt and Mahler 1989). Through exercising their assertiveness, toddlers will, by age 3 years, begin and continue to develop an autonomous identity as they increasingly demonstrate their various self-initiated competencies in exploring the world without the constant presence of their parents.

Toddlers' exploration of and curiosity about their world must be supported and not exploited. Some parents have overly ambitious aspirations for their toddler to separate and assert his or her autonomy too fast; others believe that their toddler should not be autonomous and assertively explore the world; for either type of parent, the result is the same: the toddler's own temperamentally based comfortableness with approaching the new and the unexpected while autonomously exploring will be hampered by parental aspirations or beliefs that are not attuned to his or her autonomous strivings. In both cases, a toddler's degree of separation anxiety will usually be increased. In time, these toddlers may give up exploring altogether, or they may continue to explore but stop themselves from internally perceiving their high level of separation anxiety by using the defense mechanisms of denial and projection, manifested in behaviors such as running away from the mother, pretending never to be anxious, tending to be a daredevil, and often getting hurt or into trouble.

As a toddler's autonomy develops, his or her psychologically aware parents neither overly push nor overly inhibit the toddler's autonomous excursions. They do, however, restrict the degree of autonomy by setting limits on their toddler's exploring. They thereby instill a healthy sense of doubt that eventually teaches the toddler that his or her individual will is limited by social constraints. Toddlers must slowly learn that their autonomy will bring emotional pleasure only if they follow family and societal rules.

Mastery over bodily functions: toilet training.   As mentioned above, Freud considered the period coinciding with toddlerhood as the anal and urethral stage (S. Freud 1923/1963). In so doing, he emphasized the pleasure toddlers experience in holding and letting go of urine and feces, but underemphasized toddlers' need to both have mastery of their body and interact in a loving and socially acceptable way with their parents.

Toilet training, a triggering social variable initiated by toddlers' parents, generates responses within both the biological and psychological domains. Biologically, a toddler is capable of training his or her sphincters after those muscles are maturationally ready for such training. Psychologically, a toddler's inner world (as an aspect of the psychological domain) receives new conceptions based on these experiences. Toilet-trained toddlers then possess within their self-representation a new awareness of their self-competence; within their object representations of their parents, they possess a new awareness of their parents' support and admiration for this new aspect of their autonomy.

Toddlers with a developmentally enhancing goodness of fit with empathically attuned parents and a predominance of good memories of good experiences with their parents will feel loved and valued. These toddlers will want to do things that bring further parental love and approval. If toilet training brings even more love and mirroring admiration from their parents, toddlers will try to become trained and follow their parents' social constraints. They will, in time, give up the pleasurable experience of voiding and defecating whenever and wherever the urge occurs and begin to delay the instant gratification of these wishes (M. Mason, personal communication, June 1990). The loved and valued child will be proud of accomplishing the task of toilet training and will learn that this is a highly valued social behavior. (See illustration of these factors in Figure 4–6.)

Achievement of toilet training is a body mastery experience that increases toddlers' self-esteem. Indeed, toddlers adopt the goal of becoming toilet trained as a new standard. They quickly learn from observing their parents, siblings, and others that going on the "pot" is a good behavior and going in one's underwear is a bad behavior. In seeking to do what is right and good, the child assists the parents in the process of achieving body responsibility (A. Freud 1965).

Advances and regressions in achievement of autonomy.
In every example of an advance in a toddler's capabilities, parents can describe an episode in which their toddler gave up this advance and returned to an earlier phase of development. This re-

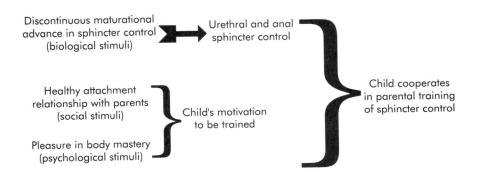

Figure 4–6. Toilet training: toward achieving mastery in body control.

turn is called a *regression* (see "Development of Adaptational Capabilities," below). The overall human developmental process is one in which regressions, progressions, and plateaus in various biological, psychological, and social competencies take place.

Regression appears to assist toddlers in consolidating recent advances (Bever 1982). For example, play can function in the service of regression when toddlers literally turn away from real life experiences because 1) they are not ready to keep demonstrating a new advance, 2) they need to practice in symbolic play a fantasy concerning what they wish the new advance will bring to them in terms of more admiration or a similar reward, or 3) they are fatigued, physically ill, or experiencing overstimulation that leads to an emotional state of fear, anxiety, or anger.

A. Freud (1965) described the developmental line that proceeds from "irresponsibility to responsibility in body management." Toddlers being raised in a healthy family learn that their parents will approve of and love them if they take care of their body. However, all children, in progressing along this line (and especially in toddlerhood), will regress when one of the three factors noted above is present. The following is an example of a toddler's experience with her developing sphincter control:

> A 2½-year-old girl was learning about controlling her urethral sphincter. She was observed often telling her dolls, "Now don't pee till I tell you to. Try hard. Hold it and I'll love you if you do it on the pot. And I'll give you toys and candy." This girl was verbalizing, in part, her fantasy that her own sphincter control would bring her new rewards more than the pleasure of her own mastery smiles and the pleasure of seeing mirroring smiles in her parents. She wished for more because her mother had just returned home with a new baby sister. The arrival of the baby had generated some separation anxiety in the girl, and along with it the wish that she be given more support and love by her mother and father. Within the same time period that she was becoming preoccupied with this doll play, she began to show regression in her previously developing sphincter control.

The rapprochement stage. Limits set on toddlers' autonomous exploration will invariably generate new emotional states in toddlers that are difficult for them to handle. As toddlers begin to experience episodes of separation anxiety, they struggle with the growing realization that their separateness and growing autonomy from their parents do not protect them from experiencing stranger and separation anxieties. In addition, parents do not always positively mirror and admire their toddler's explorations and new experiments—especially, for example, when they involve the new dining room dishes! Finally, toddlers, in their autonomous excursions, are discovering how physically little they really are and that sometimes, no matter how much they want a parent to do something, their parent says no. Thus toddlers begin to use the word "no" quite often themselves.

All of these new discoveries cause toddlers to have somewhat of a "breakup" of their loving attachment with their parents. They begin to have episodes of being quite angry at their parents. Noshpitz and King (1991) described the types of behaviors demonstrated by 2-year-old children at this time:

> For many 2-year-olds, negativism, intense demandingness, refusal to comply with routines, defiance of limits, and eruptive tantrums are common elements of behavior. More severe reactions appear occasionally and include prolonged screaming episodes, running away, refusal to eat, refusal to accept toilet training, cruelty to pets, destructiveness and other disturbing behaviors. In these extreme cases the caretaker comes to feel tormented and may become intensely provoked because everything is so negative; everything is a battle. (p. 230)

This period, which occurs approximately between ages 18 and 24 months, was labeled by Mahler (1975) as the *rapprochement subphase* of her separation-individuation developmental theory. The use of the term *rapprochement* (or its synonym, reconciliation) points to the need for toddlers to get through this relative "breakup" with their parents. Rapprochement, according to Horner (1989), is a process initiated by the toddler when he or she has gone through an episode of feeling frustrated and angry at a parent. The toddler then restores his or her sense of being secure and loved in reengaging the parent in an emotionally positive interaction.

A mother can become confused and even angry at her toddler if she does not have empathy for the toddler's dilemma: how her toddler can feel lovingly toward her when she encourages his or her autonomy and also angry at her for not making his or her autonomous excursions always anxiety free and totally pleasurable, and for not always saying yes to what the toddler wants to do or where the toddler wants to go. Toddlers' ambivalent feelings of love and anger toward their mother (and usually their father) are what fuel their whining episodes, temper tantrums, and intense separation reactions that alternate with an aloof attitude toward their parents.

As they grow older, toddlers increasingly view their mother as a separate individual whom they cannot control and who possesses and communicates feelings separate from their own. Thus toddlers are more capable than they were as infants of recognizing the feeling states within their mother when they leave her to explore and then return from their explorations. These maternal feelings become an important source of data for toddlers, who are quite preoccupied with their mother's emotional reactions to their behaviors. For example, Hamilton (1988) wrote of a 20-month-old boy, who

> repeatedly searched out his mother, interrupting her while she was reading or folding clothes or working at her desk. He would climb into her lap, overcoming all obstacles, get her attention, and snuggle warmly in her lap. When she would put her arm around him, he would push it away and wriggle away off her lap; but he would linger near her looking a bit indecisive. During the practicing subphase [i.e., Mahler's practicing phase that takes place between ages 10 months and 16 months during which episodes of emotional refueling often take place in the child's interactions with his or her mother], he had been content to play at her feet awhile [to emotionally refuel] and then dash off again, joyful and enthusiastic. Now, he seemed to need more closeness, but sought control over the closeness. (pp. 45–46)

In the above example, the toddler would also become quite attuned to his mother's responses to his ambivalent behaviors and feelings. He would be particularly affected by her emotional expressions because he is at a phase in life where emotions are taking on profound significance in his conscious awareness. One reason for this importance is that he has yet to consolidate a more emotionally constant self-representation and object representations of his mother and father.

As noted earlier, toddlers experience loving and admiring feelings toward their parents. These feelings are stored within their object representations of them. In addition, because toddlers want to view their parents as all-powerful protectors, they are slowly constructing an ideal object representation of each parent. This representation is an internal view of their parents the way toddlers wish their parents could be. These ideal object representations are "colored" by toddlers' egocentrism and supported by parents in that they allow themselves to be idealized by their toddler. For example, a son says to his dad, "You are the strongest dad of all!" and the dad, knowing he is not, nevertheless smiles and says, "Yeah, that's me!" The father knows that as his son develops he will slowly and sometimes painfully become aware of the fact that his father is not the strongest father in the world.

In conjunction with constructing ideal object representations—which exist concurrently with toddlers' more general object representations of loving, admiring, and supportive parents—toddlers also construct an ideal self-representation that exists concurrently in their representational world with their more general self-representation. Toddlers' ideal self-representation is an internal view of themselves the way they wish they could be. It is obviously colored by their egocentrism and is supported by their statements of grandiosity. For example, a toddler girl might say, "I am the fastest runner!" and then demonstrate her running for her parents. Her parents might then respond by saying, "Wow! What a runner!"

The difficulty for toddlers occurs in situations in which they feel angry toward their parents (e.g., when their parents restrict their autonomy) but at the same time love them as well as expect them to idealize them. The rapprochement crisis becomes difficult because toddlers must face their own ambivalent feelings toward their parents. Ambivalence as a fact of human experience is not easy for toddlers to tolerate and understand. When the rapprochement crisis occurs, toddlers still tend to think that each person can experience only the emotion they are evidencing at the moment. So when their mother is angry, toddlers do not understand that her loving feelings have not gone away. This is because toddlers at first segregate their loving object representations from their angry object representations of each parent. When one emotion is dominant, the other is nonexistent in their view of their parents. The angry mother becomes a great threat, because the loving mother is "gone." So when toddlers feel angry toward their mother, they act in a rejecting manner, and when toddlers feel loving toward their mother, they act affectionately. These emotionally driven ambivalent behaviors associated with the rapprochement crisis continue for some time.

If, by about age 3 years, toddlers have had more loving than angry transactions with each parent, they will mentally integrate their good and bad representations of each parent and construct an *emotionally constant positive object representation* of each (Fraiberg 1969; hereafter referred to as *positive object constancy*). In achieving this integration, they will possess an object representation of their mother and father in viewing each as loving, admiring, and supportive even when they are angry with or absent from them. Their emotionally constant object maternal and paternal representations are no longer ambivalent (Solnit and Neubauer 1986). They are used by these young children to comfort themselves and help them tolerate a delay in their parents' responding when they becomes anxious. At this point, 3-year-old children have taken into themselves the comforting and admiring presence of their parents and use these object representations for self-soothing and emotional self-regulation.

Concurrently, 3-year-old children integrate their feelings of self-love and self-hatred into a predominantly self-loving representation. They now begin to view themselves as valued and loved even though they may have angry and hateful feelings toward their parents. This *emotionally constant positive self-representation* (hereafter referred to as *positive self-constancy*) gives birth to their cohesive self (Kohut and Wolf 1978); that is, they achieve an objective self-awareness in which they believe that their admiring and valuing parents (in their functioning as selfobjects) will continue to provide these mirroring representations even though they may at times disappoint and anger them (Tolpin 1971, 1978).

The establishment of positive self-constancy and object constancy brings the rapprochement crisis to a successful solution. In normal developmental situations, positive self-constancy and object constancy prevent toddlers from resurrecting their ideal self-representation and ideal object (parent) representations to the place of prominence they once held in their relationships with their parents. Nevertheless, these ideal representations are still maintained because of children's inability to relinquish their wishes for self-perfection or for perfect parents, something that is not accomplished until late adolescence. (Even then these representations become the substance of late adolescents' ideals and allegiances to idealized figures.) In achieving the goal of constructing positive self-constancy and object constancy, toddlers do not need to deny their anger and frustration with their real parents by resorting to the fantasies of being ideally omnipotent themselves (i.e., I don't need any parents), nor do they have to generate a fantasy that their father or mother is really an impostor and somewhere in the world there exists their ideally omnipotent, all-loving father and mother who lost them when they were an infant. Positive object constancy enables 3-year-old children to more fully perceive their mother and father as autonomous individuals who at different times possess both loving and angry feelings toward them, but who are primarily constant in their valuing, loving, and protection of them. Parents are no longer viewed as being ambivalent toward their children.

Likewise, positive self-constancy enables 3-year-old children to perceive themselves more fully as autonomous individuals who at different times possess both loving and angry feelings toward their parents, but who are primarily constant in valuing and loving them. They also do not view themselves as being ambivalent toward their parents. This postambivalent, emotionally constant level of object relationship with their parents is then transferred to others (e.g., siblings, peers).

The attachment relationship that had produced an external attachment to both parents has now been internalized, and becomes a part of toddlers' representational world. Now toddlers begin to detach without overly excessive separation anxiety because they rely on an internal and mostly positive representation of their attachment to their parents. Positive self-constancy and object constancy also help 3-year-old children delay the immediate gratification of their needs and wishes. They expectantly wait, think, and remember their representational images of their good parents, whom they expect to eventually gratify them.

Although it is postulated that the presence of positive self-constancy and object constancy do not become consolidated until about age 3 years, the foundations of this process are most likely present earlier. For example, having too many overstimulating, emotionally displeasurable, bad separation experiences during which they become fearful and anxious when their parents do not soothe them will interfere with the development of toddlers' positive self-constancy and object constancy. They may develop an overall negative object representation of their parents as unloving and devaluing. This representation will be accompanied by their construction of an emotionally constant self-representation that is unloved and bad. Such toddlers will inhibit the assertive expression of their wish to achieve an autonomous identity because of their excessive separation anxiety, caused by their perception that their parents will abandon them for being bad or unvalued. Consequently, they form an attachment to their parents, even though their positive object representations of their parents are those of nonprotecting, nonsoothing, untrustworthy parents. In fact, rather than avoiding their parents, they cling to them quite strenuously. This is because it is not possible for 3-year-old toddlers to tolerate such negative object constancy; they are too dependent on their parents for basic survival and for positive mirroring responses. So what do they do? They use the defense mechanism of splitting.

In *splitting,* children retain two diametrically opposed images of a parent: one as all good and the other as all bad. Most often they automatically bar from their consciousness the displeasurable feelings they have toward the all-bad parent (e.g., hate, anger, fear) and instead consciously view the parent as being wonderful. The process of splitting their object representations of each parent is so all-encompassing that toddlers sacrifice their ability to perceive reality without significant distortion and, as Terr (1994) noted, the good and bad feelings toward a parent are sequestered, one from the other, and the child is aware of only one set of feelings at a given time. . . . As a result, they often end up with holes in their memories. (p. 126)

Splitting is a defense mechanism that is defined by some as a normal developmental mechanism in all children (Kernberg 1982); however, in my view, splitting is used only when a child has had a developmentally inhibiting poorness of fit with his or her parent in which he or she has had nonsoothing, unempathic, and covertly or overtly hostile experiences with the parent.

Children who engage in splitting often have parents who also have engaged in the same process. Parents' unempathic treatment of a child is often caused by the parents' distorted view of their child as inherently bad. Parents arrive at this conclusion through the use of splitting, through which they view one of their children as all good and another as all bad. Consequently, the child who is viewed as bad assimilates this badness into his or her self-representation and then identifies with the parent's use of splitting by viewing the parent as good and himself or herself as bad (Rosenthal 1983). To do the reverse—to view the parent as bad and himself or herself as good—would expose the child to parental hostility and further emotional abuse, physical abuse, or both.

Development of the Superego

In the process of choosing between right and wrong behaviors, toddlers are forever occupying themselves in play fantasies that involve themes of good and bad, right and wrong. In creating symbols in the play, they create situations in which they know a choice must be made, but also seem to know that they need some time to work on what choice to make. Through playing with toy dolls that symbolize themselves, their parents, and their siblings, they act out their various choices, try on various identifications with their parents' behaviors, and experience their own emotional reactions to those choices (Peller 1954). This play behavior is illustrated in the following example:

A 2¾-year-old girl is left by her mother and father in a hospital nursery while they attend to their respective medical appointments. They tell her upon leaving, "Be a good girl and play with the nice people. We'll be back in a little while." At first she is upset and stares at the door through which they have left. Suddenly, she responds to a male nursery attendant who offers her various toys. She picks a dollhouse and puppets and spontaneously assigns them the roles of a mother, father, and little girl. She then symbolically acts out some of her choices in the situation she is presently experiencing in her real world.

Initially, she has the parent puppets leave and the little girl puppet throw things around the playhouse kitchen. She then says, "She's bad," but the girl looks happy as she achieves vicarious gratification in choosing the play, which, although socially unacceptable, enables her to assert her growing independence from her parents. Thus for a while she achieves great pleasure in doing something in play that she would experience too much separation anxiety doing in reality—throwing things around the room after her parents left.

After a few minutes, however, she looks uncomfortable and has the mother puppet say to the little girl puppet, "You're no good." The little girl puppet then says, "No, Mommy, I am good," and then shows her mother she is good by cleaning up the kitchen. Next the toddler has the little girl puppet make a new choice: she plays in the backyard of the playhouse and invites the playful interaction of the male attendant. After a while, she has the parent puppets return and say to the little girl puppet, "You are a good girl," as the parent puppets look around the house, "smiling" because it has been tidied up so well.

Through this play, this toddler practiced how to be social. She can then use her play experiences, in addition to her real experiences with her parents, to construct beliefs about which behaviors are good versus which are bad. These beliefs, often called *standards* (Kagan 1984), become internal motivators that function in congruence with toddlers' innate need to engage in pleasurable emotional interactions with their parents by acting in ways that will bring parental approval, love, and admiration.

As I note in Chapter 2, Freud postulated that toddlers were exclusively motivated to seek gratification of their sexual and aggressive drives and would adopt standards only as a result of their separation anxiety about the loss of their parents or their parents' love and admiration. A second motivation, however, for toddlers' construction of standards is their own innate need to engage in, and hence maintain, an emotionally pleasurable attachment to their parents, and in the process be regarded by them as valuable and good. If toddlers did not possess some innate need to be valued and loved, their adoption of their parents' and society's standards would be based entirely on the rewards and punishments they received from their parents in reference to every one of their innate needs (which, in Freud's view, did not include any innate need to establish a loving attachment with one's parents). This is not the case, as most parents will attest. Kagan (1984) has suggested that toddlers possess an innate need to choose the good over the bad. In learning what is good and right, they want to choose good behaviors as goals in themselves, not only as a means of having their survival needs met but also because they have an innate sense of morality.

Another quality that emerges during toddlerhood that contributes to toddlers' constructing standards is the early empathic capacity to infer the emotions and thoughts of others. This quality, which I also discuss above, could support Kagan's suggestion that an innate need to choose the good over the bad is present in humans, given that it often emerges without prior specific training other than being nurtured by parents who are empathically attuned to their infant's emotions.

Development of
Adaptational Capabilities
Development of New Defense Mechanisms

As I note several times in this book, socialization exposes children to internal and external developmental conflicts. In infancy, these are only external conflicts that take place between infants' and their parents' wishes. During toddlerhood, toddlers experience not only external conflicts but also the internal conflicts of ambivalence between two of their wishes, two of their feelings, or their wishes and feelings, and prohibitions against their wishes or feelings, prohibitions that emanate from one or more of their internal object representations.

As they develop into objective self-observers, toddlers seek to rid from their consciousness any wish, belief, or fantasy that is associated with a displeasurable emotional state. Although there are many times when they will consciously suppress a thought, wish, or memory that is generating, or has generated in the past, a displeasurable emotional state, toddlers are also endowed with innate, maturationally emerging mental processes that serve to automatically—and unconsciously—either bar the disturbing mental contents from their conscious awareness or distort their perception of these contents (Rapaport 1959; see Table 4–3).

Defense mechanisms, by definition, are activated by toddlers' unconscious mental domain. As noted in Chapter 3, the self is conceptualized as having access to both the conscious and unconscious domains. Thus the unconscious aspect of the infant's self will scan all mental activity and activate a defense mechanism when a mental

---

Table 4–3.   Characteristics of defense mechanisms

- Are innate
- Evolve chronologically as an aspect of maturation in the psychological domain
- Evolve outside of voluntary control and awareness
- Produce external behaviors or certain ways of talking
- Are recognized by their systematic distortion of those events that are known to have occurred, are occurring, or are expected to occur
- Restore emotional self-regulation, allowing an unpleasurable emotional state to no longer be consciously experienced
- Are the psychological counterparts to immune mechanisms (e.g., as people differ in their immune response to inoculation with live bacilli, so they differ in their defensive responses to unpleasurable emotional states)

event is entering the infant's consciousness that will generate highly displeasurable emotions.

■ Functions of Defense Mechanisms

Defense mechanisms function as mental safety valves. Once they are in operation, a momentary state of emotional self-regulation and sense of control is regained after a turbulent event. However, these mechanisms always distort the perception of reality to some degree and, therefore, they are usually useful to toddlers only when they are fairly transient. Defense mechanisms can be viewed as at times functioning as offense mechanisms. In this view, the transient distortion of reality can enable toddlers to experience a pleasurable emotional state, and thus, through a type of self-deception, rid themselves of an awareness of an emotionally intolerable external or internal conflict. In all definitions of defense mechanisms, it is acknowledged that these mechanisms should be transient because they are mental processes that suspend toddlers' assertively addressing the resolution of an external or internal developmental conflict.

Defense mechanisms tend to be used transiently when toddlers grow up in a family where 1) verbally expressing the truth of what they believe and feel is supported by their parents and 2) the parents use their empathy and knowledge of their toddler's wishes, needs, and temperament to sense when their toddler is using a defense mechanism to deal with an external or internal conflict. In the latter situation, parents will permit their toddler to verbalize the wish, feeling, or memory that they are denying or projecting onto someone else. For parents to sense that their toddler is using a defense mechanism, they must have a certain degree of knowledge of life to appreciate when their toddler is distorting or hiding the mental or behavioral responses to an event that the parents know has occurred, is occurring, or would be expected to occur. For example, a mother will become suspicious that her son is not expressing his true feelings when he tells her he is not unhappy or angry because she has just canceled a scheduled trip with her to an amusement park so that she could take his new baby sister to the pediatrician. The mother usually would allow her son to persist in this defense mechanism for a while, but, at a later date, would help him relinquish its use and verbalize his true feelings to her.

Toddlers' use of defense mechanisms can be minimized when parents are successful in limiting the amount of distressing over- or understimulation their toddlers experience. For example, by exposing their toddler to only small doses of the frustration of hunger, parents assist their toddler in developing the capacity to gradually delay eating. In the process, the toddler learns that he or she is not always at the mercy of his or her hungry feelings.

Parents who do not adequately shield their toddlers from overly distressing situations can affect the attachment bond between themselves and their toddler. Fraiberg (1982) treated a group of depressed mothers who did not respond to their infants' cries. These mothers often looked at their infants with rage, and their infants, at these moments, showed fear. As early as age 3 months, these infants began automatically avoiding looking at their mother's face. This avoidance was selective, in that these infants sought to look at other adult faces. They did not smile at their mothers, nor did they turn toward their mothers' voices. Avoidant behavior had become a behavioral defense in that it decreased the time these infants had to gaze at their mother's face, which in turn decreased the displeasurable feelings associated with looking at an angry and depressed mother. Although all normal infants will use gaze aversion and head turning as avoidant defensive behaviors to some extent, this group of infants developed too much avoidance in their interactions with their mothers; this high degree of avoidance interfered with these infants' forming a developmentally enhancing attachment with their mother.

■ Types of Defense Mechanisms

The defense mechanisms that emerge during toddlerhood are the following:

Repression. *Repression* is the unconscious automatic barring from consciousness of those wishes, feelings, and memories that are associated with a highly displeasurable emotional state. When repression is fully effective, the repressed mental event is relegated to a toddler's unconscious, but may be stimulated by a future sensation and perception that is related to the repressed mental content. For example, such stimulation may lead to a slippage into consciousness of a piece of the repressed contents, as is manifested in a "slip of the tongue."

Projective identification. *Projective identification* is an unconsciousness automatic process that is a primitive forerunner of the future capacity for empathy. In this process, a toddler unconsciously projects onto a parent or another person an intolerable mental possession (e.g., a feeling, a wish) and then, in inferring that the other person wishes or feels the same way, attempts to manipulate that person to show the projected wish or feeling (Kernberg 1976; Meissner 1980). (For an extensive discussion of projective identification, see Sharff 1992.)

Projection. *Projection* is the unconscious and automatic barring from one's consciousness a wish or feeling with the conscious conviction that the wish or feeling is possessed by a parent or another. For example, a toddler boy is angry at his mother, but is afraid to express his anger. By using projection, he consciously believes that his mother is angry at him. He has thus projected his anger onto his mother. But unlike in projective identification, the toddler distances himself from the now undesirable angry person.

Introjection. The opposite of projection, *introjection* is the unconscious taking in of another's wish or feeling, and then consciously believing it is one's own. For example, an infant girl has a mother who hates her. The infant introjects her mother's hatred, bites her mother, and then believes she is full of hate for her. Introjection is thought to be a primitive form of identification (see below).

Turning against the self. In *turning against the self,* a person unconsciously and automatically bars from his or her consciousness a wish or feeling and then turns the wish or feeling against himself or herself. For example, a toddler girl has excessive angry feelings toward a sibling. Her anger, however, is intolerable. She begins to bang her head rhythmically on the table. At that moment, she is no longer aware of any anger toward her sibling, but only experiences a need to hit her head on the table.

Identification. *Identification* is

> changing the shape of one's self-representation to become more like the perception of an admired person or of some aspect of an admired person. The term is used to refer both to the process of making such changes and the changes themselves. (P. Tyson and Tyson 1991, p. 329)

Identification is an automatic childhood behavior that does not require specific operant conditioning. For toddlers, this process can be both an unconscious and a conscious mental operation that has both defensive and structure building functions (Compton 1981).

Using identification as a defense mechanism allows toddlers to unconsciously identify with parental behaviors that are causing them to experience repeated episodes of intensely displeasurable emotions, often at a traumatic level. When they cannot use fight-or-flight behaviors, or when their posttraumatic play fails to relieve their misery, toddlers can achieve some sense of mastery of these traumatic experiences by identifying with the aggressor (A. Freud 1936/1966). Phenomenologically, toddlers make an unconscious decision: If I can't beat him, I'll join him by acting toward others the way [the aggressor] is acting toward me. Usually the others are younger or weaker than they are. For example, a 3-year-old girl who is repeatedly slapped by her father feels less angry at her father when she gets away with slapping her 2-year-old cousin or a more passive 3-year-old playmate. However, by becoming a bully around other toddlers, this toddler girl will manifest a developmental inhibition of her assertiveness around her father.

In this example, the unconscious motivation for the father's slapping his toddler could possibly be his identification with his aggressor parent. (Fraiberg et al. [1975], in their article "Ghosts in the Nursery," described how a parent's parent can unconsciously enter the grandchild's nursery and remain within the family to motivate the parent to behave toward the grandchild the way the grandparent behaved toward the parent when he or she was a child.

When such a "ghost" remains, the attachment relationship between parent and child is invariably developmentally inhibiting.)

In addition to identification being used as a defense, it can be a mechanism for supporting toddlers' growing independence by helping toddlers explore the world away from their parents without experiencing excessive separation anxiety. It allows toddlers to assimilate into their internal world an aspect or attribute of those who gratify their needs and soothe them when they are hungry, tired, anxious, or frustrated.

Identification also aids toddlers in developing a superego (Sandler 1960). As they manifest a growing ability to generate self-imposed standards and goals, toddlers are motivated to identify with their psychologically attuned parents' behaviors in order to receive their parents' admiration and attributions of value. The superego is, for the most part, constructed by identifications with parents' prohibitions, standards, and rules. Thus when toddlers experience conflicts between their wish for their mother's (or father's) love and their other wishes that risk the loss of that love, such a conflict

> indicates the growing presence of the introject [or representation of the mother] evidenced when the child, in a kind of early imitation and role play, says "No, no" to himself, slaps his hand, or shows other identifications with the prohibiting parent such as gestures, inflections and facial expressions as preliminary phases in superego development. (P. Tyson and Tyson 1984, p. 90)

■ Effect of Parents' Use of Defense Mechanisms on Their Toddlers' Use of Defense Mechanisms

An important aspect of the maturation and development of defense mechanisms in toddlers is how often and what type of defense mechanisms are used by parents in their interactions with their children. As I note in Chapter 3, infants are ready-made "screens" on which parents can project their unwanted current or past displeasurable feelings and wishes. One certain characteristic of a toddler may trigger the toddler's parent to develop a negative transference reaction to him or her. For example, a son seeking his father's admiration for his performances unconsciously stimulates within the father repressed angry memories of his own father's avoidance of him as a child. As noted previously, the son's father may then identify with his (aggressor) father and view his son's wish for admiration with disinterest or even contempt.

Parents may also use projective identification to project unwanted negative aspects of their representational world onto their toddler, and then identify these projections as an aspect of the toddler's true self. For example, a mother who has a voracious need to overeat, and who is quite depressed and hates herself for this overeating, might project her voracious wish to overeat onto her toddler daughter. She will then "see" many signs in her daughter that indicate to her that she is hungry. One 3-year-old girl in such a situation who was told by her mother, "You're hungry again, I know," responded saying, "No, I'm not. I want to play with my toys, not eat again!"

Finally, parents can use denial in not recognizing temperamental characteristics, emotional states, wishes, and so on within their toddler that generate intensely displeasurable emotions in the parent—usually anger. The following example illustrates this process:

> A woman who had been emotionally abused by her father possessed an intense hatred for men. However, when she married, she believed that she had found a man whom she could trust and admire. When her husband eventually abandoned her with a 4-year-old boy and 1-month-old boy, her hatred for men was rekindled.
>
> This woman's older son possessed a difficult temperament. She now projected onto him her rekindled hatred for men. By the time he was age 8 years, he viewed himself as a "bad boy" and was forever in trouble with the police, as well as continually being expelled from school. The mother's younger son, now age 4 years, had grown up to be a boy who was continually teased in his preschool because other children believed he looked like a girl—his mother had never cut his hair and left it at shoulder length.
>
> The mother reluctantly followed the school's recommendation that she have her 4-year-old son evaluated by a child psychiatrist because of his tendency to withdraw from peers. She was also forced to address her strong resentment of any suggestion to cut the boy's hair.

In an evaluation interview I conducted with this family, the 8-year-old boy teased his brother for having shoulder-length hair. The younger brother thereupon got up from his chair, walked over, stood in front of his mother and said, "I look like a girl and I want my hair cut." The mother quite calmly looked at him and said, "Little boys and big boys are mean; they tease you just like your brother does. He's a boy and always gets into trouble like his father. But you don't have to be a boy or a girl and have one sex. You can be asexual; I'll help you." The child's face at that moment demonstrated intense bewilderment. He quietly sat down and hung his head.

This 4-year-old boy was apparently trying to establish, despite his mother's anger toward men, a gender identity as a boy. However, such a child will often fail in his attempts to counteract intense maternal denial unless he has another influential objective frame of reference to contrast with what he sees mirrored in the eyes of his mother. Such a frame of reference could be a child psychiatrist.

When the inner world of a parent causes the parent to view his or her toddler through the selective filter of transferentially supported denial or projection, then the parent does not really provide a mirror, but instead provides a distorted picture, to the toddler. Then, because a toddler will identify with what he or she sees reflected in his or her parent's eyes, the toddler could accept this distorted picture as his or her true mirror reflection. On the other hand, if such a toddler does not identify with his or her parent's defensively distorted view of him or her, then the toddler will forever remain in conflict with his or her parents.

All parents inevitably use some defense mechanisms in their dealings with their toddlers. For example, from what is now known about infant temperament, it is apparent that children within the same family may stimulate quite different reactions in each parent, as in the following example:

One mother tended to become angry at people who were overly assertive because, in her view, this behavior was indicative of someone who was selfish and self-centered. In the presence of such a person, the mother would become angry; however, afraid to express her anger, she unconsciously used projection to bar her anger from her consciousness. The result was that she ended up fearing an assertive person's anger. This mother did fine with her first infant, a slow-to-warm-up child who was rather inhibited in facing novel and unexpected stimuli. Thus this mother's first child did not display, in her view, any self-centered or selfish behavior. However, this mother did not do as well with her second child, a daughter, who possessed a much more normal degree of assertiveness. With this child, she manifested a negative transference: she viewed her daughter's healthy assertiveness as a sign of her being self-centered and selfish.

Parents' transference reactions that support their denial of perceiving their infant's true qualities are often operative in the first few years of an infant's life. However, more psychologically attuned parents usually manifest positive transferences to their infant, projecting and then identifying within the infant the same sense of wonder and value that they received from their own parents (i.e., non-performance-related positive mirroring; see discussion in Chapter 3). Eventually, parents must modify their transferentially motivated, extreme positive attributions as they face the truth about themselves and their child. When parents do not modify their perfectionistic views of their child, the child's true self can become just as damaged, as in the above case of the mother who did not modify her negative transferential view of her 4-year-old son's gender as a boy.

Defense mechanisms are adaptive when used transiently by both toddlers and the parents. In their transient usage, defense mechanisms give both toddlers and the parent time to consider other options when a wish, feeling, or memory has been, and still is, associated with displeasurable emotions. Just as spouses usually help each other in truthfully expressing what each wishes for, feels, remembers, and aspires to become, parents assist their toddlers in expressing the truth about their wishes and feelings and in recognizing that the truth is not always easy to face.

Parents intrinsically allow their child to develop and use defense mechanisms as one way of coping with life's demands and the inevitable external and internal conflicts with the parents and others. However, they eventually coax their child to relinquish defense mechanisms in the context of their protected and trusting relationship created by the ongoing transactional goodness of fit attachment relationship.

Progress Through Developmental Phases

Progressions and Regressions

As I discuss in Chapter 2, child development can be considered as both a continuous process—as progressing through somewhat predictable phases—and a discontinuous process—when periods of disorganization and disequilibrium are encountered. The overall developmental process is thus characterized by progressions alternating with regressions.

Regression is observed when children give up a newly developed behavioral competency (e.g., the social ability to feed themselves) or a mental ability (e.g., the ability to speak) and return to an earlier mode of functioning. Causes for regression are ubiquitous in the normal growth process. For example, regressions often occur in terms of the maturation and development of body control. When a 3-year-old girl is, for example, overtired, frightened, or sick, she may abandon her ability to walk and follow her mother, and regress and ask to occupy an old familiar place by being carried in her mother's arms. If behavior is defined as an ego function, then a transient regression is termed *regression in the service of the ego* (Bever 1982). This means that a transient regression serves the steady but slow growth of many of the child's ego functions, for example, speech, fantasy, formation, and recall and reconstructing memories.

As I noted previously, one of the functions of play in toddlerhood and childhood and into adult life is to act out, in playful fantasy, a pleasurable life experience. Many aspects of children's play are a form of regression that seems to enable them (and adults, for that matter) to remain at a certain developmental level for designated periods of time. Preschool teachers demonstrate this in allowing their students to engage in free, unrestricted play after they have been restricted by having to focus on learning something new. The free play takes place in a *play space,* which is defined as a specified physical place with certain rules of play and with certain limits on time to play (Ekstein 1966). The play space in essence helps children control their regression in play. This developing self-control of play helps children learn how to engage and disengage from regressive play.

Regression is defined, therefore, as normal if toddlers soon return to the level of development attained prior to the regression. Regression is abnormal when it becomes chronic. This occurs either because the cause for the regression makes it difficult for toddlers to return to their preregression functioning, or the developmental level reached prior to the regression was reacted to by the parents or significant others with criticism of the child's performance, disdain, physical or emotional withdrawal, or outright punishment, as in the following example:

> A severely depressed, divorced mother became quite anxious when her 3½-year-old daughter began to talk to a same-age girl playmate. The mother possessed the abnormal belief that talking to strangers was dangerous and told her daughter so. The mother was petrified that her daughter's talking to this other little girl was the beginning of her daughter's deciding to not spend time with her. Within a few weeks, her daughter had stopped talking to everyone, including her father, whom she visited on weekends. In identifying with her mother's warnings about the danger of speech, this girl regressed to a "safer" level of functioning, one that caused her to be mute to everyone but her mother.

Within a psychologically healthy parent-child attachment relationship,

> regression of functions is taken for granted as a common characteristic of infantile behavior. . . . An individual child's capacity to function on a comparatively higher level is no guarantee that the performance will be stable and continuous, . . . [for] occasional returns to more infantile behavior has to be taken as a normal sign. (A. Freud 1965, pp. 98–99)

Chapter 5

Early Childhood Phase of Mental Development

Age 3 Years to Age 6 Years

Biopsychosocial Stimuli Involved in the Mental Structural Organization of Mental Development

Six Steps in the Mental Processing of Biopsychosocial Transactions

By age 3 years, when children's representational world has begun to be constructed, their minds will use this inner world to process more complex transactions involving perceived biopsychosocial stimuli. This conceptual model of the mind is called the *information-processing model* (Berg 1992; Kail and Bisanz 1992). This model, in my view, is significant because it emphasizes that the manner in which cognition develops is a crucial variable in children's mental developmental changes. Berg (1992) emphasized that the focus of this model is not the input (i.e., biopsychosocial stimuli) or the output (i.e., resulting behaviors) but the intervening mental processing steps.

I now more fully describe how mental developmental change—as a final output of children's mental processing of biopsychosocial transactions—occurs through the following six mental processing steps:

1. The reception of biopsychosocial input stimuli
2. The generation of emotional responses and cognitive and emotional processing of transactions among biopsychosocial stimuli that generate children's representational perceptions, conceptions (i.e., wishes, fantasies, and beliefs), feelings, and memories
3. The processing of mental contents into internal motivators that lead children to generate one or more of the following initial output responses:

   a. Initiate an action or surface behavior (e.g., a 3-year-old boy walks toward his mother or decides to play with a novel game)
   b. Initiate speaking (e.g., a 3-year-old girl tells her mother, "I don't want to go to the store")
   c. Delay acting or speaking while consciously and privately contemplating their thoughts and emotions as internal "mental actions" (e.g., a boy remembers a game that is similar to the one he has been looking at and then recalls how much fun he had playing this game with his father)
   d. Delay acting or speaking while unconsciously activating a mental mechanism of defense, which usually involves behaving or talking in a certain way (e.g., a 3-year-old girl unconsciously projects her angry feelings onto her older brother and then complains to her mother that her older brother is angry at her)
   e. Delay acting or speaking while unconsciously activating the defense mechanism of somatization (e.g., a child with asthma experiences distressful overstimulation and begins to experience an asthmatic episode)

4. Activation of capacity for self-observation, which enables children to receive feedback information about the effectiveness of their initial output (one of a–e, above) in achieving their goal in their current interactions with others
5. Activation of capacity for self-reflection, which enables children to reflect on this feedback information in order to decide if they are achieving their goal at the moment and whether or not they should generate a different response
6. Construction of a new representation involving their final output responses and the responses or lack of responses from others in their social environment

In elaboration on #4, above, it should be noted that, by age 3 years, children have the ability to be objectively aware; that is, they can observe themselves in interacting with others or inanimate objects and also observe their own mental products (e.g., perceptions, fantasies, beliefs, memories). This self-observing capability is a source of feedback information on how they are doing instead of their parents being the primary source for this feedback. Also, as was the case since infancy, 3-year-old children receive not only conscious but also unconscious feedback information that influences whether their mind will activate a defense mechanism or influences their current perceptions about whether they are achieving their goals at the moment, as in the following example:

A 3-year-old girl sees a doll that she perceives as novel. Her initial response as she plays with the doll is to fantasize about being a mother. On a conscious level this fantasy is pleasurable, but on an unconscious level this fantasy (as unconscious feedback information) begins to activate a dynamic unconscious memory that is highly displeasurable. In this traumatic memory, the little girl was fed by her mother in a way that caused her to vomit. This would happen when her mother was in one of her agitated depressed moods. As this girl begins to engage in her fantasy play, she sees some play dishes and eating utensils and, without being conscious of how these perceptions stimulate her unconscious traumatic memory involving eating episodes with her mother, she abruptly suspends her doll play. In so doing, her unconscious mind protects her from recalling her traumatic eating memory.

In returning to the six processing steps listed above, once children have generated their final output response, they move on to the sixth processing step, which is the construction of a new representation or reconstruction of a preexisting representation. This representation, which may be stored as a long-term memory, will become a new mental developmental change if it represents new knowledge.

Major Developmental Tasks of Early Childhood

If their first 3 years of life have gone reasonably well, children will continue to develop the following representations, which are part of their positive self-constancy and object constancy:

- *An autonomous and valued identity,* while at the same time believing their parents can be trusted to continue to support, admire, protect, and love them
- *A gender identity* as a male or female, while at the same time believing their parents can be trusted to continue to support and admire their further development of male or female characteristics

In addition, by age 6 years, young children begin to have experiences that enable them to construct the following new additions to their self-representation that constitute new pieces of their overall identity:

- *A sexual identity*—This is a collection of beliefs, fantasies, and emotions that defines children's awareness of being able to seek sensual-sexual gratification from other individuals and that prohibits such gratification based on the rules of the family and society.
- *A peer identity*—This is a collection of beliefs, fantasies, and emotions that defines children's awareness of being able to

interact, cooperatively play, and negotiate conflicts with other children as a member of a peer group.

- *A superego or conscience*—This is children's awareness that they can control their behaviors by choosing between right and wrong behaviors relatively independently of the presence of their parents. Erikson (1959) described this as children's beginning to believe in their ability to exercise their initiative and curiosity in assertively choosing good over bad behaviors in a way that overrides their concern about feeling guilty in being assertive.

Functions of the Social Environment

Fostering Children's Healthy Narcissism in the Construction of Their Sexual and Peer Identities

As 3-year-old children's parents, siblings, and other significant acquaintances continue to provide the functions of the social environment, children demonstrate more of their own preferences as they assertively express their autonomous identity and their gender identity. As such, children more than ever before will challenge their parents in maintaining a goodness of fit.

In a mutually gratifying goodness-of-fit process, parents allow their children to gradually learn that, at times, they can achieve a certain degree of gratification of their needs in a manner that is emotionally pleasurable, but that at other times the gratification of those needs must be delayed because such gratification places them in conflict with the wishes of their parents. Parents provide appropriate instruction to assist their children in initiating delays in their actions so they can think about various behavioral solutions to these conflicts.

■ Development of a True Self

When a goodness of fit exists between children and their parents, children are said to be developing a true self-representation of their true self (Kohut 1971; Winnicott 1959/1989). A true self means children are basically true to their innate needs. They do not have to avoid perceiving and learning about their own needs. A child's true self emerges as he or she matures and develops in a family and social environment in which he or she has learned how to gratify or delay the immediate gratification of his or her needs in ways that, in most situations, please both himself or herself and the parents.

Sensitively aware parents assist their children in their struggle to develop a true self vis-à-vis their periodically resurrected wishes to be perfect or to idealize their parents as being perfect in the following two ways:

1. *Trying to be aware of their child's aspirations, both conscious and unconscious, to be perfect.* Any parental aspirations to raise a perfect child or to raise a child who will worship the parent as being perfect must, if present, be relinquished sooner rather than later. If not, children will begin to try to identify with their parents' perfect view, especially when parents do not accept their children's performances. For example, a 4-year-old girl says to her father while showing him a drawing, "This is a good drawing, huh Dad?" The father smiles weakly and says, "It's okay, but I watched you as you were drawing. You didn't take your time. You can do much better." The daughter replies somewhat angrily, "How do you know that?" The father then gets angry and says, "Because I'm your father and I know you can do much better." In time, the daughter may identify with her father's ideal or perfect view of her and resurrect her own ideal self-representation to such a position of prominence that her more true self-representation is increasingly repressed.

2. *Allowing their child to periodically see himself or herself as perfect alternating with allowing their child to see his or her parents as perfect.* Parents intuitively know that their children will periodically need to view themselves as perfect, often when they have recently been confronted with a new limitation or a disappointment; children do not take setbacks easily. For example, a 4½-year-old boy tells his parents, "Johnny said he

won't play with me because he wants to play with Freddy. I don't care. I'm the best runner. So I don't have to play with them. I'm the fastest." This boy's psychologically aware parents do not confront his grandiose fantasy but allow it to persist temporarily. They know that in time their son will want to play again with Johnny. If he did not, then his parents would become concerned about why their son was holding on to his grandiose, idealized view of himself as his primary view of himself. These parents do not tell their son, "You don't need Johnny. He's not as smart as you and he's just envious because you're great." Instead, they say, "You and Johnny got angry at each other. But Johnny and you are good friends, so maybe we should talk about why you want to think you don't need to play with him or anybody else anymore." His parents would be helping him express his true self—his true feelings of anger at Johnny and of missing him—rather than support his false grandiosity.

Psychologically aware parents also intuitively know that their young child will periodically need to view them as perfect. For example, a grandmother restricted her 4-year-old granddaughter's wish to play by telling her it was time to take a nap. In response to this limitation placed on her autonomous will by her grandmother, the girl greets her mother on her return with the statement, "Mom, you're the best mom! You always say it's okay to play and you never get mad at me." Her sensitively attuned mother knows that she is not perfect, that she must limit her daughter, and that she will often make mistakes in either overlimiting or underlimiting her daughter's assertive will. So she smiles and tells her, "Thank you for thinking I'm the best mom." She knows that eventually her daughter will have to confront her idealization of her mother and will inevitably be disappointed. In the future, as this mother allows her daughter to verbalize her disappointment, she helps her express her true feelings about not having a perfect mother.

The development and ascendancy to a position of prominence of a true self (over an ideal self), therefore, protects young children from wanting to abandon the reality of their current relationships—

conflicts and all—with their parents and others. Such abandonment leads them to seek narcissistic gratification in attempting to live the fantasy of being perfect and not needing their parents to guide and protect them, or to resurrect the fantasy of trying to find a perfect parent figure whom they can worship and who will take care of them and protect them from experiencing any developmental anxieties.

■ Developing Healthy Narcissism

Narcissism is generally defined as self-love (P. Tyson and Tyson 1984). *Healthy narcissism* is synonymous with toddlers' first objective awareness of being valued and loved by their parents. It leads to healthy self-esteem but also to children's development of esteem and love for their parents. Thus, in normal development, children's healthy narcissistic investment in themselves goes hand-in-hand with their loving investment in their parents. Stated in another way, narcissistic self-love and object love develop concurrently in children and are particularly prominent in 3-year-old children as they embark on developing the early manifestations of a sexual identity and a peer identity.

Children involved in a poorness of fit with their parents are constantly being forced to adapt to their parents' unreasonable developmental taskings that gratify the parents' needs more than the children's innate needs. In such a relationship, children experience highly displeasurable feelings because their parents' taskings are beyond their capabilities, causing them to repeatedly experience levels of stimulation outside their optimal stimulation range.

A poorness of fit existing between a 3-year-old child and his or her parents usually means that the infant attachment relationship also was a poor one. Consequently, by age 3 years, such a child inevitably will have failed to develop positive self-constancy and object constancy and will be in the process of continuing to develop a false self. As such, this child will not be true to his or her innate needs, provided he or she has already given up fighting for his or her true self. Some young children are quite defiant of their parents' unreasonable taskings of and ambivalent relationship with them.

Such defiance, however, usually brings children more displeasurable responses from their parents, leading them to figure out eventually some way of getting back at their parents, even if it means adopting the parents' ambivalent or hateful view of themselves. As one 5-year-old boy told me as he smiled, "My parents treat me like I'm always bad and now I act bad all the time. It makes them mad."

One of the innate needs that young children involved in a poorness of fit may give up is their need to engage in pleasurable interactions with their parents—specifically, to receive their parents' admiration and mirroring smiles that enhance their development of healthy narcissism. When they deny this innate need for admiration and love because it is ambivalently given or not given at all by their parents, children develop *pathologic narcissism.* According to Kohut (1971), the central mechanisms "I am perfect" and "You are perfect, but I am a part of you" are the two basic narcissistic configurations used to preserve a part of the original experience of narcissistic perfection (i.e., the early toddler's sense of experiencing no limitations in assertively exploring the world). Later, in the rapprochement phase, these toddlers must face the developmental crisis of confronting limitations. They resolve this crisis by taking the "road" of emotional self-constancy and object constancy, while still keeping within their mind a potential "detour," which is their "I am perfect" representation—their ideal self-representation—and their "You are perfect, but I am a part of you" representation—their ideal object representation. They use this "detour" to lead them to a periodic refuge from particularly tough days when they must face a limitation or a disappointment. Young children involved in a poorness of fit and developing a false self, however, can stay on the "I am perfect" or "You are perfect and I'm a part of you" road permanently as they journey through childhood. Noshpitz and King (1991) described how such a child's grandiose wishes

act as a cushion against the intolerable reality of being tiny, helpless, vulnerable and unloved; the assertions of grandeur buffer the inner uncertainty of inadequacy and emptiness, and the insistence on entitlements wards off the profound feeling of worthlessness and having no lovability whatsoever. The healthy child has no need for such adaptations because he has a great, loving, gratifying other (his mother and father) to help him past the stresses of growing up. (p. 220)

The survival of a relationship—albeit an already poor one—between 3-year-old children who have not attained a positive self-constancy and object constancy and their parents is in jeopardy because the children must live with a diminished or damaged self-constancy that leaves them with very poor self-esteem, a devalued view of themselves, and a belief that if anyone knew their true self, they would reject them if they found out that they were not living up to their ideal self. These children's self-view might be expressed as, "I am great and I don't need anyone, but people must do what I want"; this is their compensatory fantasy that supports their false self. It functions as a defense mechanism that represses their true self, which, if verbalized, might sound something like, "I feel worthless when I am not perfect and maybe I am worthless. But I am in a [narcissistic] rage at my parents for not admiring me, for ignoring me and sometimes ridiculing me, but I'm afraid that now that I've told you this that you'll also want to get rid of me." Such children treat siblings and other same-age or younger children quite sadistically as objects to unquestionably serve their desires at the moment. Their grandiosity alienates other children; they usually end up playing only with either younger or more passive same-age children whom they can control. Other children who resurrect their ideal self as their only self constantly seek admonitions of unlimited praise. When this praise is not forthcoming—or not enough, as these children often believe—the same (narcissistic) rage erupts.

Children involved in a goodness-of-fit relationship with their parents find acceptable ways to gratify each of their innate needs in an emotionally pleasurable fashion. They are true to their innate needs and attain the progressive additions to their overall true identity—their autonomous, gender, sexual, peer, and social identities—while fulfilling their parents' developmental taskings necessary for them to become socialized members of their family and society.

It is important to emphasize that, in a goodness of fit between parents and their child, both arrive at reasonable expression and gratification of their individual innate needs and reasonable expression of their true selves. In this context, the term *reasonable* indicates that they arrive at compromises between what they want and what they realize is possible while maintaining an attachment relationship with each other. Extending these ideas from the family to the societal level, each society will differ in the degree to which it permits its members to reasonably gratify their individual needs against the context of the good of the group.

The true selves developed by young children and their parents are not selves who always get what they want. Instead, these true selves are shaped by the ongoing need to adapt to the true selves of others. This is one of the important lessons of life that psychologically attuned parents are able to teach their children: personal independence, assertion, and the attainment of a true self is tempered by one's need to be dependent on and adapt to the needs of others. The increasing assertion of one's independence and the development of one's attachment relationships go hand-in-hand during normal development.

Maturation and Development of Innate Needs
The Genital Phase

At about age 3 years, children begin to focus much more on their genital region. Whereas toddlers were interested in looking at and exploring their body and genital apparatus (which served the purpose of their constructing a gender identity), young children seek sensual pleasure by manipulating their penile or vaginal area. Masturbation becomes more prominent. In addition, children become much more preoccupied with thinking about what use the genitals have in the operations of their body. These changes in children cannot be explained on the basis of learning alone. Parents do not normally encourage their 3-year-old children to learn how to masturbate. Instead, children are propelled in these behaviors by the maturation of their innate need for sensual-sexual pleasure (a psychological stimulus).

S. Freud (1923/1963) documented a progressive maturation of what he called children's sexual drive. This progression began with seeking sensual pleasure through oral mucosal stimulation (the *oral phase*), to seeking sensual pleasure through anal and urethral stimulation (the *anal phase*), to seeking sensual and truly sexual pleasure through the stimulation of the sexual organs (the *phallic phase*). (Freud named this latter phase using male genitalia because he believed that the penis—the phallus—dominated the thinking of both boys and girls. Later researchers [Galenson 1993; Kestenberg 1968; Parens et al. 1976; Roiphe and Galenson 1981] have shown, however, that girls demonstrate just as much interest in their own genitals as boys do in theirs. Both boys and girls are interested in the genitals of each other. Thus I am in agreement with some who have suggested that the phallic phase should be called the *infantile genital phase* [P. Tyson and Tyson 1991].)

Erickson (1993) speculated that children's healthy attachment relationship with their parents prepares them for maturation into their infantile genital phase. He documented how a normal attachment relationship creates a bonding called *familial bonding* between parents and their children; this bonding prevents or is a protective factor that inhibits children from seeking direct sexual contact with their parents.

In contrast to the maturation of children's innate need for sensual-sexual gratification—which is documented by observable changes in children's bodily preoccupations and self-stimulations (Galenson 1993)—the maturation of children's other innate needs is more difficult to observe and quantify. With regard to the innate need to assertively seek novel stimuli, it is speculated that this need changes only in that it takes a new direction—toward exploration of one's own body and the bodies of one's parents and others. Similarly, young children's innate need to signal distress continues to develop as they become more competent in sending external distress signals and using their own anxiety as an internal signal to alleviate their own distress (e.g., through constructing a fantasy, engaging in play).

Maturation and Development of Physical Capabilities

Maturation of Body Control and Coordination

During early childhood, there is a significant increase in children's body weight, size, and motor coordination (i.e., walking and running abilities, hand-eye coordination, and leg-eye coordination) (Ames and Ilg 1976a, 1976b, 1976c, 1979). Children age 3 years also begin to show whatever athletic abilities they possess as they show maturation of muscle mass. (The major gross motor, visual motor, and manual dexterity capabilities are listed in Table 5–1.) This latter development will further enhance their already constructed gender identity in that boys begin to show muscle development in a different distribution than girls. All of these changes become new biological stimuli in the biopsychosocial model.

Maturation and Development of Cognitive Capabilities

Gradual Decline of Egocentrism and Further Development of Reality-Based Thinking

Egocentrism predominates toddlers' thinking because they are unable to understand that their self-centered perceptions of events or people are different from others' perceptions of the same things. By age 3 years, this egocentrism is further accentuated when limitations and disappointments cause young children to resurrect their ideal self-representation or object representations. As a result, children will insist that their omnipotent view of reality is the only view or insist that their father or mother can omnipotently change reality—the reality that children say exists.

Egocentric thinking is a manifestation of toddlers' and young children's use of certain symbolic representations to develop their primary process, magically oriented thinking. Although it appears that children's use of magical thinking means they have suspended their ability to differentiate between real and unreal phenomena, on the contrary, while engaged in magical thinking, they are still able to deal with the environment in a meaningful way (Greenspan 1979).

Table 5–1. Major gross and fine motor skills that emerge between age 3½ years and age 6 years

Age	Motor skill
3½ years	Have more assured balance in walking, running, and jumping
	Can ride tricycle using the pedals
	Can catch a large ball and maintain balance in throwing a ball
4 years	Demonstrate a great increase in balance and overall coordination
	Can stand on one foot for several seconds and can skip with one foot
	Can better control the direction in which they throw a ball
	Can button and unbutton clothing, lace shoes, and direct their cutting with scissors
5 years	Demonstrate increased control of all body movements, including coordinating their eyes, head, and hands in focusing in one direction
	Display more coordinated use of the dominant hand
6 years	Can ride a bicycle with training wheels downhill
	Demonstrate greatly increased fine motor skills
	Can grasp a pencil and print legibly

Source. Adapted from Ames and Ilg (1976a, 1976b, 1976c, 1979).

This capacity to maintain a realistic perception of real events begins prior to children's developing an objective self-awareness. Infants learn by trial and error; that is, they learn by observing contingencies. These experiences lead them to construct unconscious implicit memories that become their stored record of what Greenspan (1979) called *somatic intelligence.* At about age 18 months, following the emergence of objective self-awareness, toddlers develop *representational intelligence* (Greenspan 1979). This form of intelligence entails toddlers' beginning to delay action or immediate imitation of others' actions until a later time when they evoke representations to engage in deferred action or imitation. Representational intelligence encompasses symbolic thinking and secondary process, reality-oriented thinking. (I disagree with Greenspan's dating the initiation of representational intelligence at about age 18 months, for I believe that infants build up a rich representational database of unconscious, implicit, long-term memories.)

Greenspan (1979) noted (correctly, I believe) that, between ages 18 months and 6 years, children learn to develop and differentiate their magical (primary process) thinking from their reality-oriented (secondary process) thinking. He stated that, occasionally during this period, although children will tend to talk in a magical way that suggests they have lost touch with reality, they will unconsciously be using their somatic intelligence to continue to behave in a logical manner. Leslie (1987) documented the development in children ages 2–3 years of the ability to pretend—which often incorporates primary process thinking—as an indication of their new capability to understand that people have different minds that produce different ideas, feelings, and memories.

At ages 3–4 years, children become more adept at using secondary process thinking; by age 4 years, they begin to realize that someone else can have a view of a person, object, or event that differs from their own. They can understand how one person looking at a dollhouse from a different vantage point from themselves can form a different perception of the same; furthermore, they seek to explore this novel discovery by walking over to the other person's vantage point and observing how their own perception of the dollhouse changes. Associated with this advance in understanding that they can have different perceptions of the world, children ages 3–4 years can understand the concept of belief (Leekam 1993); that is, they comprehend that beliefs will cause them and others to view people and things and behave in specific ways. Chandler et al. (1989) described *small scale deceit* in young children as indicating their understanding that people have separate minds. For example, one November morning, a 3¾-year-old boy told his mother, "It's snowing out Mom, so you need to get the snow shovel." His mother, believing him, immediately went to a window and raised the blinds, looking out on a cloudy but dry day. Her son, laughing, said, "I tricked you!"

Another manifestation of the further maturation of children's ability to use secondary process thinking is an advance in their ability to distinguish between symbols and what they symbolize. Children age 3 years endow their symbolic objects with the quality of being alive or real. Children ages 4–5 years, however, may call a puppet a cookie monster and engage in an animated play fantasy with it, but they continue to be aware that the puppet is both a symbol and an inanimate object. They no longer magically endow the cookie monster with the quality of being alive. Thus when they are asked what they are doing, they readily reply, "I'm pretending. Let's make believe the cookie monster is real and he can talk. I know he's only a puppet."

By ages 4–5 years, children will use symbolic objects in play to construct a *compensatory fantasy,* a fantasy that helps them repress or deny becoming consciously aware of a developmental anxiety they are feeling. If, for example, an observer or participant in a young child's fantasy play attempts to point out to the child the symbolic object's true meaning, the child will stop playing, as did the boy in the following example:

> A 5-year-old boy was playing that he was a mean wizard, and as-signed me the role of mean helper in his compensatory fantasy. We both were going to torture a 3-year-old girl who was a stranger, lost in the woods. When I told the 5-year-old that per-haps the 3-year-old stranger was really his 3-year-old sister, he commented, "I'm not going to play anymore if you ask me to talk about my sister. I want to play!"

This boy was, in effect, telling me that his symbols were needed to establish his emotional equilibrium, as he used play as a vehicle to achieve vicarious gratification of a wish he knew was forbidden (i.e., his wish to torture his younger sister). He used symbolic play to support the development of secondary process thinking as evidenced in his ability to deny his wish to torture his sister. In addition, his symbolic play revealed a maturation of his ability to use primary process thinking in a creative way through fantasy play. As such, he was able to manipulate his conscious symbols while keeping repressed within his unconscious the true meaning of each symbol. This process was adaptive for him in that he could vicariously gratify the forbidden wish to torture his sister without being bothered by thoughts that his symbols were real (e.g., if he was age 3 years, he might have become afraid of me as the mean helper).

In early childhood, children's play slowly contains more and more creative thinking. Modell (1988) noted that a creative attitude toward life is based in spontaneous play engaged in as a child. Intuitive parents know this and support their children's play, encouraging development of their imagination, and enthusiastically responding to their children's play creations. They also intuitively encourage their children to "play with their thoughts" to come up with their own creative solutions to their developmental conflicts. Thus the parents of a 4½-year-old son smile when he parades around the house in a cape and declares he is Superman right after his 6-year-old cousin has gotten the best of him in a brief wrestling match. Parents also support their children's creativity by providing them with toys that encourage them to create images, narrative stories, and symbols (e.g., pencil and paper, drawing materials, clay). During such creative play, children use symbolic representations to develop their primary process thinking further, and then use this thinking to create novel ideas about themselves and their place in their family and expanding social world.

Another manifestation of young children's development of their primary process thinking is seen in their dreams in which unresolved conflicts from their daily lives are replayed. Once they are able to verbalize the content of their dreams, children begin to translate the primary process characteristics of their dreams—

the disregard of time and logical connections, the presence of mutually contradictory ideas, and the use of visual imagery and symbols in place of language—into the logical rules of secondary process thinking. In so doing, they begin to gain access to what they have repressed within their unconscious domain. In this way, primary and secondary process thinking become more integrated, a development that enhances the creative thinking capability of children. This development is seen in the little girl in the following example:

> A 5-year-old girl I was seeing in psychotherapy was struggling with both an internal and an external conflict: she was enraged with her mother because her mother had angrily yelled at her for going away from her to explore when they were in a store together. At the same time, the girl felt extreme separation anxiety that her mother would abandon her if she told her of her rage. She also felt extreme anxiety that her conscience would punish her with excessive guilt if she remained severely angry with her mother.
>
> One night she had the following dream, which she reported to me as follows: "I woke up last night and a bad witch came out of my mirror on my wall. I was real afraid because she was going to take me to the woods and leave me there."
>
> In the ensuing several therapy sessions, she played out her dream. She had me play the bad witch and she played herself. She told me to come out of a pretend mirror and try to scare her. She then told the bad witch, "You can't frighten me." In time, as we replayed this game, she began to wonder more about the mirror symbol she had created in her dream. When I asked her, "What do children see when they look into a mirror?" she answered, "Themselves." And when I said, "Maybe the bad witch is really your own feelings toward your mom that you feel are too bad to ever say to me or your mom," she responded, "Yes, it's like when I'm being mad is like I'm the bad witch."

This example illustrates how this girl was able to use primary process thinking—the creation in her dream of a person living in a mirror who symbolized her own feelings—in helping herself to understand, in a creative way, her present separation anxiety. In later sessions, she was able to understand that she wanted to take her mother to the woods and abandon her mother as punishment for her mother's ambivalent feelings toward her.

Ability to manipulate category representations. In early childhood, children demonstrate another cognitive maturational advance: their ability to mentally manipulate their category representations. Earlier in life, toddlers form categories based on whether a set of objects or events share perceptual, functional, emotional, conceptual, word label, or belief-fantasy commonality (see Chapter 4). It is not until about age 4 years that they have the ability to transform knowledge from one category to another. Once they begin to be able to do this, they begin to understand the meanings of similes and metaphors. For example, a 4½-year-old boy constructs a metaphor and tells his mother, "I was a lion in soccer today." This transferring knowledge of one category to another involves children's consciously violating the boundaries of an established category (Noshpitz and King 1991). Parents of young children are often amazed to hear the results of their children's new ability to transform their current categories into new, more cognitively complex ones, like the little boy in the following example:

> Following a 1-week visit by his maternal grandmother, a 5-year-old boy constructed a simile and told his mother, "You know, Grandma is like a car that never turns off." The mother asked him to explain. He replied, "She keeps talking all the time like a car that keeps going and never needs any gasoline." The mother commented, "You know, you're right. And it's good you didn't tell Grandma this, because she likes to talk and it would hurt her feelings. But you're so smart, and thinking of Grandma as being like a car means you're a good thinker."

This example illustrates the importance of the parents' support and positive feedback for their children's use of intuitive, self-reflective thinking. Just as young children continue to give themselves a mastery smile for succeeding with a new puzzle or game and seek a mirroring smile when they demonstrate this accomplishment for their parents, they also give themselves a mastery smile when they come up with a new metaphor, joke, or story, or remember a dream and then verbalize these mental constructions to their parents to seek a mirroring smile from them. When children receive such admiring feedback, their autonomous self and positive self-constancy receive supportive nurturance. Consequently, they learn that, for most of the time, their parents encourage and admire their assertion of themselves in being self-reflective and being able to verbalize their observations about their separate and unique representational world. Children store long-term memories of these emotionally pleasurable nurturant experiences, which in the future will act as internal motivators that propel them to continue to verbalize internal perceptions of their representational world phenomena. Such a child will speak up and offer his or her own intuitive ideas or stories without having to be asked or coaxed to talk.

If, however, parents usually respond to their children's verbalization of their intuitive thoughts, feelings, and memories critically or in an uninterested manner, their children will not experience competency pleasure and will eventually store emotionally displeasurable memories of these communications. In the future, these memories will cause them to avoid being self-reflective. In effect, they say to themselves, "Why talk about what I am thinking? If I say what I think my parents don't respond much at all." Such children may become increasingly separated from their own representational world and may eventually be described as being unperceptive or unaware by people outside of their family. Alternatively, such children will increasingly carry on private conversations with themselves as their representational world assumes an ascendancy over their interactions with their external, interpersonal world.

Ability to understand analogies. In addition to young children's new capability to use intuition and self-reflection to manipulate and transform preexisting categorical knowledge into new and more abstract categories, they also become able to construct a new type of category: objects, persons, or phenomena that share analogical commonality. This becomes possible because children have attained the ability to construct an analogous representation. An example would be when a 4-year-old boy proudly tells his father, "You know, if I have a brother, then my brother has a brother, too."

Ability to recognize multiple attributes. In early childhood, children progress from *centration*—in which they focus exclusively on one attribute of an object or a person—to recognizing multiple attributes of an inanimate object or person. For example, 2-year-old children will focus on a single attribute of an inanimate object or a person that initially dominates their perceptual focus. By age 4 years, however, children will see a new inanimate object, pause, and begin to see attributes they had not seen before.

Ability to construct executive structures. In early childhood, children develop the ability to construct a new complex conception: the executive structure, which is also referred to as an executive control structure (Case et al. 1988) or structures of the executive process (Kagan 1984). The *executive structure* is a complex conception that contains knowledge of an entire experience in which children solved a problem. According to Case et al. (1988), the executive structure is initially an explicit long-term memory that contains three components: 1) the representation of a child's solving a previous problem, 2) the representation of the child's objectives if such a problem presents itself in the future, and 3) a representation of the mental strategy that the child will once again follow to bring the problem to an effective solution.

As I discuss in Chapter 4, emotional self-constancy and object constancy, which are necessary for the construction of executive structures, are not formed until about age 3 years. Greenspan (1979) described this connection between executive structure and emotional self-constancy and object constancy as follows:

> The youngster has the ability . . . to differentiate, in a relative sense, self from non-self. That this advance occurs together with the consolidation of [self- and] object constancy is not surprising; the youngster's ability to hold representations of the object, even when separated from the object . . . indicates this greater capacity for differentiation of self from non-self. . . . There is a greater flexibility to tolerate and deal with a wide range of internal [i.e., biological and psychological] and external [i.e., social] stimuli. . . . Intelligence is therefore greater than earlier in life, since a child now assimilates, accommodates, and conserves

a greater variety of stimuli, ranging over time and space, in relatively stable and permanent organizations. (pp. 309–310)

Executive structure is one such "relatively stable and permanent organization."

The ability to construct executive structures begins to emerge by age 3 years and functions well by age 5 years. For example, a 2-year-old girl who sees and wants a toy but is prevented from obtaining it by some type of barrier (e.g., some other toy, an inanimate object, a person) either tasks herself or is tasked by her parent to acquire the knowledge (i.e., through constructing an implicit representation) necessary to solve this problem. When she does so, she can use this same knowledge to solve a similar problem in the future. Although this toddler girl is cognitively capable of constructing representations of the procedures she followed, she does not yet possess the cognitive ability to advance her implicit memories to the level of an executive structure.

As another example, parents do not attempt to teach their 2-year-old children how to get home if they become lost in the neighborhood. Not only would a toddler become too anxious in thinking about being lost, but he or she also would be cognitively incapable of following all the sequences involved in solving the problem of being lost. However, when this same child begins preschool at age 4 years, his or her parents will present him or her with the following problem situation: "Let's talk about what you would do if you were waiting for me to pick you up at school and I was not there." In this way, parents ensure that their child is motivated to identify this as a problem situation and talk about not only what he or she would want to do but also how he or she would do it. Also, in assisting their child to talk about a situation in which the child would experience some separation anxiety, parents are teaching their child that he or she can take certain steps to alleviate his or her separation anxiety. This process helps the child begin to believe that he or she can exert self-control and self-soothing behaviors when experiencing separation anxiety.

Each time children remember and then activate one of their executive structures, they enhance their "faith in thought" (Kagan 1984); that is, they begin to develop confidence that they have the knowledge to solve specific problems. They recognize their ability to think and delay action in order to remember how they solved similar problems in the past. When faced with a new problem for which no executive structure yet exists in their mind, children ages 4–6 years will gradually begin to believe that they can use their thinking processes to generate a solution to the problem (Kagan 1984). Kagan illustrated this point as follows:

> I recall an unusual 5-year-old boy who was shown two identical pieces of clay that he acknowledged to be equal in quantity. I then rolled one piece of clay into a thick sausage and asked him if one piece had more clay or if the two pieces were equal. The child looked at the two pieces of clay, put his head down on the table, and remained quiet for almost two minutes. When I repeated my question impatiently, the boy looked up and said, "I'm thinking." (p. 232)

Clearly this boy had learned that he could solve problems through thinking without having to act. He was also beginning to learn that thinking about a question was an acceptable answer to a question.

Many conscious and preconsciously stored executive structures (which were originally stored as explicit memories) eventually become unconsciously stored and automatically activated implicit memories, because the explicit or declarative information (i.e., verbal and visual images) involved in originally learning the solution to the problem eventually becomes unnecessary as the procedures are practiced and become smoothly learned and then automatic. For example, a 5-year-old boy no longer has to think about how to get to kindergarten or what to do if his school bus does not come. Each morning he leaves the house and walks to the corner where his school bus picks him up; on the rare occasion when it does not come, he walks home to tell his mother that she must drive him to school. He will no longer recall how he learned these procedures, unless the acquisition of the executive structure was associated with a high level of emotion. Then the structure may remain in his preconscious memory as a declarative memory with procedural components. For example, a 6-year-old boy could easily and vividly remember the day he first was told how to go to kindergarten because it was associated with an extremely sad experience: the night before the start of kindergarten, a same-age male cousin who had been living with him since birth had been suddenly taken out of his home when the cousin's father reclaimed him.

Development of locus-of-control belief. A locus-of-control belief defines what children believe about who or what controls their life and the quality and quantity of that control (Trad 1989). Locus-of-control beliefs can be internal or external.

Children who have an *internal locus-of-control belief* believe for the most part that they can gratify their innate needs and meet their goals while also accommodating to their parents' taskings and rules. These children become motivated to assertively master tasks and problems with the generally optimistic expectation that they will eventually experience a mastery smile and receive support and admiring mirroring smiles from their parents, even if they do not always succeed in their endeavors. Perceiving their own limitations and inevitable failures does not cause them to give up being assertive, even though at times they may temporarily resurrect their ideal self-representation, which contains their grandiose belief in being omnipotent, as a response to perceiving their limitations and failures.

Children who have an *external locus-of-control belief* believe that events in their life are external to anything they can do; that is, they believe that what happens in their life is caused by chance, luck, fate, or forces outside their control. This belief causes them to inhibit their assertiveness as they are dominated by the negative expectancies associated with their negative transference reactions to others. They transferentially expect that being assertive will not bring any pleasurable outcomes. When these children do not modify their external locus-of-control beliefs by having new experiences in which they assertively master novel stimuli and developmental conflicts, by ages 5–6 years they may develop a new view of themselves as having a helpless, not an autonomous, identity. Seligman (1975) coined the term *learned helplessness* to describe the belief that one has tried all possible solutions to a problem or conflict and concluded that nothing can be done to produce an effective solution.

Both internal and external locus-of-control beliefs have two main sources in a child's life: 1) parents' beliefs about their child's power to influence themselves and others and 2) the child's experiences with his or her mastery of novel stimuli and developmental conflicts.

Parents hold certain beliefs about their children's ability to influence their environment that they subsequently attempt to instill in their children. Parents can possess two independent internal locus-of-control beliefs: they can believe that 1) they have the power to influence the behaviors of their child and 2) their child has the power to influence their (parental) behavioral interactions with the child. The second parental belief comes through parents' attempts to instill an internal locus-of-control belief in their child. When parents hold these two beliefs, they can truly engage in a transactional attachment relationship with their child.

In some circumstances, parents may instill external locus-of-control beliefs in a child rather than more developmentally enhancing internal locus-of-control beliefs that fuel their child's positive expectancies that his or her assertiveness will bring desirable outcomes. Kagan (1984), for example, observed that many working-class parents believe their children will be unable to surmount the barriers to their success present in adult American society. Thus they attempt to instill a belief within their children that they will do well only by focusing on acquiring a highly secure job, even if the job inhibits their assertiveness. A boy growing up in such a family may be told by his parents when he is entering high school, "Always remember to look for a job with a pension and security. Don't take chances or aim too high." In addition, these parents instill within their children the belief that they must maintain close family ties that will assist in protecting them from being exploited by affluent and wealthy people in America.

In contrast, Kagan (1984) speculated that college-educated parents tend to believe that their children, through education, have the power to change their place in society and achieve success. Consequently, they believe that their children will do well only if they believe in the power of their own assertiveness and autonomy to choose from many potentially successful careers. These parents emphasize that a career that develops their child's unique potential is more important than finding a job that grants employment security. Such parental messages are more likely to instill internal locus-of-control beliefs in children, but only if their capabilities fit their parents' taskings and aspirations. Children of limited intellectual endowment can be made to feel quite helpless if their parents deny their limited capabilities and continually tell them that graduate education is the only way to do well.

This takes us to the second source of children's locus-of-control beliefs: their overall life experiences with mastering novel stimuli. Parents fuel the development of internal locus-of-control beliefs in their children when they fulfill their functions of 1) protecting their children from experiencing too many distressfully over- or under-stimulating events, 2) answering their children's behavioral, emotional, and verbal signals of distress, 3) tuning in to their children's temperament as indicating a need for more or less assistance in being assertive (see below), and 4) setting up appropriate-level, novel tasks for their children to master and thereby achieve a measure of competency pleasure.

In contrast, parents who 1) expose their children to danger, 2) do not answer their children's distress signals, 3) do not tune in to their children's temperamental characteristics with regard to their level of assertiveness, and 4) do not provide their children with tasks that they can master fuel the development within their children of external locus-of-control beliefs. As noted above, these beliefs motivate children to inhibit their assertion and autonomy because they believe they will be helpless to deal with developmental conflicts in a way that will bring them any degree of emotional pleasure. In time, these children may develop a learned helplessness, leading them to become passive rather than feeling empowered in their ability to create opportunities.

Maturation and Development of Temperamental Characteristics

Temporal Stability of Behavioral Inhibition to the Unfamiliar

More research has been done on infants' innate temperament and how their temperament matures throughout toddlerhood than has been done on temperamental changes in early and later childhood. Longitudinal studies of infant and child temperament (Chess and Thomas 1986; Kagan 1989) have demonstrated that some children will show continuity or *temporal stability* in certain temperamental characteristics they exhibited in infancy into their sixth year of life, whereas other children will show discontinuity or *temporal instability* between their infant temperamental characteristics and the temperamental characteristics they manifest by age 6 years.

One factor that affects temporal stability of any temperamental characteristic over time is the parenting received by a child. For example, Hirshfeld et al. (1992) reported that 75% of children who exhibited behavioral inhibition to the unfamiliar at age 21 months retained this classification through age 7½ years (labeled the *stable inhibited group*). Within this group, there was a high association of anxiety disorders within both children and their mothers. In the *unstable inhibited group* (i.e., children who were initially inhibited but were no longer inhibited at age 7½ years), there was not a significant occurrence of anxiety disorders in them or in their mothers. The authors, in speculating as to why the stable inhibited group remained inhibited and had a high degree of anxiety disorders, offered three possibilities:

1. *A temperamental trait–like predisposition to develop anxiety disorders may be genetically transmitted from parent to child.* In this possibility, a child's behavioral inhibition to the unfamiliar and his or her parents' anxiously inhibited view of the world have a combined effect. Neither the child nor his or her parents are viewed as being able to be active in influencing the other's innate or anxious inhibition.
2. *Exposure to a parent's anxious symptoms might induce an inhibited child to remain cautious and fearful in situations of uncertainty.* In this second possibility, a mother is active and her child is reactively passive in identifying with and adopting the mother's anxiously inhibited view of the world, which reinforces the child's inhibition.
3. *A combination of genetically influenced and environmental factors interact in a reciprocal manner to lead to stability of behavioral inhibition.* For example, a child's early tendency to

be inhibited might elicit protective behavior on the part of a parent (particularly an anxious one) or aggressive behavior on the part of the other parent or an older sibling, which might increase the child's hesitancy to approach unfamiliar objects. This would lead to more protection by the anxious parent, ending in a self-perpetuating cycle. In this third possibility, a child's innate behavioral inhibition to the unfamiliar is the active variable in producing the kind of parenting and sibling responses he or she receives. In this case, the child is active and the parenting environment is reactively passive.

It is interesting that, in all three possibilities, what is omitted is the possibility that children who possess an innate behavioral inhibition to the unfamiliar can enter into a transactional process with their parents in which both they and their parents are active and reactive. For example, a child born with a behavioral inhibition to the unfamiliar may enter into a transactional process with a mother who is anxiously inhibited. In addition to the possibility that this child will become more inhibited or the mother will become more anxiously inhibited, the child and the mother may both become less inhibited because of the effect each has on the other—that is, each could activate potential resources in the other. For example, an anxious mother, concerned that her child might be growing up as anxiously inhibited as she, seeks psychiatric treatment for her anxiety disturbance. As her condition improves, she is able to help her son become less inhibited.

In summary, temperamental characteristics, like any other innate and maturing capacity in children, will mature and develop within the context of the transactional relationship with children's parents. The relative goodness or poorness of the fit between children and their parents does not remain stable throughout the children's life cycle but is dependent on how new maturational changes in children and new responses in the parents affect the transactions between them.

Currently, temperamental research is hampered by difficulties in 1) defining temperamental characteristics in infancy and how these characteristics change over time (Chess and Thomas 1986) and 2) understanding which behaviors in children are attributable to maturation of other aspects of their mental nature (e.g., innate needs, emotions, cognitive abilities) and which behaviors reflect maturation in temperamental characteristics (Dunn 1981). What is lacking in research is a focus on children's other characteristics (i.e., emotions, innate needs, and cognitive and physical abilities) as well as their own constructed representations, which affect the goodness or poorness of fit between children and their parents.

Maturation and Development of Emotions

Construction of Emotional Display Rules

In early childhood, children's emotions undergo significant maturation and development. As I initially presented in Chapter 3, these maturational and developmental changes can be conceptualized within the framework of how emotions continue to be children's main organizers for achieving 1) energy mobilization, 2) self-regulation, and 3) social adaptation.

■ Emotions as Energy Mobilizers

By age 3 years, children have already stored many emotional memories within their preconscious and unconscious mental domains. *Emotional memories* are memories that have emotional components in addition to whatever ideational components they may possess (e.g., olfactory, visual, auditory, or kinesthetic perceptions; fantasies; beliefs; behavioral responses, skills, or procedures). As I discuss in Chapter 1, most memories up until about age 2½ years are implicit memories. Those that contain emotional components are classified as *emotional implicit memories*. All implicit memories contain information about procedures or learned skills, but, as noted in Chapter 1, the content of those memories or how they were formed cannot be consciously recalled.

For example, a 1-year-old boy begins to walk away from his parents to explore his environment. His parents are encouraging and begin to give him their mirroring smiles in response to his own mastery smiles as he achieves competency in using walking to assertively explore. In time, he will store an emotional implicit memory of these walking experiences within his unconscious. In the future, this emotional implicit memory will be activated unconsciously and automatically when his innate need to explore his environment assertively is stimulated. The memory is an energy mobilizer that motivates this toddler to repeat the previous pleasure he experienced in walking. He does not need to remember consciously his past feelings of pleasure in walking before deciding to walk. Walking has become an automatic behavior that is unconsciously motivated by emotionally pleasurable implicit memories. An automatic behavior can also be unconsciously motivated by emotionally displeasurable implicit memories. A toddler boy who has experienced displeasurable emotions with regard to his walking may begin to avoid walking away from his parents to explore so that he can avoid repeating his past experiences of being scolded. He will begin to become inhibited and also begin to construct external locus-of-control beliefs. It is important to note how unconscious emotionally pleasurable and displeasurable implicit memories exert a silent energy-mobilizing influence on children's motivation to behave.

By age 2½ years, in addition to previously stored unconscious implicit memories, explicit memories will begin to be constructed and stored as unconscious, preconscious, and conscious explicit memories. These memories are stored through declarative knowledge, explained by Clyman (1991) as

> information that can be learned, stored in memory and later recalled. [Declarative knowledge] stores memories for facts or events that have been experienced, and it is represented either in language or in sensory images, such as mental pictures. Declarative knowledge is symbolic, in that the thought always refers to something else, its meaning, or referent. Declarative knowledge, however, may be conscious, preconscious, or unconscious. (p. 351)

For example, a mother introduces her 3-year-old daughter to the task of learning how to tie shoes. Initially, the daughter begins to construct executive control structures in learning this task; she engages in controlled procedures (Clyman 1991) through a trial-and-error learning process of assimilation and accommodation. If this shoe-tying task is within her capabilities, she will have fun learning how to tie her shoes. After a few weeks, she masters the task. The emotional memory she constructs of the entire experience contains explicit knowledge (i.e., her words and her mother's words of instruction, her pleasurable feelings in mastering the task of tying her shoes, and what tying her own shoes symbolically means to her, both in what she believes it means to be able to tie her shoes and what she may fantasize about what it means to possess this new procedural skill). In time, this emotional explicit memory will be slowly transformed into an emotional implicit memory and be relegated to the girl's unconscious. This occurs, as Clyman (1991) has stated, because,

> when controlled emotional procedures have become automatic with practice, the conscious feeling no longer needs to be experienced in order to execute the procedure, as conscious attention is no longer required. (p. 361)

Thus a well-learned task that originally required explicit knowledge in its learning has now become an unconscious emotional implicit memory. When this girl reaches age 6 years and is asked, "What do you remember about what happened when you learned to tie your shoes?" she might reply, "I don't remember. I just know how to do it. I guess my mom and dad showed me. Now I just do it. I don't have to think about how to do it anymore." This child is illustrating another fact about the storage and expression of emotional memories: whereas explicit knowledge can be remembered, implicit knowledge can only be enacted (Clyman 1991; Fivush 1993; Graf 1990; Terr 1994).

Not all explicit memories constructed by a child are equal in importance or significance in a child's life. Those constructed explicit memories that involve experiences in which children experienced and continue to experience a high intensity of emotions, either highly pleasurable or somewhat displeasurable, will tend to be stored and retained as preconscious—and hence recallable—emotional explicit memories. As I describe in Chapter 4, explicit memories can be episodic (i.e., they do not involve a high degree of emotionality or any particular personal meaning) or autobiographical (i.e., they contain a high degree of emotionality and usually contain a personal meaning both in what the event meant in the child's life and in how the child views himself or herself). Autobiographical memories become the sum and substance of a child's self-representation. They give the child a conscious awareness of his or her temporal stability as an emotional being with an identity that exists over time. These highly symbolic, emotional autobiographical memories remain intact and do not lose their explicit content to become unconscious implicit memories. In fact, many of these autobiographical memories are revised and added to as the developmental process unfolds. It also needs to be noted, as I discuss in Chapter 1, that explicit memories with a highly displeasurable emotional content will invariably be repressed into a child's unconscious (see below).

In early childhood, children will tend to store emotional explicit autobiographical memories within their preconscious when they have a certain degree of emotion, either pleasurable (e.g., the day a child hit a home run on the little league team) or displeasurable (e.g., experiences with a teacher who always made mean and derogatory comments). Just like unconscious emotional implicit memories, the recall of these explicit memories will function as energy mobilizers (or internal motivators) that propel children to seek to repeat emotionally pleasurable experiences (e.g., telephone a little league teammate) or seek to avoid repeating emotional displeasurable experiences (e.g., avoid talking to the teacher after class).

For example, a 4-year-old girl began to ask her mother if she could learn to dress herself. The mother, who was a psychotherapy patient of mine, reported to me, "I just don't like how she is becoming so independent so fast. Each morning we have a battle: I dress her one way, then she takes off her clothes and demands to dress herself another way." The mother was a single parent, recently divorced, and was clinging to her only daughter, whom she viewed as wanting to get away from her. Although this mother's psycho-therapy eventually helped her to become less inhibiting of her daughter's healthy development of an autonomous identity, it is easy to imagine how in another scenario such a mother would make her daughter's overall experience of dressing herself an emotion-ally displeasurable one. If this girl's emotional displeasure was not so excessive that it led her to feel a sense of rage, intense anxiety, and helplessness—characteristics of a traumatic experience—then her emotional explicit autobiographical memory would be stored as a preconscious memory of high symbolic significance: it would symbolize this girl's struggle with her mother to win her autonomy and assert her need to take over more management of her own body. The girl might construct a highly emotional autobiographical belief such as, "I hated to get dressed in the morning because my mother never liked what I wore."

But what about the emotional explicit autobiographical mem-ory of a traumatic experience? This type of emotional explicit mem-ory will be relegated to a child's unconscious. In Chapter 1, I designate this type of emotional explicit memory as an *uncon-scious dynamic memory,* where dynamic refers to the mind's use of defense mechanisms, notably repression, to push the emotional explicit autobiographical memory out of the conscious domain and into the unconscious domain. The unconscious dynamic explicit memory does not lose its explicit content but becomes incorpo-rated into the primary process thinking mode of the unconscious (Person 1995; Terr 1994). These types of memories exert a silent influence on children's perceptions of their current experiences and will lead them to unconsciously enact certain behaviors in an attempt to re-create aspects of and repeat the trauma in a new, more masterful way. (This tendency to repeat trauma-related be-haviors and attempt to re-create the trauma in order to achieve more feelings of competency pleasure and a sense of control—known as the *repetition principle*—is discussed more fully in Chap-ter 4 in the section on the functions of play.) In this case, the intensely displeasurable unconscious emotions associated with the repressed memory act as an unconscious energy mobilizer. It is as if a child's mind does not tolerate a repressed unconscious dynamic memory by just storing it away in the recesses of a child's unconscious. In effect, the unconscious mind causes a child to repeat certain behaviors associated with the trauma as a way of remembering in action, not in thought.

Three factors seem to assist children in their attempt not just to re-create the traumatic situation but to repeat trauma-related behaviors and achieve a sense of mastery by constructing a fantasy and eventually a new belief that fuels their positive expectancy that in the future they will be the active victor over frightening experiences:

1. *Their relationship with their parents and others*—Parents' ability, after the occurrence of the original trauma, to continue to provide an environment of safety, protection, and admiring feedback will assist a child in eventually reaffirming his or her pretrauma belief in the parents' ability to protect him or her from future traumatic episodes. This reaffirmation also prevents the child from resurrecting and maintaining his or her wish for an ideal self or ideal object representation as a denial in fantasy that he or she will never be again exposed to a frightening experience.
2. *Their advances in cognitive thinking*—Children who have recently developed a new cognitive ability may be able to use this new ability to come up with a new creative solution to a past traumatic event (e.g., they realize something now that they could have done at the time of the original trauma that would have protected them or enabled them to flee in some way).
3. *Their capacity to extract resources from their environment*—Children who are able to seek and find more psychologically attuned and empathic people (e.g., relatives, friends, teachers, coaches) to associate with assist themselves in working through past traumas as well as protect themselves from being retraumatized.

As young children use both their unconscious implicit memories and their unconsciously repressed dynamic explicit memories as energy mobilizers in deciding to act or not act, they begin to learn more about what specific behavioral strategies they can use to express or withhold their emotions. In early childhood, they begin to construct *emotional display rules* (Maletesta and Haviland

1982; these are what Clyman [1991] called *emotional control structures*). These are the emotional rules and procedures learned by children about 1) whether it is permissible to consciously feel their different emotions and 2) whether it is permissible to verbally express their different emotions and how each emotion is allowed to be expressed.

In psychologically attuned families, children learn developmentally enhancing emotional display rules in two ways. First, they learn them automatically (e.g., learning whether it is permissible to say when they are sad), after which the emotional display rules become automatically activated unconscious procedural memories. For example, a 5-year-old boy is asked, "Is it okay to say you are sad in your family?" He says, "Sure it is." He then is asked, "How do you know that?" He answers, "I just know it. I can say I'm sad and my dad and mom will listen to me and say it's okay that I'm telling them." This child does not have to ponder whether it is permissible to feel sad and verbalize those sad feelings. He just enacts the procedures of verbalizing his sad feelings and generates a positive expectation that he will feel better after having verbalized them.

On the other hand, a child may grow up in a family where he or she learns that he or she must not consciously feel a certain emotion and definitely not express it verbally or even, in some cases, behaviorally. The following example illustrates this:

> I interviewed a 6-year-old child as part of an evaluation for his inattention in the first grade and for his periodic severe stuttering problem. During most of the interview in my office playroom, his stuttering was barely noticeable until I asked how he felt when his dog had to be put to sleep 1 month earlier (the dog had been in the family since before his birth). He began to stutter severely as he said, "I felt okay." The following week when I asked his father, "Tell me what you and your wife have told your two sons about being sad," the father quite angrily told me, "In our family, we have no time for sadness. It's a useless feeling and I don't tolerate it. My sons know that if they feel sad or depressed that I'll send them to their room until they get those feelings out of their mind."
>
> Because it was so dangerous to feel and express sadness in his family, the boy had learned and then repressed this emotional

display rule into his dynamic unconscious. Now quite automatically, as when I asked him about how he felt about his dog (obviously he must have felt sad as well as perhaps angry), he activated the procedures in his repressed emotional display rule: he denied having any feelings and automatically used stuttering as a somatizing defense mechanism to bar his unconscious sadness from entering his consciousness.

The second way children learn developmentally enhancing emotional display rules is by being consciously motivated to learn which behaviors trigger their parents' approval and which do not. For example, a 4½-year-old girl gets angry at her younger brother and throws a toy at him, saying, "You shit!" Her mother takes her aside and says, "Okay. Let's go through what we do in this house when we get angry. We don't hit or throw, but we talk. And when we talk, we don't use curse words, but it's okay to say you're angry." If this girl has a goodness of fit with her mother, she will be motivated to listen to what her mother is teaching her is the emotional display rule for the expression of anger in her family. The mother is also helping her daughter go from action dominance to speech dominance. Thus emotional display rules help children learn to use their emotions as energy mobilizers in a manner that adapts their innate needs to the needs of their parents.

■ Emotions as Self-Regulators

In early childhood, children also use their emotions as organizers for developing their capacity for self-regulation. In this respect, they are assisted by a maturational advance occurring at about age 3 or 4 years, when they are able to consciously experience not only a wider range of emotions but also different shades of emotions (Lane and Schwartz 1987). Being happy is no longer one state; children can now perceive within themselves and in others that there are degrees of happiness. In being better able to internally and externally perceive and discriminate many more emotions than they were able to before age 3 years, children become better able to self-regulate their own emotions. For example, with their emerging capacity to differentiate when they are slightly angry versus being very angry, they are able to act or speak in certain ways that will regulate their own anger and often prevent it from becoming excessive. They also become more capable of perceiving shades of emotions in their parents, which allows them to assess better what to do to keep the interaction with their parents in a mutually pleasurable range and what to do to return the interaction to a pleasurable range when it has becoming displeasurable. They now begin to become more proficient at using their emotions as internal signals of distress and using the displeasurable emotions of their parents as their possible external signals of distress.

When 3-year-old children who have attained positive self-constancy and object constancy experience distress, this distress can be ameliorated when they experience the internal sense of their parents' love and protection. When they cannot resolve their own internal emotional distress, they desire to believe that their parents will. Parents validate their children's belief when they use empathy in verbalizing what their children may be distressed about or teach them other behaviors that will alleviate their feelings of distress. Subsequently, young children begin to achieve a new type of competency pleasure—which further develops their autonomous self—when they are able to talk or act, often in identifying with their parents, and alleviate their internal distress. When they are successful, they gain experience in believing they can regulate their own feelings more than when they were younger.

One feeling in particular that becomes important for them to regulate is anxiety. Young children gradually become more proficient not only in recognizing when they feel anxious but also in discriminating what they are anxious about. In becoming increasingly able to perceive anxiety as a signal, they become able to recognize that they may be anxious about one of the following possible developmental calamities befalling them if they do not alleviate their anxiety: the loss of their parents' love and value for them (i.e., Kohut's [1971] disintegration anxiety), abandonment (i.e., S. Freud's [1923/1963] separation anxiety), and physical punishment (i.e., S. Freud's [1923/1963] body damage anxiety; this is discussed further under "Development of the Self and Object Relationships," below). The following illustrates a little girl's being motivated by her anxiety that she would lose her mother's love:

A 4½-year-old girl was in her kindergarten class when her teacher stated there would be no playing outside that day. She became acutely anxious and abruptly wanted to leave the class. She did not leave, however, but remained in the room. Later that day, I interviewed her as part of a study on normally developing children. She told me, "I'm real proud. I wanted to leave kindergarten when my teacher said 'No playing outside today' because it was raining. Big deal! So what if it was raining? I wanted to just go outside myself. But then I got a little afraid [i.e., anxious] when I remembered that my mom said she'd be angry at me if I didn't obey the teacher. So I stayed. I didn't want to get punished."

■ Emotions as Facilitators of Social Adaptation

In early childhood, children use their emotions as they continue to improve their social adaptation. In so doing, they attempt to achieve an internal adaptation to their innate needs and an external adaptation to the developmental taskings and rules of their parents and society.

Young children usually achieve self-regulation and social adaptation concurrently. More often than not, their internal adaptation is not achieved at the expense of their external adaptation. For example, children do not adapt to their innate need to be assertive while completely disregarding their external adaptation to their parents' rules about limits on their assertive will. Unbridled assertion might momentarily make children feel good inside, but they would then have to deal with others in their social world (e.g., their angry parents) if their assertive behaviors disregarded family or societal rules. Unless children's parents are not teaching their children about limits—thus producing an extremely self-centered child whose ideal representation of being omnipotent with no restrictions becomes their prominent self-representation—children's unbridled joyful assertion will turn into anxiety about their parents' angry displeasure. Children's continued ability and need to engage in emotional referencing enables them to use their parents' emotions (and shades of those emotions) to help them achieve social adaptation. As Zajonic (1980) noted, "It is much less important for us to know whether someone has just said 'you are a friend' or 'you are a fiend' than to know whether it was spoken in contempt or with affection" (p. 153).

Although children's social adaptation will suffer when they are attempting to achieve internal adaptation at the expense of external adaptation (and ignore their parents' signals of emotional displeasure in response to their behaviors), their social adaptation will also suffer when their parents' taskings and rules are excessive. A poorness of fit will then develop that children will forever be achieving external adaptation while giving up achieving a healthy degree of internal adaptation. To adapt to their parents' unreasonable tasks and rules, children automatically begin to internally flee from perceiving one or more of their innate needs, because the gratification of these needs brings intense criticism, physical punishment, or something similar. This hypertrophy of external adaptation at the expense of internal adaptation is called *developmentally inhibiting social adaptation*. It leads children to develop a false self, false in that they are not being true to their own emotions. They silently experience anger, sadness, and anxiety when they adapt to their parents' taskings and rules while their own innate needs go unanswered. To achieve social adaptation in their family, such children's emotions eventually become unconscious signals of distress, propelling them to use their own defense mechanisms to eventually keep them from perceiving their own frustrated innate needs and associated displeasurable emotions. They must defend against experiencing their own emotions, especially when the emotional display rules in their family prohibit their angry rebellion in response to their parents' neglect of their innate needs. After a while, a family's emotional display rules—here, its emotional nondisplay rules—will become relegated to the children's unconscious, and these children will begin to automatically do and say things to not feel angry or sad about their lack of gratification. In time, such children will begin to believe that they do not have a need, for example, to assert themselves and will never become angry when their assertion is restricted. The boy in the following example was such a child:

> The parents of a 4-year-old boy being evaluated for his passive and intense behavioral inhibition told me, "We are ashamed to

say how much we both hated him in the first few years of his life because we blamed him for all the problems we were having in being married to each other. If we had not had him, we would have split up." In an interview with the boy, he sat almost motionless in a chair despite my telling him he could explore the playroom. When I asked if he wanted to play with any of the many toys he could easily see, he said "No," sounding very sad. When I commented, "How are you feeling today?" he said, "Just fine."

Maturation and Development of Verbal Language Abilities

Development of Verbal Language for Script or Story Expression

In early childhood, children's maturationally emerging abilities to acquire new vocabulary, new syntax rules, and new complex sentence structures all contribute to the development of their use of verbal language to further enhance their 1) self-esteem, 2) self-assertion and autonomy, 3) self and object interdependence, and 4) self-regulation and social adaptation.

In particular, children's words begin to become as important as their play actions in expressing their fantasies. Young children's fantasies are a combination of their current thoughts, recalled memories, and predictions of the future (Garvey and Kramer 1989). Beginning around age 3 years, children try to use thought, speech, and behaviors to achieve some belief in anticipating and predicting what will happen in the future. Also, they begin to remember their past—known as *reproductive memory*—and ask questions of themselves and their parents about why things happened in the past. In this process, they begin to engage in *reconstructive memory* (Perry 1992; Piaget and Inhelder 1973), which is when they generate a fantasy based on their recalling a memory and reconstruct the memory to enhance its pleasurable emotionality in some way or change its displeasurable emotionality into a pleasurable one. Many of these memories and their reconstructions are expressed in children's stories (Beal and Flavell 1984; Hudson 1990, 1993).

During early childhood, children increasingly improve their ability to express their wishes, fantasies, beliefs, and memories in spoken and written stories (Pitcher and Prelinger 1963) or scripts (Slackman and Nelson 1984; Trad 1992). Hudson (1993) defined *scripts* as "mental structures which organize information about the sequence of predictable actions, locations, roles and props that constitute events" (p. 142). For example, by the time a 4-year-old child has attended his or her preschool class on a daily basis for a few months, the child will have constructed scripts for what happens when he or she enters the classroom, when lunchtime arrives, and how he or she meets his or her mother in the carpool line. Children also use verbal language to reveal many aspects of their conscious, preconscious, and unconscious representational worlds. In this respect, their stories contain elements of both primary process and secondary process thinking (Gobnik and Graft 1988). In composing stories and verbalizing them to their parents and others, children learn to differentiate between magical and reality-based thinking. Stories, therefore, help children develop the ego function of reality testing.

In early childhood, storytelling performs many of the functions that play did in toddlerhood (see Chapter 4). These functions include the following:

1. *To verbalize and enhance a pleasurable life experience by assigning various roles to characters who symbolize the children themselves, their parents, or others, and their emotions or wishes.* Although these pleasurable stories may, and often do, contain some of children's developmental anxieties, in the end the storyteller usually achieves a certain kind of competency pleasure in that he or she has achieved a feeling of pleasure in creating a story that is pleasing. The following is an example of such a story told to me by a 5-year-old girl after she had spent the preceding day on a special visit to the zoo with her father. It is notable that she had the positive expectation that I would enjoy her story:

> Today, here's the story. I want to tell you [smiling], you are my father and I'm me. We are going to the zoo but then we

> will go to Disney World on a special plane. We will have so much fun. And Mom and my brother won't care, because they will do something fun together. When we get home, Dad says, "What a great idea to go to Disney World!"

Although there is the hidden element in this story of this girl's wish for an exclusive relationship with her father and her worry about her mother's reactive envy and retaliation, she creates a story that brings her much pleasure—even more pleasure than her real trip to the zoo with her father had the day before.

2. *To verbalize those wishes and emotions that are causing both internal and external conflicts, and compose various creative solutions to these conflicts that are different from reality.* Because stories express children's fantasies, their wishes and feelings are often disguised in symbolic representations. For example, Pitcher and Prelinger (1963) reported this story told by a 4¾-year-old boy:

> Once there was a baby eagle and a mother eagle. One day, the mother eagle went into the store. The baby eagle flew away. The mother eagle came back. The baby wasn't there. So the mother eagle flew away to find the baby eagle. She found the baby eagle. He came back to his nest. Then at night the father came back. (p. 86)

The story contains elements of this boy's work on his separation anxiety, which is stimulated when his mother leaves him. In his story, he flies away when his mother goes into the store. This may be his repressed wish to test his mother's love by leaving her and then seeing if she will come after him. At the end of the story, the family is back together.

3. *To rewrite a previous traumatic experience into a new story in which the child is not the victim but the victor.* As I note in this and other chapters, children who have experienced a trauma invariably repress the emotional explicit autobiographical memory of the experience. In the future, they will tend to unconsciously enact certain trauma-related behaviors and experience trauma-related fears (Terr 1990). When the

traumatic memory is stimulated by a current perception that is related to the original trauma, children become motivated to tell a story without realizing how the story is an attempt to rewrite the original trauma in which they experienced themselves as a helpless victim, undo the intensely displeasurable feelings they have stored within their unconscious, and construct a new, developmentally enhancing memory in which they view themselves as an assertive victor; in this way, they replace the grim, developmentally inhibiting memory of the traumatic experience. The story is often fragmented, and the theme is often difficult to decipher unless the listener knows the facts of the original trauma. Terr (1991) gave an example of such a story:

> Three and a half years after experiencing a series of traumatic events, a 5-year-old was discovered [through pornographic photographs confiscated by U.S. Customs agents] to have been sexually misused in a day care home between the ages of 15 and 18 months. The girl's parents did not dare speak to her about what they had learned from the investigators. They, in retrospect, realized that she had been sketching hundreds of nude adults beginning from the time when she had first begun to draw. . . . Despite the fact that the little girl's only verbal memory of the events was "I think there was grave danger at a lady's—Mary Beth's—house," her volumes of drawings represented strongly visualized elements that she had retained and had needed to re-create from these very early, nonverbal experiences. (p. 12)

Continuing Influence of Preexisting Representational World

Development of Accommodation-Transformation and Hierarchical-Restructuring Processes

In early childhood, as young children's cognitive capabilities continue to develop to process all the maturational changes in their innate needs, physical capabilities, temperamental characteristics, emotions, and language, they begin to increasingly engage in hierarchical reorganizations of their preexisting and ever-developing representational world (Werner 1940). This prioritization will be based on their ability to think about which people in their life are most important in helping them both gratify their innate needs and maintain their self-esteem.

At this time, children's developing·capacity for self-reflection fuels their mind's use of the accommodation-transformation principle. In learning more about what others will and will not do to help them meet their innate needs, children transform some of their object representations of their parents, siblings, and others. Accordingly, certain beliefs about their parents will be transformed into new beliefs, based not only on new experiences with their parents but also on children's new cognitive ability to transform preexistent object representations.

For example, in coming to understand the concept of reversibility of actions, children begin to realize that if they are currently angry at their mother, they will be able to reverse this angry experience into a loving experience at a later time. Such an appreciation of a future in which they can wish, feel, or act in a manner opposite to their current one toward their parents gives them the capacity to transform and reconstruct their object representations to include the concept of inverse relationships (Greenspan 1979).

Development of the Self and Object Relationships

As I note in Chapter 4, by age 3 years, children have begun to construct the sequence of subidentities that make up their overall identity. Thus, by the time they reach early childhood, they have constructed an autonomous identity that enables them to explore away from their parents without intense separation anxiety. They have also already constructed a gender identity and have attained positive self-constancy and object constancy in that they know their parents are not ambivalent about whether to love them in their autonomous excursions and in their gender development. They know their parents are emotionally constant in their love for them and that their episodes of anger toward them do not make their parents reassess whether they truly love them and do not make children reassess whether they truly love their parents. Thus, although children's continuing autonomous development may make their parents angry at them (e.g., when they disobey a rule), and parents likewise make their children angry at them (e.g., when they refuse their children's wishes), 3-year-old children are beginning to worry no longer about losing their parents' fundamental love and admiration during these "angry ripples," nor are they excessively worried that they will stop loving their parents.

The attainment of an positive self-constancy enables young children to begin to value and love themselves as their parents value and love them. In other words, in beginning to carry within their representational world a primarily positive self-constancy, they confidently look outside of their primary relationship with their parents and toward their own body and social world of siblings, peers, and others.

■ Development of a Sexual Identity: Emergence of the Genital-Narcissistic Phase

In addition to continuing to learn what it means to be a boy or a girl in their society (in continuing to develop their gender identity), 3-year-old children begin to construct a sexual identity. A *sexual identity* is one's view of oneself that has to do with all the emotions, fantasies, beliefs, and behaviors that are involved in the stimulation and gratification of one's innate need to seek pleasurable sensual-sexual gratification. (Some developmentalists follow Stoller's [1976, 1985] classification. He defined *core gender identity*, established by age 3 years, as children's "unquestioned, unthinking conviction—a piece of identity—that they are male or female" [p. 55]. He then defined *gender identity* as all the beliefs and fantasies children possess about what it means to be masculine or feminine. However, I find it less confusing to separate gender identity from sexual identity for this reason: a boy, for example, can possess a firm set of beliefs that define himself as being a man, while possessing a sexual identity can be either heterosexual or homosexual. His gender identity, therefore, does not dictate his sexual identity. The same holds for girls.)

Precursors of a sexual identity take place during the oral phase (in infancy) and anal phase (in toddlerhood) (S. Freud 1923/1963). Parents shape their children's oral and anal gratification and do not overly stimulate their oral or anal mucosa. As I discuss under "Maturation and Development of Innate Needs," above, around age 3 years, the primary focus of children's sensual stimulation shifts to the genital region (Galenson 1993). In constructing a beginning sexual identity, children ages 3–4 years construct two new category representations: sensual-sexual behaviors of boys and sensual-sexual behaviors of girls. They begin to construct these categories as they concentrate more on learning how to achieve genital pleasure and how their genitals may be involved in their relationships with the parents and others. The beginning construction of these categories ushers in the *(infantile) genital-narcissistic phase* (Edgecumbe and Burgner 1975). This phase, which occurs at about ages 3–4 years, is so named because children develop much self-love, or narcissistic preoccupation, with their genitals. Two components of this body narcissism are exhibitionism and curiosity.

Exhibitionism of genitals. The exhibitionism of the genital-narcissistic phase becomes evident in children's prideful manner of showing off their genitals. This behavior indicates that children have begun to construct a sexual identity (Edgecumbe and Burgner 1975). In the initial unfoldings of the genital-narcissistic phase, children are quite intensely exhibitionistic. They admire their own body and are intensely joyous in receiving mirroring smiles of admiration from both parents. The need for admiration is without shame. For example, a 4-year-old boy entered his parents' bedroom one morning and proudly showed his erect penis, stating, "See, Dad, mine goes up just like yours!" In another example, a 4-year-old girl was being interviewed as she took part in a study on normal development. As I played at building a block tower with her, she periodically got up to dance and spin around until she was satisfied that I could see her underwear beneath her dress. Suddenly she commented, "I have beautiful legs like a ballerina. I wish I could take my dress off so you could see my whole body."

The examples above illustrate, however, a basic difference in the exhibitionism of boys versus that of girls in the genital-narcissistic phase. Boys have a ready organ on which to focus. The penis is outside, visible, and manipulatable; boys can make it "grow" by making it erect. They seek the admiration of their parents for their beautiful penis and like to show how erect they can make it become. However, their need to be curious, particularly in looking at the genitals of their parents and siblings, makes them eventually aware that their father's or another man's penis is much bigger than theirs.

Although girls do not have such an externally visible organ on which to focus, their genital region is as easily accessible and manipulated. Girls eventually learn that their vagina is an organ that is primarily a cavity, and that their reproductive organs are internal in contrast to boys' external penis and scrotum with its testicles. Girls ages 3–4 years slowly learn that they have a clitoris, primarily through learning how to manipulate their genital region, but initially do not have a clear sense of its shape and stimulation properties. In the process of establishing her gender identity (by age 2½ years),

> a girl's genitals and their associated diffuse, whole body sensations, are experienced as integral and protected, yet easily located and stimulated, part of her body from the beginning; they are not experienced as an appendage seemingly vulnerable to loss as is the case with the male. Therefore, defining a sense of body integrity is normally a smooth process for the girl, despite certain difficulties in mentally representing her genitals [within her self-representation]. (P. Tyson 1994, p. 422)

As girls learn about breasts, they begin to value their mother's breasts, while knowing that boys can never develop them the way girls can. Edgecumbe and Burgner (1975) have theorized that, because of the lack of one organizing organ on which to focus their genital preoccupations, girls tend to view their entire body as boys view their penis alone. Thus, as in the above example, 4-year-old girls may want to exhibit their entire body.

Curiosity about genitals. Boys' and girls' intense curiosity about their sexual organs is really an outgrowth of normal 3- to 4-year-old children's assertive innate need to continue to explore their body and their parents' bodies, particularly both parents' genitals and the mother's breasts. Young children want to follow their mother, father, and siblings into the bathroom to watch them undress, take showers with them, watch their mother change a baby sibling, engage in pretend play of being a doctor so they can examine the genitals of another child (Noshpitz and King 1991), and attempt to look at and touch the genitals of their parents or the breasts of their mother. For example, one 3½-year-old boy, concurrent with his repeatedly telling his mother that he was a "big boy" who stood up "like the boys to do pee-pee in the pot," began to periodically attempt to fondle his mother's breasts whenever she held him in her arms. Freidrich et al. (1991) assessed the frequency of sexually related behaviors in children ages 4–6 years. They reported that these children engaged in the following behaviors: scratching their crotches, touching their genitals at home and in public, masturbating with their hands or by rubbing against their parents, undressing in front of others and attempting to see parents and siblings undress, exposing their underwear or genitals while sitting, and attempting to touch their mothers' breasts.

As for previous manifestations of their children's assertive will, parents begin to teach their children about the limits on their sexual curiosity; in the process, they teach them about a developmental task associated with constructing a sexual identity: the necessity of learning about body privacy. Children eventually learn that they can masturbate, but in private; that bathroom time is private; and that they must sleep alone while their parents can sleep together, bathe together, and stay in the bathroom at the same time. Obviously, children become intrigued with these facts about their parents, particularly the fact that their parents have a physically intimate relationship that excludes children. For example, the mother of the 3½-year-old boy noted above gently but firmly would remove his hands from her breasts, telling him that he should not touch her there. After a few more times when he attempted to touch her breasts, followed by her punishing him by making him sit in a corner for several minutes, he adopted this restriction into his conscience and ceased this behavior.

Children's curiosity about their genitals, the rules about exhibiting them within the family, and the use and function of their parents' genitals raise questions that become quite important to children. Parents must answer their children's questions with empathy for their children's feelings lest they cause their children to begin to think that they are doing something bad in taking the initiative to be curious in asking such questions. For example, 3- to 4-year-old children will ask their parents many questions about where babies come from, who can have babies, what are the family rules about nudity, and so on. Erikson (1963) labeled the psychosocial task in early childhood as the need for children to attain a belief that they can be able to express initiative and curiosity without an overriding feeling of guilt. Erikson was discussing the danger of guilt feelings that may be evoked if children's genital-narcissistic interests and actions are not supported and protected by their parents. (Here "protected" refers to parents' setting limits on their children's initiative and curiosity, lest their children's developing autonomous, gender, and sexual identities lead them into highly displeasurable situations.)

Body damage anxiety. Although parents provide encouragement for and at the same time protect their young children in asserting their genital exhibitionism and curiosity about genital issues, they will begin to hear them talk about a new developmental anxiety: body damage anxiety. *Body damage anxiety* is another of the developmental anxieties that S. Freud (1923/1963) defined as inevitable. It results from children's fearing the possibility of a new developmental calamity in which their body is damaged, particularly their genitals or genital area. Freud, in emphasizing the penis as the predominant body part that both boys and girls highly value, called this latter specific body damage anxiety as *castration anxiety*. (I believe the term *body damage anxiety* better reflects a more generic anxiety in the boy and the girl.)

As 3- to 4-year-old children explore their body and social world, they make new discoveries about the vulnerability of their body. The normal hurts, scrapes, and falls inherent in their experimentations and explorations create a worry in children about possible damage to their body, as is illustrated in the following example:

> A 3-year-old girl begins playing with a beetle. In her moving the bug with a stick she accidentally crushes it. She tells the bug, "Move!" but the bug does not move. She seeks her mother and tells her about the squashed bug. The mother says, "The bug is dead; it can't move anymore." This girl will begin to transfer this scenario between herself and the bug as a possible scenario between herself and another person bigger than her (e.g., her mother). She may stop exploring for a day or two as she worries, "Can I be stepped on too?" Suddenly, a new interest will emerge in her: she becomes preoccupied with using band-aids to reassure herself that she can be assertive in "fixing" herself if her body becomes damaged in some way.

Parents need to ensure that their children's genital-narcissistic–motivated curiosity and exhibitionism are limited to prevent them from frequently physically hurting themselves, which only increases the frequency and intensity of episodes of body damage anxiety. Sometimes it is not easy to maintain limits on behaviors that may be dangerous, as, for example, when a son is enjoying himself immensely in running around the backyard with a stick between his legs (as a possible symbol for his erect penis). Parents also need to ensure that their children are protected from having too many body damage experiences inflicted by others (e.g., not choose a pediatrician who is abrupt and unempathic but choose one who is gentle and patient and tries to minimize children's body damage anxiety).

However, some events that will increase children's body damage anxiety may occur, despite parents' best efforts. For example, the death of an important person in the life of children ages 3–6 years will provoke both separation and body damage anxieties, particularly in stimulating children's anxieties that one or both of their parents will die. As a result, these children will often activate the defense mechanism of denial. This denial is usually manifested in fantasy, wherein children's play and story composition will reveal some variant of the following compensatory fantasy: "I am not afraid of being left alone if my parents die, and I'm not even afraid of ever getting hurt." This fantasy signals their resurrection of their ideal self to the position of prominence. Thus, for a while, their behavior may be characterized by daredevilish deeds or by their not heeding their parents' rules (e.g., be careful of strangers, do not ride a bike in the street).

Another response children may have to a death or some other event that stimulates intense body damage anxiety (e.g., a physical accident) is to regress to behaviors and ways of talking that were prominent at an earlier developmental age. Regression may occur immediately after the event but can also develop gradually when other initially activated defense mechanisms (e.g., denial in fantasy) do not alleviate children's high level of separation and body damage anxieties. In either case, the regressive behaviors that result are often designated as symptoms of a childhood adjustment disorder. This is a diagnosis made retrospectively after a physician has observed that a child's regressive symptoms occurred following a stressful event and were short-lived.

The struggle against resurrecting an ideal self-representation and object representations to a position of prominence. As I mention above, young children will respond to events that generate high levels of body damage anxiety by resurrecting their ideal self-representation and ideal parent representations, at least to some degree. However, it needs to be emphasized that this occurs less often after age 3 years—when they have developed positive self-constancy and object constancy—than before that age. Thus the angry feelings children have toward their parents for not protecting them from experiencing intense body damage anxiety will not dominate their loving feelings for their parents. No matter how angry children may become at their parents, they still believe that their parents will be able to protect them from experiencing excessive body damage anxiety in the future. This belief is justified only to the extent that parents can prevent their children from being exposed to too many intense body damage anxiety experiences; any child's positive self-constancy and object constancy will likely be disrupted if that child is exposed to too many separation and body damage events. If this occurs, the child will no longer believe in his or her parents' ability to protect him or her; the child's resultant level of anxiety is so severe that it affects his or her development. Even young children who are being raised in a psychologically aware family and have their positive self-constancy and object constancy in place may still respond to body damage experiences with some degree of wishing that they were omnipotent (their ideal self-fantasy) or their parents were omnipotent (their ideal parent fantasies).

In early childhood, children are still struggling with accepting the limitations and imperfections in their parents and themselves (Herzog 1982, 1984). With regard to their parents, they do not immediately accept the limitations of their parents in not always being able to respond and soothe them empathically. However, parents intuitively know that they cannot always empathically respond to their children's distress signals (they could if they were perfect with perfect empathy). Also, parents intuitively know that when they gradually do not respond to their children's every distress signal, they invite them to develop their ego function of self-soothing and self-regulating their emotions. With regard to themselves, children do not accept this invitation without a fight, so to speak. They resurrect their fantasy of possessing an ideal self-representation in response to their parents' asking them to accept their limitations and immediately and effectively soothe themselves. They tell their parents that they are perfect and wonderful and want to have their parents tell them the same thing. (For example, the child depicted in the cartoon in Figure 5–1 wants his father to support his wish to view himself as a perfect young baseball player.)

According to self psychology theory (Kohut 1971), when children resurrect these ideal representations, their parents' role is to respect and tolerate these images; at the same time, parents know that as their children contend with life's inevitable distresses using their growing cognitive, emotional, and self-reflective capabilities, thereby becoming more aware of their and their parents' imperfections, they will relinquish these ideal representations. This occurs as children internalize their parents' ongoing realistic admiration and support of their performances, including children's experiences of soothing themselves when they experience anxiety. This internalization leads to children's constructing realistic ambitions (Kohut 1971). The development of healthy ambitions and ideals is a long process that goes on all during childhood and into adolescence (see Chapter 7, on adolescence).

THE FAMILY CIRCUS ®   **By Bil Keane**

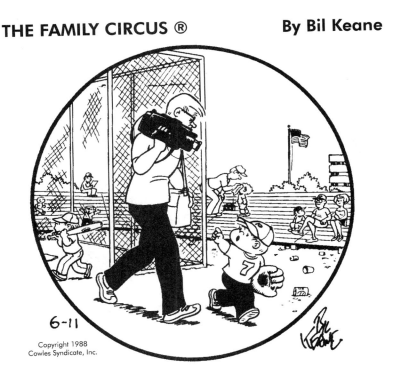

6-11

Copyright 1988
Cowles Syndicate, Inc.

"Daddy! You've gotta erase my strikeouts and errors from that tape."

Figure 5–1. Cartoon depicting a boy's need to resurrect his ideal self-representation to a position of prominence in viewing himself.
Source. Reprinted with special permission of Cowles Syndicate, Inc., New York, New York.

Parents of young children can inhibit rather than assist the process through which their children relinquish their wishes to have perfect parents and to be perfect. One way is when parents are uncomfortable with their children's idealization of them and do not allow them to view them—albeit transiently—as perfect, as in the following example:

> A 4-year-old boy experiences severe body damage anxiety when he is hit in the eye with a baseball by his older brother. He then seeks out his father and tells him, "I only want to play baseball with you, Dad. You throw the ball the best and never hurt me with the ball. I'll always catch it and never get hurt." The father, however, is quite uncomfortable with this ideal view of himself as bestowed on him by his son and tells his son, "You are stupid; I can't throw that good. Besides, it takes a long time before you can catch well enough so you won't get hit in the head by a baseball. So don't act so wimpy." The son immediately becomes both sad and angry at his father.

If similar situations with the father continue to occur, this little boy might begin to feel the sense of helplessness, rage, and loss of control associated with a traumatic experience—in this case, the trauma is the boy's too abrupt loss of his belief in his father's being able to protect him from all body damage. The traumatic, emotional explicit autobiographical memory that this boy will ultimately construct of these experiences will involve his ideal image of his father that has been "fractured" too fast. In such a situation, this child will not eventually relinquish his ideal father image, but will repress it—with his associated intense sadness and rageful feelings—into his dynamic unconscious. If this boy's later experiences with his father, mother, or even others do not help him to resurrect and subsequently express his sadness and rage and his refusal to give up his wish for an ideal parent or parent figure, he may go through childhood and adolescence looking for the "perfect parent" he lost in childhood. Consequently, he will be prone to transferring the idealization meant for his father onto other people in authority. Inevitably, however, he will become quite angry when this newly idealized person "fails" him by manifesting a normal limitation to this idealization. For example, a teacher whom he idealized scolds him; in response, he feels rage because, in idealizing the teacher, he believed that he would be idealized in return (i.e., that he would never be scolded). This boy now experiences *narcissistic rage,* which is rage felt toward a person from whom one wanted unlimited love, admiration, and protection from limitations and from experiencing anxiety. This boy's narcissistic rage causes him to devalue the teacher; he then seeks a new person to idealize.

This process of idealization and devaluation will be repeated many times in his life as, in accordance with the repetition principle, he becomes unconsciously motivated to attempt to re-create and undo the original traumatic situation he experienced with his father. In his behavioral or procedural reenactments, he automatically engages in an *idealizing transference* to new symbolic father figures, with the unconscious goal of making each person accept some degree of his idealization. When that occurs, he momentarily undoes his father's rejection and recaptures the feeling of competency pleasure he lost when his father's rejection of his idealization produced so much narcissistic rage and sadness and a sense of helplessness. Inevitably, however, the idealized person is rejected and devalued when he or she shows his or her imperfections.

When children become locked into compulsively seeking to repeat a maladaptive behavior—in this case, idealizing transferences to new people but inevitably rejecting each of them because each is found to be imperfect—they most often require a psychotherapist to assist them in becoming aware of how they are not willing to give up the wish for a perfect father or mother figure in their life.

Parents can also interfere with the process of assisting their children in gradually relinquishing their reactive wishes to have perfect parents or be perfect themselves when they do not provide empathically attuned mirroring responses of admiration and support in response to their children's demonstrated competencies and abilities. This can begin from earliest infancy when the infant does not receive positive mirroring and parental attributions of being intrinsically valued. When such children reach age 3 years, they may more intensely resurrect their wishes to be perfect as a way of compensating for the lack of admiring mirroring from the parents, which has left the child with the sadness associated with possessing negative self-constancy and object constancy.

Like the wish for a perfect parent, the wish for an ideal self is viewed as a compensatory mental structure. The term *compensatory* reflects how children's wishes and need to be perfect and have their perfection mirrored by others are an aspect of their false self— false in that they are no longer able to risk exposing any of their normal imperfections because of the narcissistic rage that is generated when they are not responded to with profound admiration and perfect empathy. They tell themselves that they do not need anyone else to tell them they are perfect. In these situations, children use a *narcissistic defense mechanism,* which is some variant of children telling themselves and others, "I'm perfect and I don't need anyone to tell me so. In fact, I don't need anybody because I don't have any worries or anxieties." When children maintain narcissistic defenses to hide the narcissistic rage they experience when they are not profoundly admired, they can become quite isolated. They will not relinquish these narcissistic defenses until they find a new person to give them idealized or unlimited admiration.

There is another family scenario that can lead children to becoming preoccupied with being perfect and seeking the idealization of another: when parents provide admiring mirroring that is not based in reality. In this situation, parents demonstrate an idealized, grandiose, and perfectionistic view of their children, regardless of their children's revealing, through their performances, their normal limitations. The parents simply refuse to "see" their child's normally imperfect true self. They support the development of a false self in their child when they insist that their child is, can, and should be perfect. Such a child will not fully comprehend such a faulty parental belief until he or she reaches age 3 or 4 years and manifests a normal reactive wish for self and parental perfection when he or she experiences a high degree of separation or body damage anxiety. This situation is illustrated in the following example:

A 4-year-old girl tells her parents, "I am the best on the soccer team, all the time!" The parents make it quite difficult for her to gradually accept her limitations and gradually relinquish her resurrected ideal self-representation when they tell her, "That's right. We always knew you could be the best. If you practice a lot you will be the best." Through this message—which the parents truly believe and repeat to her—the girl begins to believe this ideal view that her parents have of her and eventually adopts it herself. Consequently, she begins to become intolerable of any of her normal age-adequate imperfections. She then goes through her childhood and adolescence very critical of her successes, always asking more of herself than anyone else does—other than her parents—and tending to believe that all the important figures in her life expect her to be perfect and will become very disappointed in her when she does not perform perfectly. (These expectations about how others will view and react to her is a negative transference—that is, she expects important people in her life to feel narcissistic rage at her when she does not perform perfectly for them.)

Children's wish for perfection in their sexual identity.

The periodic resurrection in early childhood of perfectionistic wishes is a ubiquitous occurrence during this phase of sexual identity development. Young children's beginning awareness of their body vulnerability, coupled with their curiosity about the differences in the body makeup of boys versus girls, leads them to come up with intuitive guesses or inferential ideas about why boys have penises and girls have vaginas. In the genital-narcissistic phase, boys react to their acknowledgment of the anatomical differences between girls and boys by becoming more aggressive toward girls, by demonstrating a tendency to deny the differences and the presence of a female vagina, and by continuing to manipulate their genitals (Galenson 1993).

In wanting both parents to admire his penis, a boy develops some body damage anxiety in reference to

1. His fear that his father will retaliate against him when his father senses the boy's wish to steal his father's larger penis for himself
2. His fear that his mother will retaliate against him for having a penis because of his inferential idea that maybe she had a penis and lost it or wants a penis instead of a vagina (Edgecumbe and Burgner 1975)

3. His fear that his mother will withdraw her love because of his inferential idea that his mother is not pleased with his being different from her and his wanting to identify with his father and other males

In normally developing boys, these fears do not generate so much body damage anxiety that they stop exhibiting themselves and withdraw from their parents or from girls. Neither do they resurrect their wish to be perfect and then deny having any need to exhibit their penis. They do worry, however, about demonstrating their erections to their mother and other women, including same-age girls, when they become concerned that girls will retaliate against them out of envy or that their mother will withdraw her love. At this stage, they respond by seeking out their father and being proud to walk with and imitate him, and being reassured to know that their father has a penis just as they do (P. Tyson 1982b). Through these more positive experiences, boys further develop their gender identity as they begin to feel good about belonging to the category of "males."

During the genital-narcissistic phase, girls ages 3–4 years react to their acknowledgment of the anatomical differences between boys and girls by changing from direct manipulation of their genital region to indirect manipulation of it by rocking or pressure. Some girls may show a period of play in which they hold pencils or other objects to their genital area and claim they have a penis, thus exhibiting a short-lived *castration reaction.* Not fully comprehending how her vagina can be as valuable as the easily visible and manipulatable penis, girls may become to some degree angry at their mothers for not giving them a penis. For a while, they view their genital region as one that is barren; in other words, they experience some *penis envy.* However, normally developing 3- to 4-year-old girls have experienced the ongoing admiration and valuing communications from both of their parents since infancy. They have already established positive self-constancy and object constancy and continue to develop their autonomous gender identities. They also have already viewed their genitals as valued, in some ways more valuable than boys':

> Narcissistically valuing femininity, the girl's comparison of her body with that of the opposite sex optimally brings pride and exhibitionism. . . . If the girl can find a narcissistically valued sense of femininity in identification with her mother, this paves the way for triadic object relations. (P. Tyson 1994, pp. 460–461)

The triadic object relations Tyson referred to is the girl's eventual entrance into the oedipal phase (see below).

At this age, girls turn to their mothers, who continue to communicate to them that being a woman and having a woman's body are good things. Girls want to identify with their mothers, wishing that they could have breasts like them. Their play will now involve their becoming mothers to their dolls and developing the ability to have babies. They add to their positive self-constancy a new "coloring" within their gender identity: they feel valued and admired in being able to produce babies within their internal, but special, vagina and uterus. They may now return boys' teasing them that they do not have a penis with, "Oh, yeah, well I can make babies and you can't even make one!" It is interesting that many normal boys ages 3–4 years will have a short-lived "womb envy" reaction, in which they envy this baby-producing ability that they will never have.

A girl's fantasizing about having breasts and being able to produce babies like her mother usually includes her wish to steal her mother's more beautiful breasts and genitals for herself. These fantasy wishes generate body damage anxiety in her because of her fear that her mother will retaliate against her when she senses her daughter's wishes to take her larger breasts and more beautiful genitals for herself. As is true for boys, however, girls' body damage anxiety is not so excessive as to stop them from seeking admiration from their fathers at the same time. As one 4-year-old girl, in the midst of her genital-narcissistic phase, told me, "My mother looks in the mirror, and wants to be the prettiest. But I am getting prettier and Mom may want to hurt my vagina so she has the prettiest [vagina]."

Psychologically attuned mothers who are not threatened by their daughter's emerging femininity continue to support and love their daughters and reassure them that they will not retaliate when their daughters exhibit their feminine appearance to their father, even at times when their daughter is quite provocative in inviting their father's praise (e.g., praise of a new dress). Gradually, girls sense their mother's support and then reaffirm their previously developed sense of valuing their own genital anatomy, thus wanting to identify more with their mother. Girls further develop their gender identity and feel pleasure in belonging to the category of "females." Hence, in this genital-narcissistic phase, imitation and identification with the same-gender parent helps define gender roles for boys and girls.

The society in which children live also defines gender role behaviors for them. Toys for young children differ based on their gender. Girls tend to be interested, especially by age 5 years, in playing with dolls, whereas boys are attracted to building blocks (e.g., Legos), action figures, cars, boats, planes, and video games. Girls' preoccupation with dolls is not completely understood, other than as an identification with their mother's nurturant actions and reproductive capabilities.

Boys' and girls' continuing need to identify with the same-gender parent to consolidate and develop their gender identity lessens their body damage anxieties because, in identifying with their parent, they have a same-gender ally who helps them feel less anxious about their wish to belong to the gender category. Thus identification with the same-gender parent also helps children accept their anatomical features. Consequently, girls can tolerate some penis envy and boys can tolerate some womb envy. In essence, both can accept certain valuable aspects of the other's genital equipment.

Choice of sexual object. Between ages 3 or 4 years, children begin to make a sexual object choice. This occurs as they begin to expand on their earlier masturbatory fantasies, which contained their early attractions to either the same gender or the opposite gender for sexual gratification. If the former, they begin to make a homosexual object choice; if the latter, they begin to make a heterosexual object choice.

As noted earlier, a child's sexual attraction to a parent—whether it be a homosexual or heterosexual attraction—is considerably lessened when there has been a normal attachment process in the first

3 years of the child's life (Erickson 1993). In addition, a developmentally enhancing, predominantly "goodness-of-fit" attachment relationship enhances altruistic behavior in children toward their parents (altruistic in the sense that children develop a specific need to be concerned about the safety and well-being of their parents). In reviewing anthropological and cross-cultural research, Erickson (1993) explained these phenomena as follows:

> In sum, it is now known that attachment bonding in early life, and later on sexual avoidance and preferential altruism, occur almost exclusively between immediate kin. In contrast, sexual behavior typically occurs between distantly related or unrelated individuals. (p. 413)

Children ages 3½–5 years become quite preoccupied with their sexual object choice. They experience sexual attraction for one or the other parent and others of the same gender as the parent to whom they are attracted. Children with a heterosexual object choice are sexually aroused by their opposite-gender parent. An example of a heterosexual young boy's experiences was provided by a medical student taking part in an investigation on normal development. He reported the following:

> I recall when I was just about 5 years old. When I was in kindergarten, I used to sneak under my teacher's desk. She had the most beautiful legs and a few times when I looked up her dress I remember getting all aroused and feeling an erection.

Children with a homosexual object choice experience sexual excitation in being physically close to their same-gender parent. A 28-year-old homosexual psychiatrist, with a firm gender identity as an autonomous and competent male, described this process as follows:

> From about 4 years old, I recall becoming aroused by my father's smell, his big arms and how he looked. I remember rubbing the hair on his arms and getting an erection. I knew then, from being around other boys, that I was different in reference to sexual attraction. Not different in terms of being a boy; I played sports and

liked looking like a boy. But my sexual preference was not like theirs. I knew I liked men in a way that they liked women.

■ The Oedipal Phase

Emergence of the oedipal phase. Young children's sexual object choice becomes the main organizer for their developing sexual identity, as well as a basic aspect of 4- to 5-year-old children's progression into the oedipal phase (Mayer 1995; P. Tyson 1982a). The *oedipal phase* is the phase during which the heterosexual child fantasizes about replacing his or her same-gender parent and engaging in an exclusive, sexually tinged relationship with his or her opposite-gender parent. The term *oedipal* was selected by S. Freud (1905/1963) based on the story in Greek mythology in which Oedipus unknowingly marries his mother and then is blinded as punishment for his incestuous deed.

This phase comprises a mixture of behaviors based on what children have learned—and carry within their object representations of their parents and others—about what constitutes being a man and a woman. It is also based on what inferences children make about what it means to be a husband or wife, father or mother. For example, children will construct their own fantasies of what it means for their mother and father to sleep together.

In children who have made a heterosexual object choice, their sexual object choice is the same as that of their same-gender parent. For example, for the heterosexual boy with a heterosexual father, his gender identity and sexual identity are congruent in the sense that being a boy means pursuing a person of the same gender as does his father for sensual-sexual gratification—that is, a woman. For example, he sees his father hug and kiss his mother and he knows his father is able to look at his mother when she showers and in other intimate settings. He begins to pretend and fantasize that he is like his father and wishes he could possess a wife for sensual-sexual gratification; in essence, he wishes to possess what his father has. He begins to ask his mother, "Will you go to the movies with me alone the way you go with Dad?" He may ask to sleep in his father's place in his parents' bed. He fantasizes about giving his mother a baby, not really clear about the physical process this would entail. He seeks his mother's and other women's admiring smiles in relation to his sexual advances. For example, a 4½-year-old boy pinched his teacher on her buttocks when she turned her back to him during kindergarten class. When the teacher turned with a shocked look on her face, he smiled and winked at her (Vivian O'Neill, personal communication, November 1993). The heterosexual boy's burgeoning sexual identity in being attractive to women develops from what he perceives in the eyes of his mother and other important women in his life.

When 3½- to 5-year-old children view their parents engaged in sexual intercourse, they may become extremely anxious, tending to view sex as an aggressive act because the parents' active sexual movements seem to signify fighting or wrestling to them. In such a situation, the boy may begin to stop wanting to be like his father if he sees his father "hurting" his beloved mother in the sexual act; similarly, a girl may begin to stop wanting to be like her mother if she sees her mother letting herself be "hurt" by her father. For this reason, observations of sexual intercourse between their parents are quite disruptive for heterosexual children in their oedipal phase.

In the psychologically attuned family, the parents' bedroom is private, leaving heterosexual boys and girls to continue to fantasize about what it means to be excluded from this private relationship that takes place between the parents. Children begin to construct their conception of marriage, and their fantasy life becomes dominated by wishes about being married.

Oedipal behavior in the heterosexual boy culminates in his wish to "marry Mom" or at least have an exclusive relationship with her that excludes Dad (as depicted in the cartoon in Figure 5–2). The hallmark of the oedipal phase for children is their conviction that their same-gender parent is their rival and their wish that this rival parent would leave or otherwise relinquish their authority over them. A heterosexual boy may verbalize his wish to marry, or have an exclusive special relationship with, his mother or keep this wish hidden and fantasize about it in his play and stories. Often the symbols a boy uses in his play and stories hide his wishes to marry his mother as he struggles with his worries about his father's response. However, some boys will be quite open in declaring their sexual intentions toward their mother (as depicted in Figure 5–3).

When children experience an overwhelming need to hide their oedipal wishes, it may signal the presence of excessive body damage anxiety within them. They may have had a less-than-adequate attachment relationship with their parents that has not led them to attain an adequate degree of positive self-constancy and object constancy.

Oedipal behavior in heterosexual girls takes a similar form to such behavior in boys. P. Tyson (1994) described the transition for the heterosexual girl from the genital-narcissistic phase to the oedipal phase as follows:

> Instead of simply wishing for an exclusive relationship with one or the other parent in efforts to be the center of attention, the girl's fantasy now is to replace and to play the role of mother with her father. This requires a change in role in relation to father— from baby to fantasized lover and possibly mother of father's baby. (p. 461)

The heterosexual little girl who is beginning to include herself in the category of "women who seek men for sensual-sexual plea-

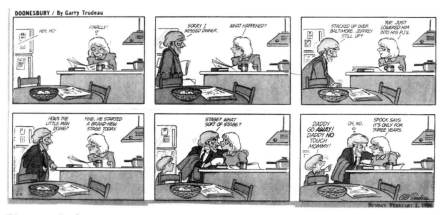

Figure 5–2. Typical behavior of a boy age 3½–5 years in the oedipal phase wishing for an exclusive relationship with his mother.
Source.   Copyright 1986 G. B. Trudeau. Reprinted with permission of Universal Press Syndicate. All rights reserved.

sure" now views her mother as a rival for her father's affections. She wants her father to admire her new dress and make a fuss over her hairstyle, and wants him to exclude her mother from her and her father's special times together. She fantasizes about marrying her father, of having a baby with him, and of sending her mother away. However, it is unclear in her mind just how she and her father will physically produce a baby. The heterosexual girl's burgeoning sexual identity in being attractive to men develops, for the

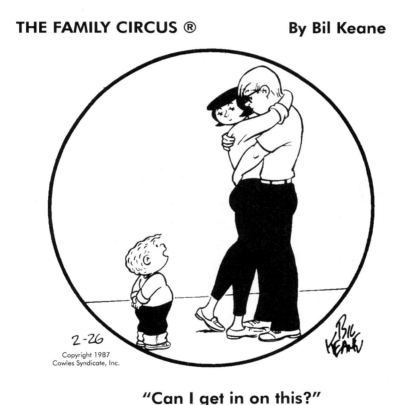

THE FAMILY CIRCUS ®   **By Bil Keane**

2-26
Copyright 1987
Cowles Syndicate, Inc.

"Can I get in on this?"

Figure 5–3. A young boy's possibly disguised expression of his sexual intentions toward his mother.
Source. Reprinted with special permission of Cowles Syndicate, Inc., New York, New York.

most part, in what she perceives in the eyes of her father and other important men in her life (e.g., her uncles, male teachers). At the height of her oedipal phase, she wants to look like her mother but then wants to see the proud gleam in her father's eye when she shows her new dress, hoping he will say, "You look more beautiful than Mom. Let's you and I go to the movies without Mom."

Psychologically attuned parents need to react to their children's oedipal wishes in the same fashion in which they respond to their children's resurrected wishes to be perfect or have perfect parents: by tolerating and limiting the expression of these oedipal wishes—when the parent is envious of or threatened by the child's oedipal behaviors toward the parent, and without overly criticizing them or without overly encouraging them—when the parent is experiencing some need to push the child into an overly close, incestuously tinged relationship with the parent (P. Tyson 1989).

At the height of heterosexual children's awareness of their oedipal wishes, they are experiencing the displeasurable emotions of both separation and body damage anxiety. These are generated because of their fear of retaliation, through both the withdrawal of the love of and the infliction of physical harm by the rival same-gender parent. For the boy with a heterosexual identity, the content of his body damage anxiety is his fear that his father will hurt or in some way decrease his capacity to generate pleasurable penile sensations. Thus a boy may have a series of dreams (or even nightmares) wherein he is being chased by angry animals who simultaneously symbolize both himself (as the angry child who wants to drive his father from the family) and his father (as an angry man whose wife is being stolen from him). A boy also may suddenly fear the dark, worrying about a "big monster man" in his closet waiting to attack and hurt him. A heterosexual girl also worries about abandonment and body damage anxiety perpetuated by her mother. The content of her body damage anxiety is her fear that her mother will 1) painfully penetrate her vagina, 2) decrease her capacity for pleasurable vaginal sensations, and 3) take away her reproductive ability to have a baby (Richards 1994). A girl also may have dreams, nightmares, and fears of monsters as do boys. However, for her it is the "witch mother" who is after her. She may, for example, be mesmerized, excited, and scared by a classic story such as *Cinder-*

ella and a more modern story such as *Annie,* in which she identifies with the girl who is trying to stay away from evil stepmothers, evil monster women, or evil women in general.

Relative relinquishment of oedipal wishes. Oedipal wishes in heterosexual children decrease when they begin to put aside, but not completely give up, their wishes to both have what their same-gender parent has and do what their same-gender parent does. Because boys love their mother and father, they are helped in relinquishing their wish to replace their father and are encouraged in identifying with and wanting to grow up like their father when their father is respected and loved by their mother and their mother is respected and loved by their father. Similar dynamics need to exist for girls; they are helped in identifying with and growing up like their mother when their father respects and loves their mother and their mother respects and loves their father.

This decreased intensity of children's oedipal wishes does not resolve them forever. This is only their first and relative relinquishment; oedipal wishes return when children enter puberty at about age 12 or 13 years. Etchegoyen (1993) remarked how oedipal wishes at each stage of development "are partly operative and partly worked through and defended against" (p. 349). And Loewald (1979) noted that there is no definite destruction of the complex (i.e., the oedipal conflict), but that the child and future adult must repeatedly attempt to master any urges toward an incestual relationship with a parent. This first relinquishment and internal turning away from oedipal wishes is also much easier when children's periodic resurrection of their wishes to be perfect and to have perfect parents are not unduly strong and have not become prominent and persistent. Children who are wishing to be perfect and omnipotent rebel against accepting that they must accept the limitation that they cannot claim an exclusive relationship with the opposite-gender parent.

A healthy resolution of the oedipal phase in heterosexual children will enhance their identification process with same-gender individuals. Their gender identity becomes more consolidated as they become comfortable in demonstrating their correct gender role behaviors. In essence, heterosexual children with heterosexual parents end up where they began: their genital-narcissistic phase identification with the same-gender parent propels them into their oedipal phase, and their continued wish to maintain this same-gender identification helps them resolve their oedipal phase. This wish to identify with their same-gender parent significantly decreases their preoccupation with body damage anxiety.

Many adults often find it difficult to believe the normal heterosexual oedipal phase exists for one of two reasons. First, the examples they have heard to illustrate the presence of normal oedipal wishes are examples from abnormally developing children who had intense body damage anxiety and intense behavioral reactions to their parents during their oedipal phase. In my view, children who manifest an intense level of conflict about possessing the ir oedipal wishes are the exception, not the norm. Most pare do hear about their child's wishes to replace the parent, sleep in bed with the opposite-gender parent, and even explore the same-gender parent's body in a physically intimate manner. All these wishes are present in normally developing children, but not in the extreme and not in a prolonged temporal manifestation.

Second, many adults cannot remember any aspects of their own oedipal phase—or of their lives before ages 5–6 years, for that manner. One reason is that, for many adults, their oedipal phase was not associated with high emotional content, either displeasurable or pleasurable. As such, many of the oedipal experiences were not major events in their life. For example, if a boy asked his mother, "Can I sleep with you because I am a boy like Dad?" and his mother responded, "No," the boy would probably be angry with his mother, but the intensity of his anger would not approach an intolerable level.

Alternatively, many adults cannot remember their childhood oedipal wishes and feelings because they experienced childhood amnesia pertaining to many autobiographical memories of events that occurred before age 6 years. This amnesia would encompass oedipal wishes to replace the same-gender parent. The reason for this childhood amnesia is presently not well understood (K. Nelson 1993a). It may be that certain childhood memories undergo a *normal developmental repression*. This type of repression may be a slightly different form of repression that functions in small part as a defense but in large part as a maturational advance that allows continued developmental progress. For developmental repression to be normal, however, it must occur after the oedipal phase has been adequately dealt with. If repression occurs before a heterosexual child turns away from trying to establish an exclusive relationship with the opposite-gender parent and turns toward reinforcing his or her identifications with the same-gender parent, then that child's oedipal wishes are never fully turned away from; they may be decreased in intensity, but they remain quite active within the child's unconscious and will interfere with his or her development in the next phase of childhood (i.e., between ages 6 and 11 years).

Recently, M. L. Lewis (1995) described alternative possibilities to the above explanations for normal developmental repression. He suggested the following:

1. Memories that are forgotten can not only be relegated to the child's unconscious but also may be forgotten and lost. Lewis quotes Squire (1987), who states, "All forgetting, whether it occurs in a few hours or over a period of years, reflects in part an actual loss of information from storage" (p. 38).
2. New learning may alter prior learning encoded in existing memories.
3. "The memory system that enables long-lasting declarative memory (as opposed to nonconscious, procedural memory) is not yet established in the infant" (p. 412).
4. "Different memory processes may operate at different stages of development," (p. 412) so that much of what is "forgotten" at around age 6 years was never encoded into verbal memories in the first place.
5. As the developing child accommodates to new experiences, he or she restructures and changes many existing memories.

■ Development of a Peer Identity

It is during early childhood that children's need for peer intervention first becomes manifest. Peer identity is another piece of children's overall identity that is formed during this phase.

Initially, when toddlers' self-awareness dawns at around age 18 months, they engage in simple reciprocal play with other children with no sharing of play; they will get toys from each other in order to play alone and conduct their "experiments" on novel objects. By age 2½ years, parallel play between children begins in which there is still no common goal between their play activities but there is more of an awareness of each other's play. By age 3 years, however, children engage in social play where there is cooperation, a common goal, and a burgeoning interaction. Peers are now beginning to be acknowledged as other individuals with whom one can develop a relationship. In social play, children consolidate their concepts of "mine" and "not mine." Their need to assert their independent wishes and claim newly discovered articles as their own leads to inevitable fights and clashes.

The social play with peers and siblings that is characteristic of early childhood involves children's gradually learning about the concept of sharing. Often, at first, sharing seems like a ridiculous idea to children, especially when they are told to share what they have with another child who has nothing to share. The child doing the sharing always gets less than what he or she began with. However, if children trust their parents, they will accept their parents' promise that sharing will eventually become reciprocal and enjoyable and they will gradually risk sharing with other children. Also, it helps children to learn to share when their parents are good arbitrators. For example, if two children are fighting over ownership of a toy, a mother might help them solve their conflict by presenting them with the idea that they take turns "giving the orders" about how they will both play with the toy.

By age 4 years, many children are in a preschool for at least 2–3 hours per day. Now peers become a way for children to practice the parental standards and moral values they have been trying to adopt as their own. These standards and moral values are either reinforced or extinguished by the teacher's edicts, standards, and moral values.

The play of children ages 4–5 years with peers and siblings often involves children's playing out those adult roles with which they are trying to identify. These identifications do not usually become permanent parts of their overall identity, but function more as pleasurable activities in which they assertively exercise their growing ability to use their imagination in pretend play. In pretending, children take on different adult roles and expand their knowledge of categories. For example, after a family friend who was a priest visited his home, a 5-year-old boy dressed himself after school for the next several days in the robes of a priest and walked around his house blessing each room with holy water.

Sometimes, however, when adults observe children's roleplaying, they may use this play to manipulate children into believing the role is one they should adopt in reality. For example, the neighborhood priest might say that the 5-year-old boy described above is showing his true vocation to become a priest. This attempt by adults to strictly interpret children's creative play will restrict children's use of play to learn about their social world.

Play with younger peers and siblings can also enable 4- to 6-year-old children to assume adult roles in which they imitate being the adult and, through their play, reaffirm an adult edict or standard they are trying to adopt as one of their own. For example, a 5-year-old girl was struggling with a conflict between her wish to bite people when she is angry at them and her parents' edict that she should talk when she is angry and not bite. In an attempt to use play to help resolve her conflict, she was observed playing with her younger brother where she spontaneously stated, "I am showing my little brother how to learn things. He bites the way I did as a baby; but now I know that biting is only what babies do, not big girls."

Development of the Superego

Beginning Operation of the Superego as an Internal Structure

■ The Superego

In Chapter 2, I define the conscience, or superego, as one of a group of four complex organizational structures (the others being the id, the ego, and the self). The *superego* is a metaphorical mental construct that comprises specific mental functions that share the common quality of providing an inner source of children's, society's, and families' standards, ethical rules, and moral values. Thus it can be thought of as a collection of children's standards, ethical rules, and moral values categorized into two global categories: what is viewed and permitted by children as right, ethical, and moral, and what is viewed and not permitted by children as wrong, unethical, and immoral.

Each of children's standards—their shoulds and should nots—is an aspect of the numerous object representations they hold of the important people in their past and present life. Thus the superego also holds the collection of all the shoulds and should nots that are contained in children's object representations. For example, if a 5-year-old girl is asked, "Is spitting a good thing to do?" she might answer with an object representation, "My parents have taught me it's wrong." However, children's standards of right and wrong are not the result of only their identification with their parents. They also emerge as the result of operant conditioning as well as children's own ability to make inferences about what is right and wrong. In summary, children will be motivated to construct standards and activate them 1) in the automatic process of identification, 2) to avoid punishment, or 3) to assertively fulfill their wish to maintain a goodness-of-fit, healthy attachment relationship with their parents and act in a way that will please their parents and trigger their mirroring admiration for them.

■ Development of the Superego

Modeling and eventually identifying with parents' standards or rules of conduct is fueled and supported by 1) children's receiving love, 2) parents making demands on children that do not exceed the children's capabilities, and 3) parents making demands on children that do not interfere too abruptly with children's need for play. In the earliest beginnings of superego, children remember past punishments for breaking rules. Consequently, one of their motivations for following standards of behavior is to avoid their parents' anger and disapproval. Toddlers, however, who have been overpunished for breaking a family rule will begin to have significant trouble in developing positive self-constancy and object constancy. They will begin to obey more through identification with the aggressor (i.e., the overly aggressive parent). These children obey out of fear of punishment, not out of fear of losing their parents' love and mirroring admiration.

By ages 2–3 years, the normally disciplined child's motivation to obey to avoid punishment has minimal carryover (Damon 1988). At about age 3 years, conventional morality begins (Kohlberg 1981). If the establishment of positive self-constancy and object constancy has led to children's construction of primarily loving object representations of their parents, children will be motivated to obey their parents' rules to keep receiving the love they have learned to expect. However, all children regress and break rules if the parent is away. It is not until around age 4 years that children's construction of both new object representations and categories of standards enable them to retain their parents' standards within their representational world.

Once children begin to believe in their own rules, the superego comes into being. Children experience guilt when they do or say something that their conscience now tells them is wrong or forbidden. Guilt occurs when children 1) know what is a right and what is a wrong behavior, 2) believe they have a choice between the two behaviors, and 3) have made the bad choice. Children do not like guilt; it makes them feel they are bad and potentially unloved. In their first experiences of feeling guilty, they will try to blame someone else for their own wrong statement or behavior.

In the normal development of a conscience, children will do or say things that their conscience forbids. They then must gradually modify the concrete "eye-for-an-eye" nature of the early conscience so that the guilt is less severe and more tolerable. Parents help this modification process when they empathically sense their children's guilty feeling, verbally identify the feeling for them, and point out that guilt is often a healthy feeling that children can admit to and one that is not associated with being bad. Parents teach their children that guilt is their internal signal that they have done something wrong.

When children's guilt becomes less intense, they will then develop tolerance of their *superego anxiety*—that is, the anxiety they experience when they think about doing or saying something that is forbidden by their conscience. This superego anxiety is another internal distress signal that warns the child that guilt will ensue if the forbidden action or verbalization occurs.

When children verbalize their wishes and standards, they are considering their options aloud. By encouraging such verbalization, parents further teach their children about standards. In time, parents encourage their children to stop, think, and listen to and use their conscience signals in deciding upon their actions or words.

When not excessive or extreme, guilt can gradually become an emotion that does not have to be denied or repressed; it can become an internal response to misdeeds from which children can learn. On the other hand, children are who are immediately spanked or slapped after a misdeed, thereby making a quick payment for their "crime," soon forget their transgression; they are not given the necessary time to focus consciously on and experience their guilty feelings. They then learn that, when they do something wrong, they receive a physical punishment. In this interaction, they are passive and their parents are active. They do not learn how to perceive their guilt actively, acknowledge it, and then enact certain behaviors, as directed by their parents, that will make amends or symbolically undo the misdeed.

Psychologically aware parents know that their children need to be proactive in undoing an action in which they obviously disobeyed a rule. For example, if children are punished only by having things or activities taken away (e.g., not being allowed to watch television), they are being punished in a way that does not allow them a chance to learn that active, completed good deeds can undo bad deeds. Even their saying "I'm sorry" is not enough. Parents help their child by giving them an "undoing task," such as cleaning up the yard; when this task is completed, they can then ask their child to say "I'm sorry." This verbal apology after completing an "undoing" deed reinforces within children their becoming aware of their intrinsic wish to be moral and good. The apology helps children reaffirm the authority they gave to their parents when they turned away from their oedipal wishes and recognized both of their parents' authority as the source of moral values.

An important part of conscience development is the role of *inner speech,* also called *private speech* (Berk 1994; Diaz and Berk

1992). This entails children's verbalizations to influence them-selves, not others. Children talk to themselves, especially during solitary play, in an attempt to self-direct themselves in stating rules or standards that they are considering about making a part of their representational world of conscience. Inner speech helps them de-velop an internalized set of rules and is another way of viewing one function of the conscience.

Children's interpersonal play also assists them in developing their conscience. Children will engage in play in particular as a way of delaying an immediate action and thinking about the choice they have to make between two behaviors, as in the following example:

> A 5-year-old girl was angry with her mother because her mother had spent a lot of time that day with her new baby sister. The mother then told her that she would take her to the store with her later in the day. The girl loved her mother and wanted to take advantage of what time her mother had offered to spend with her in going to the store. She delayed acting mean toward her sister as was her inclination and began playing with her dolls.
>
> An uncle visiting the family sat with her and she told him about this fantasy: She was a mother who had a daughter who had a problem. She told the uncle, "My daughter can't make up her mind whether to go to the store with me or be angry and stay at home. She'd be happier if she could make up her mind and go with me." After a while she told her uncle, "I like helping Mom. She says when I help her, I'm a good girl." She had made a choice to do what she considered right and used her ability to engage in playful fantasy to give her conscience a chance to be heard. When her mother entered the room she told her, "Mom, I want to go to the store with you."

Development of Adaptational Capabilities

Repression as a Defense Mechanism

Repression is defined as an automatic unconscious mental pro-cess, viewed as an activity of children's ego under the direction of their self, which bars from their conscious awareness 1) those wishes and feelings that, if gratified, would produce either parental (external) disapproval or superego (internal) disapproval (once the superego becomes an internal structure), and 2) those memories of experiences that are associated with an intensely displeasurable emotional state.

Repression begins to emerge at around age 18 months, but does not become a predominant defense mechanism until children reach about age 3 years. At that age, children's superego begins to function more as an internal structure, and children must begin to deal with the rules or standards that their superego brings to bear. When their superego generates guilt in response to a forbidden wish, feeling, verbalization, action, or recalled memory that is so excessive that it generates a level of displeasure that exceeds a child's stimulation threshold, then the forbidden wish, feeling, verbalization, action, or recalled memory and associated guilt will be repressed. The emotion of guilt and the aspect of the superego that is stimulating that guilt will both remain unconscious (Blum 1985).

In Chapter 4, I describe abnormal (or pathological) beliefs as those beliefs that inhibit development. Guilt that is excessive and consciously intolerable is often attributable to the influence of an abnormal belief about a standard that a child possesses. As such, abnormal beliefs become part of an unhealthy or abnormal superego. These abnormal beliefs generate such excessive, and often consciously intolerable, guilt that the child will repress these beliefs. These unconscious abnormal beliefs then exert a silent and inhibiting influence on the child's progress in developing his or her true self, for the true self comprising the child's wishes and feelings has to be repressed or denied because the child believes that those wishes and feelings are bad. Subsequently, the child will activate unconscious superego anxiety whenever certain feelings or wishes are stimulated (either through memory or by external stimuli). This unconscious superego anxiety (generated before the action) and guilt (generated after the action) will cause him or her to engage in automatic actions that cause him or her to avoid the expression of his or her own innate needs and emotions as well as avoid interacting with others.

Repression, as with all defense mechanisms, is adaptive when used transiently. It gives children time in that, once repression is activated, a conflict has been temporarily put on hold. Subsequently, children will find themselves, without conscious forethought, generating play in which the fantasy (or compensatory fantasy) is directly related to their repressed wish, feeling, or memory. In the safe world of play, children will give up the use of repression as they use symbolic play objects to create their story dramas. These dramas symbolize their need to eventually resolve their real life conflicts.

Repression helps children adapt and is used all throughout life. However, it can be used too much—that is, it can be used to repress those childhood wishes (e.g., oedipal wishes) that should normally be partially relinquished during development or to repress wishes and feelings associated with traumatic events that need to be worked through and eventually mastered. The following gives an example of repression being used nonadaptively to deal with a trauma:

A 5½-year-old boy who was hit in his eye developed a cyst that required surgery. This boy's body damage anxiety was at a consciously tolerable level when he was given his preoperative sedation. However, because of an operating room mistake in scheduling, he waited 3 hours for surgery, by which time the sedation wore off. To compound the problem, he was left in a surgery instrument room where he watched various technicians handling all sorts of surgical instruments (e.g., scissors, clamps, scalpels). His body damage anxiety increased markedly as he stayed quiet but wide eyed and well aware of what was going on around him. When he was wheeled into the operating room, he very anxiously told the doctor, "Please don't hurt me with all those tools."

Two weeks later he was discharged, and when his mother asked what he remembered about the operation, he said that he could not remember what had happened before his operation. He had repressed all that had happened in the instrument room and in the operating room. However, this repression was not adaptive. He subsequently began to cry excessively (an automatic behavioral enactment) whenever he had a pediatric appointment, but he could not understand his excessive fear. As time went by, this boy began to become anxious whenever he entered a hospital. Eventually he needed the help of a child psychiatrist to unrepress the memory of the trauma he had experienced in the hospital.

Permitting his shame about possessing such a high degree of body damage anxiety to enter his consciousness was not easy. Prior to admitting to his shame about being so afraid before his operation, he complained to his child psychiatrist, "I am feeling things I don't want to think about." However, in the process of conscious elaboration, he was able, along with his empathically attuned child psychiatrist (and the empathy of his parents), to expose his pathogenic beliefs (i.e., that doctors would damage his body and that it was cowardly to admit to being so afraid of doctors and hospitals) and associated emotions to the cognitive reappraisal of his current ability to understand. Consequently, he was able to reconstruct his traumatic memory about what had happened to him. In time, his irrational level of body damage anxiety around doctors and hospitals was extinguished. He was left with an understanding that when he saw a doctor he would experience some extra anxiety because of what he had experienced before his operation, but he now recognized his current internal anxiety distress signal around doctors and hospitals in a new way: he recognized that it was a signal of a possible developmental calamity (i.e., being "cut on" while awake) that he once worried would occur in the past but that would not occur in the present.

Repression can also be used to bar from consciousness childhood developmental wishes that caused excessive anxiety and were "handled" through repression. Once repressed, these wishes are not given up and, consequently, produce fixations in the developmental process, as in the following example:

A boy had repressed his developmental oedipal wishes and so had never given them up, with the result that, throughout childhood and adolescence, he never relinquished his unconscious wish to marry his mother. At age 25 years, he began seeing a psychiatrist with the complaint that he always found himself drawn to married women who were depressed about being involved in a bad marriage. However, when these women would want to leave their husband for him, he would abruptly become extremely anxious and abandon them. At those times, he was unaware of never having given up his childhood oedipal wish to marry his mother. Once when his oedipal wish came true (i.e., when he could marry a woman who was very much like his mother), he experienced intense unconscious superego anxiety, which caused his abrupt abandonment of the woman.

This man's developmental history revealed that his mother was often depressed, complaining to her son that she was unhappy being married to his father. His father was overly strict with his son and did not admire and support the boy. When the boy's mother would become depressed, the father would encourage his son and wife to spend time together as the father absented himself from both of them. Now in adulthood, the son recalled his father often telling him, "Talk to your mother. You're better at cheering her up when she is down in the dumps; at these times she would rather be with you than with me." In effect, his father was offering his son an "oedipal victory."

This boy's normal oedipal wish to replace his father had been overly encouraged by his father and mother. In addition, this man still possessed a strong wish to be perfect and continually admired. As a boy, he had turned to his mother for this admiration when he did not receive it from his father. However, seeking such admiring closeness from his mother caused him to experience excessive body damage anxiety (i.e., he feared his father would punish him for becoming too physically close to his mother and for receiving his mother's admiration when his father did not). His father's strictness and unavailability as a mirroring empathic parent also made it difficult for him to identify more with his father, which made it difficult for him to give up his oedipal wishes to replace his father.

In summary, repression is another defense mechanism that helps children keep highly anxiety-provoking wishes or traumatic events out of conscious awareness. Like all defense mechanisms, if repression is not used for too long a time, it will serve an adaptive purpose. However, if repression is used for an excessive amount of time, it will produce developmental inhibitions and fixations in the developmental process. Chronic repressions are caused by, and subsequently maintained by, pathogenic beliefs.

At times, parents may need their children to excessively use a defense mechanism. Psychologically aware parents, however, eventually recognize their children's defense mechanisms. When they do, they help their children gradually give up the defense mechanism, as this father did in the following example:

> A 6-year-old boy spent the weekend at his grandparents' home. They were overly strict with him and, although he became angry at them, he repressed his anger because his father had issued an edict that he "be nice at your grandparents' house." When he returned home, although he told his father all went well, his father empathically sensed his son's inner, repressed anger. The father suggested that his son tell him how he felt about the visit, even though he might feel some of his feelings were not so nice. The son eventually told his father he was angry at his father for telling him that he had to "be nice" at his grandparents' house no matter what feelings they caused him to have, but also stated that he felt it was wrong to be angry at his grandparents. This father could empathize with his son because he could remember how hard it was for him as a child to get angry at his parents because his father wanted him to always be nice to his overly strict grandfather. Now, the father, in being able to empathize with his son, was able to encourage his son to talk. This considerably lessened his son's need for the defense of repression to deal with his anger.

One other defense related to repression that emerges in early childhood is *reaction formation.* This is an automatic, unconscious mental operation that bars from consciousness an unacceptable wish or feeling, and produces in consciousness the opposite wish or feeling. For example, a 5½-year-old girl is afraid of her hateful feelings toward another child. If she were to use projection to deal with her feelings, her hate would remain unconscious while consciously she became convinced that the other person hated her. If, however, she were to use reaction formation, her hate would remain unconscious, while she consciously felt affection and even love for the other child.

Chapter 6

Late Childhood (Latency) Phase of Mental Development
Age 6 Years to Age 11 Years

Major Developmental Tasks of Late Childhood

The major developmental tasks for late childhood are as follows:

1. To continue to add to and reconstruct one's peer identity, particularly in being able to begin to relate cooperatively and competitively to peers in the formal grade school setting
2. To construct a beginning social identity (the beginning belief that one is a member of various categories within one's society as a whole)

During late childhood, children undergo many developmental changes, but with less of the commotion characteristic of either the earlier childhood years or the later years of adolescence. However, their cognitive abilities and representational world develop signifi-

375

cantly during this period. Traditionally, age 7 years was thought of as the age at which children were capable of true reasoning and learning true social responsibility. This was because children ages 6–7 years were found to be able to use secondary process thinking more consistently than primary process thinking. Late childhood is the stage at which children leave their families for a considerable time each day and begin to learn a great deal of what they will have to know to function effectively in their society. It is also the time that they spend much time with other representatives of their culture: teachers, neighbors, peers, and so on. Thus, children ages 6–7 years are beginning to truly construct and develop a social identity.

By ages 6–7 years, children have developed the following components of their overall identity:

1. *Autonomous identity*—They are able to see themselves as being separate while maintaining their positive self-constancy and object constancy.
2. *Gender identity*—They are able to view themselves as a boy or a girl and have already constructed many beliefs, fantasies, and categories that define what it means to be masculine or feminine. They seek to continue to identify with both parents and others in learning more about their masculinity or femininity.
3. *Sexual identity*—They have made their sexual object choice and are sexually attracted to same-gender or opposite-gender individuals. Heterosexual children have "put aside" their heterosexual oedipal wishes toward sexually stimulating objects. At the same time, both heterosexual and homosexual children look toward both parents and others in authority for more information about the social rules pertaining to sexual stimulation and gratification, and are permitted some measure of sexual gratification through masturbation (see "Maturation and Development of Innate Needs," below).
4. *Peer identity*—They have already begun to construct a peer identity in viewing themselves as being a member of the category of "children." This peer identity was constructed during the first 6 years of life from being in the company of and eventually learning to play with children. This early peer identity

has already introduced them to an understanding of peer co-operation, competition, and the seeking of positive mirroring smiles from their peers.

Erikson (1963, 1968) proposed that, during late childhood, a major developmental task is for children to develop a belief in their ability to be industrious instead of a belief of being inferior to others, specifically their peers. He described this as the conflict between achieving industry versus inferiority. Erikson believed that children construct this belief in being industrious by performing and producing competently—both academically and in physical accomplishments—within their peer group in formal grade school. In achieving these successes, they further develop their peer identity and begin to construct a social identity. These aspects of children's overall identity will be enhanced or inhibited by children's parents and extended social environment.

■ Further Development of a Peer Identity

The development of children's peer identity further develops their 1) autonomous identity, in being able to assertively perform and produce in front of their peers and expect and receive a certain degree of admiration and affirmation from them; 2) gender identity, in being able to act like others of their gender and be accepted by their peers; and 3) sexual identity, in being able to continue to learn about the social rules between peers in terms of sexual stimulation and sexual gratification.

In children's further development of the above aspects of their autonomous, gender, sexual, and peer identity, they increasingly expand their interactions with people outside of their immediate family. This leads children to accomplish the next major developmental task of constructing a social identity.

■ Development of a Social Identity

In developing a social identity, children begin to believe that they are a member of various categories within their society as a whole (e.g., a citizen, an American, a New Yorker). In addition, children

construct other representations that define many of the procedures and skills that are required to function in their society outside of the family home.

The forerunners of children's social identity include their experiences during infancy (e.g., emotional referencing) and toddlerhood (e.g., learning which behaviors pleased and did not please
their parents). These experiences begin to be consolidated into a
social identity when children construct a superego in early childhood. I consider the construction of a superego a forerunner of
children's social identity, given that family and societal standards
and rules are the substance of children's constructed superego.
Once children (at ages 6–7 years) begin to use their superego anxiety signals as the "voice" of their parents when their parents are
not around, they are truly becoming autonomously social. When
they do not construct a superego that operates normally, they are
often described as being, at the least, asocial and, at the most, so-
ciopathic (i.e., children whose social identity is pathologically underdeveloped or malformed).

Functions of the Social Environment

Parents' Role in Developing Their Children's Peer and Social Identities

The dominant triggering social variable in the biopsychosocial
model of mental development in late childhood is the cultural requirement for all children to attend school. In essence, going to
school is the "job" of late childhood.

Beginning around age 3 years, children hear of the day when
they will go to "regular" or "big boys' and girls'" school, something
that initially occurs between ages 3 and 4 years when children go
to a 2–3 hour/day preschool class. This is followed between ages
5 and 6 years by children attending a half-day or full day of kindergarten class. Finally, children begin formal grade school between
ages 6 and 7 years. However, even before children walk into their

first day of first grade, they will have constructed both conceptual beliefs and fantasies about what they believe grade school to be and what it will mean to them, and they will have expectations about their acceptance versus nonacceptance by teachers and peers.

Beginning with preschool, children begin to learn what their particular society promulgates as the minimum or basic fund of knowledge it desires them to possess, in terms not only of knowledge about the inanimate world (e.g., mathematics, geography), but also of knowledge about how peers and adults interact in society. In many ways, school is a "classroom" for the development of both a peer and a social identity. Sarnoff (1987) emphasized this function of school (his term *latency* refers to the phase of late childhood):

> From the standpoint of culture, latency is necessary for the formation of civilization. Latency provides the period of time in which children can learn the complicated skills needed in society. . . . Sexual gratification and oedipal feelings are allayed so that the child can live in peace with those who love him. This is vital at a time when it is necessary to have someone care for him because of his economic dependence and his need to learn social skills, attitudes, and manners of living. The child can remain within the family as an accepted part of the family, and is still able to accept the authority of the parents. It is a period when the child consolidates his image of himself in relation to the world. (p. 72)

This developing social identity gives children a new understanding of their place in what was heretofore their parents' society.

In entering grade school, children are 1) leaving home for at least 5–7 hours/day; 2) joining a peer group and a social group of teachers, gym instructors, coaches, and others; 3) experiencing their first sustained exposure to authority figures other than their parents; and 4) gaining firsthand experience with how their family has been preparing them for life's challenges and how well their own views and their parents' views match the views—as manifested in the mirroring responses they will now begin to receive—of their peers and other adults they encounter at school. For children to achieve the developmental tasks of this phase of life, they must be supported by their parents as they continue to provide the five functions of the social environment.

Psychologically attuned parents possess a developmentally enhancing conscious belief that their children should enthusiastically assert themselves in being industrious with peers, teachers, ministers, coaches, and other adults outside of the family. In addition, their fantasies about their children's experiences with peer activities, school activities, and other outside-of-the-family activities cause parents to view each of these activities with positive expectations and greet their children's aspirations with admiring and supportive smiles—as emotional signaling information of their positive expectations. For example, when a boy tells his parents, somewhat hesitantly, "I think I want to play baseball after school. Okay?" his parents will probably answer, "Great! You'll meet new friends and like it." Their son hears both the words of encouragement and the pleasurable emotions in his parents' voice.

Sometimes, however, parents possess either a conscious or an unconscious pathogenic belief that will negatively affect their children's interactions with peers and adults outside of the family and may lead to their children's becoming criticized, rejected, unhappy, or rageful. When such a pathogenic belief is consciously experienced and verbalized by a parent, that parent is often viewed by other adults as being highly suspicious, distrustful, and avoidant of others. However, a parent possessing such a pathogenic belief may unconsciously repress the related belief that his or her children will be better off to stay at home and avoid peers and other adults.

Any new perception, emotion, wish, thought, conception, or behavior displayed by children attempting to achieve a new developmental task will engender, in most parents, a mixture of interest and excitement, as well as some degree of uncertainty. This uncertainty is attributable, in part, to parents' knowledgeable appraisal that they might not know how to react to this new behavior or verbalization.

Another cause of their uncertainty can be that their child's new behavior or other manifestation can unconsciously stimulate one or more repressed emotionally displeasurable memories of how their own parents negatively reacted when they showed this same behavior. If the displeasurable feelings contained within the memories are not too severe, the parents will be able to remember the events and feelings surrounding their own parents' response to this same behavior, and use that memory to avoid repeating the same behavior with their own child. For example, a mother may recall how her mother failed to admire her when she attained certain achievements in life; her memory of her sadness at the lack of her mother's response would prevent her from failing to admire her own children. Her memories, therefore, would not significantly interfere with her present response to her children's new behaviors or verbalizations, given that she can consciously recall the memories and make a connection with the past.

If, however, a parent's memories are too emotionally displeasurable, then the parent's unconscious mind will continue to attempt to repress all conscious awareness of them. Those memories may then exert an unconscious influence on the parent's subsequent perceptions, thoughts, feelings, wishes, emotions, conceptions, and behaviors toward his or her children's new verbalizations or surface behaviors. A rather sudden behavioral change—as an unconscious behavioral enactment—can ensue in the manner in which the parent treats his or her children. This is illustrated in the following example:

> A 7-year-old boy joins his first baseball team and becomes more aware of his need for close involvement with his peer group so that he can perform and receive admiring feedback from them. As a major developmental task of late childhood, it now becomes just as important for him to develop his peer identity through receiving the approval and acceptance of his baseball performances from his baseball chums as it is to get the continued approval from his parents.
>
> When he comes home after one game and tells his father about hitting a home run, he initially sees the old familiar gleam of admiration in his father's eyes. However, when he then tells his father how excited he is to go out and find his friends and celebrate his home run, he notices that his father suddenly becomes uneasy and quiet. The father then tells his son, "If you depend on the opinions of your friends, you'll be setting yourself up for disappointment. You show a lack of confidence in yourself if you really need and want your friends' approval."

This boy's father, who is a second-generation American, truly loves his son and has always enjoyed showing him how to play baseball. He is not consciously aware, however, of how his son's statement about needing his peer group's approval instantly stimulated a high level of uncertainty and uneasiness present within the father's unconscious mind. This father's father had reacted with criticism, suspicion, and disdain to his normal latency age wishes to be part of and receive admiration from his peer group. As an immigrant to the United States, the father's father was quite critical of his son's need for approval from anyone other than his family members, and discouraged his son's development of his peer and social identities. When his second-generation son initially reacted with anger, not only was he physically whipped, but his father withdrew his entire emotional support and love until his son began to view things the father's way.

In the above-described situation, the concept of normality I discuss in Chapter 4 arises again. The foreign-born father's idea of raising a normal son was to instill in his son a belief in the overwhelming need for his family and to extinguish any belief that his son needed the emotional support and admiration of his peers or any individuals outside of the family.

The 7-year-old, third-generation son subsequently has a true developmental conflict to resolve. His normal developmental wish and need for a supportive and admiring peer group—an aspect of his true self or truly developing overall identity—opposes his concurrent wish to maintain a close relationship with his father. His second-generation father's pathogenic belief (Weiss 1993; Weiss et al. 1986) that his son should relinquish his wish to develop an admiring and supportive relationship with his peer group ultimately causes the boy to construct a developmentally inhibiting, pathogenic belief, one that is necessary to stay out of conflict with his father. His external adaptation to his father's edict now takes precedence over his internal adaptation to his own innate needs to 1) engage in pleasurable interactions with his peers and 2) assertively explore his peer group environment for novel stimuli and acquire new knowledgeable additions to his peer identity and social identity.

The second-generation son (the boy's father), through the defense mechanism of identification with the aggressor (see discussion in Chapter 4), has taken into his representational world his foreign-born father's contemptible view of peers and makes it his own. Miller (1981) noted that children in such a situation take within their representational world the same contempt for their own normal developmental wish—in this case for an approving and sustaining relationship with their peer group—that their parent possesses. Once they believe that their normal wishes are contemptible and bad, they can be said to be developing more a false self than one that is true to their innate needs. In this example, a developmentally inhibiting poorness of fit now settles in between the son and his father.

This second-generation father's belief about friends was pathogenic: it maintained, or became his personal justification for, his distancing, distrustful, and suspicious behavior and attitude toward his own peers. His pathogenic belief that he neither needed nor could trust anyone outside his family had remained unmodified. Consequently, as an adult, he was very uncomfortable and uncertain in a group of peers, always expecting criticism. His immediate family was his primary source of self-esteem, and he did not cultivate any male or female friends. He never sought any type of assistance from men or women outside of his immediate and extended family. (As I note in Chapter 5, Fraiberg et al. [1975] conceptualized a similar situation in which "whisperings" regarding expected behaviors were passed down through three generations of a Hungarian family. Her treatise *Ghosts in the Nursery* is recommended.)

I now return to the example of the boy and his need for increased contact with his peer group.

This second-generation father was fortunate to have a concerned and empathic outside observer—his wife. He also possessed a good ability to reflect on his representational world, a world that contained more normal than pathogenic beliefs. His wife gently told him that she had noticed a recent change in his usual sensitivity to their son's needs, after their son had told him of the admiration and support he now wanted from his friends. The father initially listened to his wife, and then put her off, reacting quite defensively. His wife, however, was not afraid to speak her mind. She told him that he was acting as self-centered as she had seen her father-in-law act on many occasions. Nonplussed, but still motivated by love for his wife and son, the father reflected during the next few days on his wife's emotionally painful observation. Gradually he realized that in some way he was not empathically tuning in to himself or to his son.

The father gradually achieved the self-awareness that something automatic had occurred within him when his son began talking about his new need for an ongoing admiring relationship with his baseball chums. In using his capacity for empathy, this father was able to intuit his son's disappointment and anger when he had told him that the boy should abandon any need for his friends as a source of positive self-regard. Also, the father made a causal connection between his own contemptuous feelings toward his father and the contemptuous feelings he had toward his son when he told him about wanting to be with his friends after hitting a home run. He now achieved empathy for another little boy—himself. He recalled his own father giving him the same message he had recently given to his own son. He now felt sad for himself. In achieving this empathic self-awareness, he was also able to consciously recall his anger at his father and how lonely he felt when his mother did not ask him how he felt in response to his father's edict to give up developing his peer friendships.

This father now realized that he had the choice that all parents have when they realize that their belief of what constitutes normality is based on a behavioral pattern, edict, moral standard, or disciplinary measure taught to them by their own parents that they now perceive as wrong: to continue to maintain that old belief or to transform it into a new conceptual belief about what are normal developmental tasks for their children. To transform the belief would require him to engage in some mental restructuring and transformation of his representational world, a process that would create some feelings of uncertainty, given that his preexisting beliefs were the underpinnings of his understanding of himself and others. Changing old beliefs is like venturing into the unknown, and the feeling of anxiety is the mind's internal distress signal to the internal perception that one may not know what will occur in one's relationships with others if old beliefs are relinquished, restructured, or both.

In restructuring his representational world, this father was, in effect, telling the "voice" of his own father—carried around in many emotionally charged memories within his internal object representation of his father—that the message in that voice was wrong. This was tantamount to the second-generation father's telling himself that something in his mind needed to be changed. In addition to feeling anxious, the father would also feel a certain degree of guilt in disobeying a long-held belief in reference to someone in authority in the father's life (i.e., his own father). These beliefs—or "whisperings"—were the voice, in great part, of his superego. In one sense, a new potential internal "voice" came from this father's wife, who was telling her husband that his first-generation father's guilt-induced whisperings were wrong. I now return to the example.

> Eventually, a conflict ensued when the first-generation father, who was still alive, the second-generation father, and the 7-year-old boy were all together one day. The boy, in the midst of telling his grandfather about several events, proudly announced that his baseball teammates thought he was great and that they were very important to him. After his grandchild left the room, the grandfather told his son, "What is this stuff about thinking his friends are more important than his family? Remember you can only trust your family." The second-generation father then told his father, "You're wrong, Dad. You told me the same thing when I was growing up, and I ended up believing you. I didn't trust my friends and grew up more lonely than I had to be without making any good friends. And now I realize how I lost many good friendships. I am not going to tell my son the same thing you told me." The first-generation father looked disapprovingly at his son and said, "You're saying I was wrong and that I should change what I believe is right?"
>
> The first-generation father was angry at his son for several weeks. But in further conversations with his son, he agreed that perhaps what he believed to be true for him in raising his children was no longer true today. The second-generation father also gained a better appreciation for why his father felt so strongly about the family trusting only each other when he revealed to him his own anxiety and fear about venturing forth in the United States as a young immigrant.

The above example illustrates one of the many possible unconscious parental pathogenic beliefs that may interfere with a child's normal enthusiasm about entering elementary school and developing peer and social identities. By ages 6–7 years, children have already developed an autonomous identity that stimulates them to want to leave home for most of the day and be with other children and people, but that autonomy is still vulnerable to a lack of parental support and admiration. It is as if a young girl beginning grade school enthusiastically boards the school bus, but still looks over her shoulder to search for the encouraging, supportive, and positively expectant smile of her mother. She still needs that parental smile to fuel her continued passage from the rather exclusive dependence on her parents when she was younger to a more independent relationship with them as she becomes a grade school student.

Maturation and Development of Innate Needs

Children's Asserting Their Autonomy, Curiosity, and Industriousness While Restricting Sexual Gratification

Each of children's five innate needs (Lichtenberg 1989) continues to develop in late childhood. Whether each need undergoes maturation during this phase of life is a current area of speculation. I discuss each innate need separately.

Need for gratification of physiological requirements that maintain bodily regulation and physical survival. In the developmental phase between ages 6 and 11 years, no maturational advances are thought to take place in this need. But this need continues to undergo development as children learn better executive control and emotional control procedures to gratify this need in a manner that keeps them out of conflict with their parents, teachers, and others. In fact, one requirement for attending first grade is for children to be able to take over the proper gratification of their physiological requirements (e.g., dress warmly if it is winter, regulate their level of stimulation while playing in the schoolyard, take care of their need for food in eating lunch and snacks at the designated times, ensuring they get enough sleep so they will not be drowsy in class).

Need to assertively explore the social environment in seeking novel stimulation in order to learn to differentiate these stimuli and generate adaptive responses.   At about age 6 or 7 years, normally developing children appear to undergo what Shapiro and Hertzig (1988) called a *biodevelopmental shift.* This refers to children's maturation of physical, cognitive, language, emotional, and defense mechanisms that appear to fuel children's development of their innate need to exhibit their autonomous identity in the social world.

Need to attach to at least one other human in a predominantly emotionally pleasurable interaction.   Children ages 6–7 years have developed this need through their attachment relationship with their parents and siblings and with children and adults outside of their family. Their attaining positive self-constancy and object constancy provides them with a representational world in which they are able to comfort themselves during separations from the family based on their internal image of being a valued and loved child and having supportive and loving parents. These parental representations also lead them to generate positive transference reactions to new peers and teachers at school. As such, they transfer their inner expectations that their innate need to relate in an emotionally pleasurable way with new people will be gratified.

In late childhood, children enthusiastically begin new attachments and future friendships while they concurrently revel in demonstrating new autonomous behaviors. In normally developing children—as in normally developing adolescents and adults—attachment and autonomy simultaneously enhance the development of each other. Stated in another way, a child's true self develops in the context of his or her maintaining attachment relationships. When both attachment and autonomy needs are gratified concurrently, children develop more normally than when one develops at the expense of the other. Quite often, children who maintain attachments to their parents at the expense of their autonomous development have parents who are overprotective and biased against their children's autonomous growth. Such children will often develop the belief that if they manifest any autonomy, their parents will not protect them or will abandon them. On the other hand, children who emphasize autonomy over attachment may have identified with the aggressor; that is, their parents may have treated their innate need to attach to them with some mixture of emotional distance, disinterest, lack of protection, contempt, or a similar reaction. Children then develop the belief that maintaining attachments is not important in asserting their autonomous self, and will often treat others with an attitude that those others should support their autonomy; at the same time, they treat both their and other children's need to attach to each other with disinterest or even contempt.

Need for emotionally pleasurable sensory-sexual stimulation and gratification. S. Freud (1905/1963) labeled the period between ages 6 and 11 years as the period of latency—specifically, sexual latency. He was particularly impressed with the relative "quietness" of sexual instinctual wishes in children. Freud said that this is the phase of a child's life when oedipal wishes are beginning to be mastered and remain "quiet" until puberty (ages 11–13 years) when some oedipal wishes return and must be relinquished once again. Freud (1905/1963) wrote, "It is during this period of total or only partial latency that are built up the mental forces which are later to impede the course of the sexual instinct" (p. 130). By "mental forces," Freud meant the mechanisms of defense.

At about age 6 years, defense mechanisms are activated by heterosexual children in the service of their desire to turn away from their oedipal wishes of wanting to obtain an exclusive relationship with the opposite-gender parent. Children ages 6–7 years turn toward their social world of peers, school, and all the interpersonal activities generated by both. In so doing, they are using the defense mechanism of displacement (see "Development of Adaptational Capabilities," below) to switch some of their emotional and potential sexually stimulating involvement with their parents onto their peers and others outside of the family.

Other researchers (Clower 1976; Fraiberg 1972; Galenson 1993) have demonstrated that genital self-stimulation and gratification takes place during latency in both boys and girls, although it is, as Freud suggested, relatively less blatant than in any other phase of the life cycle. At this age, boys will directly stimulate their penis and girls will either directly stimulate their clitoris manually or more often engage in indirect clitoral stimulation by rubbing their genital region against objects.

Because children between ages 6 and 11 years—especially between ages 6 and 8 years—are trying hard to live up to the standards they have taken into their superego (see "Development of the Superego," below), they are usually quite strict in obeying their internalized standards. In addition, they are continuing to develop a sexual identity by learning more about how to express their needs for sexual stimulation and gratification. However, they have already learned that, at their age (as least in American society), they are not permitted by their parents or society to engage in any sexual stimulation or gratification with each other or with adults. This societal rule makes them avoid excessive masturbation because such excessive sexual stimulation makes it more difficult for them to be around their peers. Thus many developmental researchers (Galenson 1993; Kramer and Rudolf 1991; Noshpitz and King 1991; P. Tyson and Tyson 1991) have documented how masturbation during latency is present but is not a dominant preoccupation of children. When masturbation does occur, it is in the privacy of children's rooms. Also, heterosexual children's fantasies do not contain sexual images of the opposite-gender parent, nor do homosexual children's fantasies contain sexual images of the same-gender parent. (However, this is true only if children have not put aside their heterosexual or homosexual oedipal wishes at ages 6–7 years.)

Need to signal distress when experiencing an emotionally displeasurable over- or understimulating experience, and initiate other fight-or-flight behavioral and mental responses. In late childhood, children become more able to organize how they activate distress signals and how they can tolerate more of a delay before activating a fight-or-flight response.

Children's defense mechanisms years undergo considerable maturational growth between ages 6 and 11 years, particularly their aggressive fight response to a perceived threat. Isolation of emotion, sublimation, reaction formation, and displacement all emerge. Fantasy formation also undergoes considerable development (see "Development of Adaptational Capabilities," below). In addition, 6- to 11-year-old children's ability to use both conscious thinking and unconscious defense mechanisms to delay action and ponder responses makes their representational world of stored knowledge more available to them than ever before.

Maturation and Development of Physical Capabilities

Maturation of Gross and Fine Motor Skills and Visual-Auditory, Visual-Spatial, and Temporal-Spatial Capabilities

In late childhood, there are significant maturational advances in children's physical capabilities, including advances in their 1) self-regulatory and self-soothing capabilities, 2) gross motor capabilities, 3) fine motor capabilities, and (4) temporal-spatial capabilities.

Self-regulatory and self-soothing capabilities are mediated through the maturational growth of the frontal lobes of children's brain. At birth, infants' total brain volume is only 10% of the volume it will be at age 20 years. By age 7 years, children's brain volume is at 90% of the volume it will be at age 20 years (Schechter and Combrinck-Graham 1991; Shapiro and Perry 1976). The maturation of the frontal lobes of children ages 6–7 years enables them to better use their own verbalizations to achieve self-regulation of their feelings (Shapiro and Perry 1976). Specifically, frontal lobe maturation is associated with an increase in children's ability to recall and activate both executive and emotional control structures, which in turn allows them to be more proficient in selecting verbal and behavioral procedures to achieve self-regulation of their feelings. When this self-regulation is achieved, children have developed their self-soothing ability.

Advances in gross and fine motor capabilities are mediated by the completion of the myelination process for major nerve tracts in the central nervous system (Brodal 1969). Maturational advances in gross motor abilities at around ages 6–7 years include children's becoming more adept at controlling large muscle groups. Thus they have better balance and are much better runners, jumpers, bicycle riders, and tumblers than they were at age 5 years (Schechter and Combrinck-Graham 1991).

Myelination of nerve tracts also enhances 6- to 7-year-old children's fine motor abilities as well as their visual-auditory and visual-motor coordination. These maturational advances enable them to use a pincer's grasp of the fingers, draw geometric figures or a six-part person (i.e., head, body, arms, and legs), develop printing and even elementary cursive writing skills, and follow visual and auditory cues, among other fine motor skills (Schechter and Combrinck-Graham 1991).

Maturation of temporal-spatial capabilities enables children ages 6–7 years to discriminate right from left more easily, to know the day and year, and to begin to understand that past, present, and future are different points along a temporal continuum. These maturational advances assist them in further developing their positive self-constancy. As Buxbaum (1991) expressed it, "He is today what he was yesterday and what he will be tomorrow" (p. 343).

Children will at first perceive their new physical capabilities as novel events. Their emergence will encourage children to experiment in exhibiting and using them in interaction with others, particularly peers. Whereas during their genital-narcissistic and oedipal phases (between ages 3 and 6 years) children were preoccupied to a large degree with the genital area of their body, at ages 6–7 years they begin to exhibit much more of an awareness of an integrated body image. In having put aside their oedipal wishes, they now begin to enjoy their new ability to draw their own body images and their images of their parents and siblings without being overly focused on the genitals (e.g., their size, their presence or lack thereof) (Noshpitz and King 1991).

Maturation and Development of Cognitive Capabilities

■ Emergence of More Complex Mental Operations

At around ages 6–7 years, children's cognitive maturation makes it possible for them to do more complex mental operations. Piaget labeled the period between ages 6 and 11 years as the *concrete operational phase of cognitive development,* referring to children's ability to carry out complex thinking processes only about concrete events and not about abstract phenomena. (Children do not think abstractly until they reach adolescence, when they can understand events that might occur in addition to those that do occur.)

Whenever children are able to figure out the solutions to various problems presented to them—both those they are given in school and those they formulate themselves—their ability to solve those problems leads to the construction of new executive control and emotional control structures. Further, with their increasing adeptness at performing mental operations, they begin to do all sorts of "mental experiments" to solve problems that they formerly had to use action to solve.

Ability to understand others' perspectives. Children's ability to take another person's perspective undergoes a gradual change during late childhood, when the egocentrism of early childhood is greatly diminished. For example, a 3½-year-old boy stood in the doorway of a restaurant with his 7-year-old brother and their mother. The younger brother looked into the restaurant and said, "It's too crowded. I don't want to go in." The older brother agreed. The mother then told both boys, "Stand over here [motioning to a corner of the entrance that gave another view of the restaurant] and you'll see it looks crowded only from where you are." The 7-year-old was motivated to walk to the corner of the room his mother had indicated because he could now understand that his perspective was at times not the only perspective. His 3½-year-old brother refused to move to view the restaurant from that corner. Because he was unable to consider that another perspective could differ from his own, he only restated, "It's too crowded!"

Ability to develop more complex categories.   Children also have a new ability to classify objects according to their logical or reasonable similarities or differences. When a 5-year-old girl is shown a bouquet of flowers that contains two-thirds roses and one-third daisies and is asked, "Are there more roses or flowers?" she will want to handle and separate the flowers. She will not realize that she cannot solve the problem by physically matching what she sees. However, when a 7-year-old girl is presented with the same problem, she can classify objects in her mind according to logical similarities and differences. She has already learned what a flower is (a representation) and also has constructed the category of "flowers" and knows that some flowers are roses and others are daisies. Presented with the same problem, she answers, "There are more flowers than roses, but roses are flowers too!"

Children learn new categories that apply to themselves through comparing themselves with others. For example, Kagan (1984) observed how 6- to 7-year-old children will begin to view themselves as smaller than a bigger sibling and bigger than a smaller sibling. In so doing, they are viewing themselves as being members of the category of "sibling" and of the physical, relational categories of both big objects and small objects.

Kagan (1984) also observed that many of the qualities children ascribe to themselves as defining their peer and social identities come from their automatic and intuitive comparisons with peers and others. One example is the conceptual quality called courage. Based on their peer group's and their parents' view of them, by ages 8–9 years, children will generally put themselves in the category of being either "brave" or "not brave." In this case, they are defining themselves by defining what they are not. Thus a boy will define himself as a boy by saying and doing things that he believes girls do not say or do.

In their construction of categories, 6- to 7-year-old children tend to believe that the categories they belong to more reasonably define the characteristics of children themselves. Thus 6-year-old girls have much to learn about how girls think and behave in a peer group of boys and girls, and how girls behave in society at large. Early in the process, a girl will believe that she should possess all the qualities she hears and sees are possessed by girls in general, including all those qualities that boys do not possess.

By age 9 or 10 years, children begin to define a more personal peer and social identity as they continue to discover themselves in the eyes of their peer group. Whereas pre-self-aware infants and self-aware toddlers discover many of the mental and behavioral qualities they possess by looking into the eyes of their parents, latency-age children slowly develop their peer and social identity through seeing themselves as others see them and then using these reflections to construct new representational peer and social identity additions to their growing self-representation.

Ability to reason logically.   Children ages 6–11 years gradually develop the capacity to construct a conception and solve a problem that has a logical solution. Wesley and Sullivan (1980) defined a conception as "a rule that requires constancy in the 'mind' but nonconstancy in the physical environment" (p. 120). They illustrate this definition by presenting the following two problems:

> *Select the odd one from each group of items:*
> 1. O X O O O   X   . . . X . . .
>   *Answer:*   X
> 2. O X O O O   , , , , .   * * / * *
>   *Answers:*   X   .   /

Children younger than age 6 years can solve problem #1 by merely using their mental processing ability to perform simple pattern matching. Problem #2, however, as Wesley and Sullivan (1980) noted,

> cannot be solved by the mere matching of a certain pattern. The "physical" aspect or the visual pattern of the correct solution

changes from X to . to /. Such a problem can only be solved by a mental rule; "the odd one is out." It is truly a conceptual problem. (p. 200)

Thus the second problem can be solved only by children who are older than age 6 years. Such children have attained the cognitive level of conceptual thinking that will enable them to study the problem and solve it by constructing the conception "the odd one is out."

Ability to understand relational terms. Another cognitive advance that emerges in 6- to 7-year-old children is the ability to understand relational terms. Before this age, they do not comprehend that terms such as taller and bigger are related. After age 6 years, however, they begin to comprehend and classify the terms into a new constructed category named "physical qualities." They now know that bigger and taller are linked through the common relation of height. After age 6 years, children are constructing more and more categories as they acquire knowledge about how objects and events can be classified according to shared qualities. Without this new ability, their acquisition of language and its use would be greatly impaired.

Increased use of secondary process thinking. As 6- to 7-year-old children's cognitive abilities enable them to think more and act less, they begin to use more secondary process thinking in reacting to novel perceptions (see Figure 6–1). They compare new perceptions with preexisting representations and analyze them completely within their mind. They can now understand an assignment that might be given by their teacher such as, "You were just cutting up boxes and making them into different shapes. Now imagine and think about what shapes you made and which other ones you can think of making before you do any more cutting."

Ability to understand concept of reversibility. In late childhood, children's cognitive ability to understand reversible (mental) operations (i.e., that for every action or mental operation there is one that cancels it) emerges. For example, they can understand the following equations:

$$8 \times 6 = 48, \text{ and}$$
$$48 \div 8 = 6$$

The ability to solve these simple arithmetic problems stems from children's acquisition of the concept of reversibility. Children also begin to use this concept to understand new situations that do not involve math problems. For example, understanding reversibility helps them realize that, when they do something wrong, they can "undo" the wrong by doing something good. Grasping this concept also helps them understand that their body is "reversible"; for example, before age 6 years, they would have a hard time realizing that a broken bone

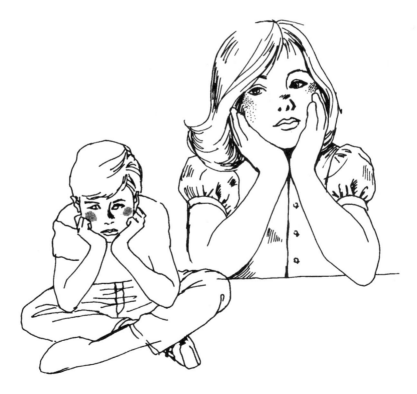

Figure 6–1. The importance of thinking and utilizing fantasy in latency-age children.

can heal. Once children can apply this principle to their body, their developmental body damage anxiety, when stimulated by environmental events or their memories, will be less intense.

Ability to compare past and present. More so than at any previous age, children in the concrete operational stage reevaluate and achieve new understandings of their memories (i.e., their previously acquired knowledge). In a process of ongoing reconstruction of prior representations, they acquire new knowledge through the internal process of comparing present and past knowledge, or, as Piaget (1967) put it, a "reshaping through thought of previous material." The resulting newly constructed representations will give rise to new motivations, new emotional responses to previous memories, and new abilities to understand developmental anxieties.

Ability to understand conservation of quantity and number. Children ages 6–7 years develop an understanding of the concept of conservation of both quantity (mass) and number. The concept of conservation of quantity states that a property or an attribute of an object remains the same despite some transformation in the object's appearance. For example, when shown two same-size pies, one cut in 4 pieces and the other cut in 12 pieces, a 4-year-old child will tell you that there is more pie in the 12-piece pie. A 7- to 8-year-old child, however, will be able to recognize that both pies have similar quantities.

With the emergence of children's maturation and development of the cognitive ability to construct the concept of conservation, they forever know that the quantity of a liquid (or a solid) remains constant despite changes in the shape of the container holding the liquid substance or a change in the conditions in which the substance exists (e.g., whether water is in the form of ice or liquid). In understanding this latter concept, children will also call on their recently acquired concept of reversibility, as Gleitman (1987) noted:

> For every transformation that changes the way the liquid looks, there is another that restores its original appearance. Given this insight, children at this age recognize that there is an underlying

attribute of reality, the quantity of liquid that remains constant (is *conserved*), throughout the various perceptual changes. (p. 376; italics and parentheses in original)

Children will begin to apply the principle of conservation of mass in further understanding themselves and others. Thus they learn that each person remains a whole person, unique and separate, despite changes in his or her appearance and emotional state.

Children age 6 years also develop an understanding of the concept of conservation of number, which states that a number of objects stay the same regardless of their perceptual configuration. A 4-year-old child can be fooled into thinking that a 2-foot row of six bottles evenly spaced has more bottles than a 1-foot row of six glasses evenly spaced has glasses. However, by ages 5–6 years, children easily notice that there are an equal number of bottles and glasses, even though the perceptual configurations are different.

Another maturational advance emerging in late childhood that is related to conservation of number is called *serialization*. This concept enables children to arrange objects according to some quantified dimension (e.g., height, size, weight).

■ Differentiation of Primary and Secondary Process Thinking: Development of Masking and Latent Symbols

As children's cognitive advances that emerge at ages 6–7 years continue to develop, children become increasingly able to use their mental abilities to modify their actions in order to better fit the demands and developmental taskings of their parents, teachers, and others. This process further helps them to distinguish their primary process, magically oriented thinking from their secondary process, logical and reality-oriented thinking.

In late childhood, children's primary process thinking remains "alive and well" in the way they use symbolic thinking, remember night dreams and daytime fantasies, write and verbalize scripts or stories, and develop new interest in activities such as drawing, painting, and building models. With regard to their symbolic thinking, there is a maturational change in how they use and apply their symbolic representations. They add many new symbols to their symbolic representational "database." Each society possesses a number of specific symbols that children must learn in order to adapt their innate needs to the parents' and society's developmental taskings. For example, a diploma from grammar school is a symbol. The particular meaning children give to this symbol will be based on how they process the transactions between the information they receive about a diploma (social stimuli) and their cognitive processing of this information (psychological stimuli).

In addition to children's giving their own personal meaning to society's symbols, they construct their own symbols. One can observe how, in late childhood, there is a gradual masking of primary process magical thinking within children's symbolic representations, whether through speech, play, fantasies, written stories, drawings, paintings, or models. Before ages 6–7 years, children could not distinguish between their symbols and what they symbolized. Also, they were unable to be aware of how transparent their symbols were to a more cognitively advanced observer (e.g., a child older than age 7 years, a parent). At around ages 6–7 years, however, children's use of their own constructed symbols begins to change. Because they are becoming more capable of figuring out other children's or their parent's symbols, they then make the logical assumption that others can decipher their own constructed symbols. Children subsequently become much more aware of how their use of symbols may reveal aspects about their wishes and feelings that they 1) do not want to acknowledge themselves and 2) do not want to reveal to their parents or others.

With regard to the first point above, although 6- to 7-year-old children continue to symbolize aspects of themselves, others, and events that involve thoughts and memories that generate displeasurable feelings, their symbols are less transparent than symbols formed before age 6 years. Beginning at age 6 or 7 years, the symbols children form not only prevent them from acknowledging something that they would rather put out of their conscious mind, but also prevent others from figuring out what the child is avoiding. The symbol in effect allows them to express certain aspects of a thought, feeling, or memory in a pleasurable, creative, yet disguised, symbolic fantasy when its direct expression would have been highly displeasurable. These *masking symbols* (Sarnoff 1987) are adaptive in that they allow children a means to mask certain facts of their life that they would be anxious about revealing directly to themselves or others in either speech or behavior. As Sarnoff (1987) noted, "It is characteristic of the thinking of children in early latency that they develop a masked way of thinking and fantasizing about experiences and observations they are trying to master" (p. 120). On the other hand, when children are unable to create adaptive symbols to "express" emotionally displeasurable facts of life, they invariably repress the thoughts and feelings associated with the situation; this repression can become maladaptive if prolonged.

Children ages 6–7 years are motivated to develop more masked ways of thinking and fantasizing by their increasing recognition that they may use pretense and deception to mask anxiety-provoking wishes, feelings, or memories of others. The anxiety is associated with their expectation that the truthful verbalization of a wish, feeling, or memory will be met with some degree of disapproval. This expectation of disapproval is one of the motivations for 6- to 7-year-old children's interest in developing secrets. Through a secret, they can consciously suppress thoughts, feelings, or memories until they are less anxious about verbally revealing them. Children also take pleasure in knowing that a secret is something they know and their parents and others do not. Thus, in addition to being adaptive in their suppression of anxiety-provoking mental contents, secrets also enhance the development of children's appreciation of having a unique mind.

In addition to forming secrets—which is a conscious action—6- to 7-year-old children also begin to mask their thoughts, feelings, or memories through their unconscious ability to form more complex symbols. As Sarnoff observed,

> Through the use of such symbols, *latent fantasies* can be expressed in the form of *distorted manifest fantasies*. Treasured loved ones can thus be spared the role of targets of forbidden drives [or forbidden wishes emanating from children's innate needs]. (p. 120; italics added)

When faced with an internal or external conflict about a wish, feeling, or memory that is generating a consciously intolerable degree of developmental anxiety, children's minds will generate an unconscious latent fantasy. If their latent fantasy remains completely unconscious, they have no chance to work on it and resolve the conflict that originally generated it. More often, however, their unconscious mind generates a new, more disguised and much less threatening fantasy that uses masking symbols, which then enters the conscious mind and is subsequently expressed in play, daydreams, stories, model building, paintings, and so on.

In the following examples, Sarnoff (1987) illustrated the difference in how a 4-year-old child spontaneously expresses a wish that, in a 9-year-old child, would generate a consciously intolerable degree of one or more developmental anxieties. The 9-year-old would repress the original wish and the fantasy associated with it, and ultimately express a symbolic fantasy that would be quite difficult to decipher in its latent meaning unless the child's parent or someone else who knew the child used empathy, patience, listening, and playful engagement to "look" beneath the child's manifest fantasy to discover its latent meanings.

> A 4-year-old girl looked at her grandmother. She admired aloud a beautiful pin that the grandmother was wearing. The grandmother then stated in a rather direct and matter-of-fact fashion, "When I die, I'll leave it to you." The child responded in equally direct fashion, in a manner typical of the prelatency child, "Oh, Grandma, I know it's wrong to say, but I can hardly wait!"
>
> The latency-age child, when confronted with such a thought, activates defensive processes to hide it from his own sight. The following vignette illustrates this.

> A 9-year-old boy was in treatment for disruptive behavior in school. His mother reported that his father had scolded and slapped the boy on the day of the session here described. When the child arrived for his session, I had expected that he would tell of this experience and of his anger at his father. Instead, the youngster spoke proudly of his father's new car, emphasizing its technical advances (e.g., wide track). None of the father's scolding or beating was mentioned. The youngster eventually turned the content of his session to a description of a fantasy of a war in which he killed the general. (Sarnoff 1987, p. 135)

This 9-year-old boy's unconscious self had activated the ego defense mechanisms of displacement (his focus of interest on his father's new car) and of resurrecting his manifest wish for a perfect father. (As I note in Chapters 4 and 5, children periodically resurrect their normal idealizing wishes to be perfect or to have perfect parents in response to certain developmental conflicts that generate intolerable levels of anxiety).

What is true about latent and manifest fantasies also holds for children's pathogenic beliefs. Pathogenic beliefs are not wishful but "compelling, grim and maladaptive" (Weiss 1993). Pathogenic beliefs inhibit the development of children's overall identity— specifically, children's development of a true self-representation. A pathogenic belief is constructed from experiences in which children's wishes and feelings have led to highly displeasurable levels of developmental anxiety, rage, and so on. Children's inferences— that is, their personal meaning for why the emotionally painful experience occurred to them—become the substance of their pathogenic belief. For example, the pathogenic belief that the above 9-year-old boy might construct if his father continues to physically hit him, and he is not helped in expressing his anger toward and disappointment in his father, could be something like, "My father hits me a lot because he hates me; he hates me because he believes I am more like my mother. However, my father loves my brother, because he's more like my dad." Here the boy's inference that his father hates him is being fueled by 1) the father's physical abuse, 2) the boy's view that his father believes he is more like his mother, and 3) the boy's hatred of his father that he has unconsciously projected onto his father.

If this boy is asked, however, what he thinks of his father, this pathogenic belief will not emerge. The answer he would give would be the *manifest pathogenic belief,* and the belief that he represses from his consciousness would be the *latent pathogenic belief.* A manifest pathogenic belief is actually the latent pathogenic belief modified and distorted as a result of the unconscious use of defense mechanisms. Thus the manifest pathogenic belief could contain elements of splitting, denial, displacement, projection, reaction formation, and so on. For example, in response to the question of how he thinks of his father, this 9-year-old boy might say, "He does a lot of things for me, he really cares a lot." His answer reveals either 1) his use of the defense of splitting in expressing only his conscious affection for his father, while the other side of his ambivalence (i.e., his anger) is consciously repressed, or 2) his use of the defense of reaction formation in expressing conscious affection, which is the opposite of his repressed unconscious hatred for his father.

At about age 9 years, children begin to abandon their use of symbols to express manifest fantasies involving their conflicted wishes and feelings. They recognize that symbols, specifically as contained within their symbolic manifest fantasies, do not truly express a latent wish the way the expression of the wish does. They, therefore, take another step in being more able to "see" their latent wishes and feelings in their manifest fantasies and begin to wonder, "Why use them to disguise wishes and feelings?"

Thus children ages 6–9 years verbalize elaborate manifest fantasies and act them out in their symbolic play, tell stories, discuss favorite motion pictures, and so on, whereas children ages 9–11 years are oriented toward playing board games, discussing rules, and sharing various collections (e.g., marbles, baseball cards, antique dolls) while keeping their fantasies, for the most part, secret. These older children often become suspicious and anxious if they are offered a story and asked to give their thoughts about it. They know that thoughts about the story will reveal much about their representational world. Because they have established thought dominance—and thus most often think before immediately acting or speaking—they take solace in believing that they can disguise their thinking through speech and less symbolic play.

Maturation and Development of Temperamental Characteristics
Stability of Temperament

As I note in earlier chapters, temperament is now accepted as part of infants' innately endowed characteristics (Thomas and Chess

1977). Behavioral inhibition to the unfamiliar, for example, is a characteristic that shows temporal stability from infancy through age 7 years (Kagan 1989). Although inhibition to unfamiliar or novel events may be an innate pattern of behavior that is unmodifiable by infants' attachment relationship with their parents, Kagan found that some infants' inhibition to the unfamiliar could be eventually modified by their attachment relationship with their parents (Kagan 1989). For example, parents of a 2-year-old boy who showed behavioral inhibition to the unfamiliar gently encouraged him to explore. When he took the risk to explore away from them, they made themselves very available on his return. Such a goodness of fit produced a 6-year-old whose prior inhibition to the unfamiliar had changed to a joyful excitement in exploring the unfamiliar. Thus an infant's behavioral inhibition to the unfamiliar can show temporal instability in some families.

Despite Kagan's research, the continuity or discontinuity of temperamental characteristics is an area of ongoing controversy (Buss and Plomin 1975; Goldsmith et al. 1987). Rutter (1986) found little stability in temperamental characteristics in longitudinal studies of temperament from infancy to ages 9–11 years. He cited evidence suggesting that a child's attachment relationship may 1) maintain stability of temperament, 2) accentuate certain temperamental traits, or 3) change a child's temperament from infancy to late childhood. Chess and Thomas (1989) have suggested that alterations in children's temperament may be attributable not only to the parenting they receive but also to maturational changes in the children's temperament in the context of the parenting environment. (However, as I note in previous chapters, the measurement of changes in temperamental characteristics is another area of controversy.)

Of Thomas and Chess's (1977) temperamental clusters (i.e., easy child, slow-to-warm-up child, and difficult child), the difficult child has been studied more than the other two, primarily in an attempt to determine whether having a temperament so classified is a risk factor for the development of behavioral problems in late childhood and adolescence. The difficult child is the one who experiences displeasurable emotions to the unfamiliar, activates fight-flight behaviors quickly, sustains his or her avoidance of novel situations for prolonged periods, and is slow to develop self-soothing behaviors or to be soothed by others.

Researchers have found that the difficult child classification shows stability from infancy to ages 8–10 years (Kingston and Prior 1995). In addition, the following differences between boys and girls have been found: whereas difficult temperament is not different in boys and girls (Bezirganian and Cohen 1992), boys who manifest a difficult temperament by age 7 years tend to remain difficult well into adolescence, whereas girls who manifest a difficult temperament by age 7 years are more prone to change their temperamental classification from difficult to easy by early adolescence (Maziade et al. 1985). The reason for this difference in temporal stability of a difficult temperament is unclear. The hypotheses explaining this difference include 1) that a boy inherits an innate difficult temperament that is genetically different from a girl's innate difficult temperament, and 2) that a boy's stability of difficult temperament is primarily attributable to his attachment relationship with his parents.

With regard to the second hypothesis, Bezirganian and Cohen (1992) found the following:

1. A girl's difficult temperament becomes unstable from infancy to early adolescence when her relationship with her father is one of "closeness, involvement, and identification" and when her mother reacts quite negatively to her difficult temperament. The close relationship with her father served as a protective factor that prevents her difficult temperament from remaining stable. The authors speculated about this finding, saying,

   > Fathers are particularly important in daughters' sex typing, and provide a model whereby daughters can learn to respond to males in general in a sex appropriate way. . . . It could be when daughters' sex-typed behavior is positively reinforced by fathers, there is a concomitant decrease in difficult temperament, which includes much sex-inappropriate anger and aggression. When daughters do not receive parental encouragement of their sex-typed behavior, they may show a worsening in their difficult temperament. (pp. 798–799)

2. A boy's difficult temperament remains stable from infancy to early adolescence when the boy's relationship with his mother is one of excessive punishment and control. The authors speculated that boys, especially between ages 6 and 11 years, may have a more negative response to female aggression than to male aggression. They found that, in the boys they studied, "closeness, involvement, and identification" with their father did not serve as a protective factor that prevented their difficult temperament from remaining stable. One possible reason for this is that a boy, in turning to his father for protection from his mother's negative responses to his behavior, does not experience the father as a protector and hence someone with which to identify. This difficulty in identifying with his father would make any 6- to 11-year-old boy have more body damage anxiety in reference to his mother's aggression toward him, which in turn becomes a catalyst for the boy's using his difficult temperamental traits in an attempt to ward off and distance himself from his mother.

Maturation and Development of Emotions

Further Development of Emotions in Assisting Energy Mobilization, Self-Regulation, and Social Adaptation

In late childhood, children gradually become aware of "blends" of feelings and can inwardly perceive how new emotions can block out old ones (Lane and Schwartz 1987). Children also discover their capacity to have ambivalent feelings. Finally, they begin to use their intuition and empathy more fully in appreciating the emotional states of others based on their own similar wishes and experiences. This increased capacity for empathy results in part from their new cognitive ability to recognize that others can have perspectives different from their own. As P. Tyson and Tyson (1991) expressed it,

Because a latency child has the capacity to imagine how she [her mother] would feel in her mother's situation and can understand that her mother has a reality separate from herself, she can empathize with her mother apart from whether or not her own wishes are affected. (p. 184)

Because older children have the capacity to reflect on much more of their complicated emotional representational world than ever before, their rules for displaying those emotions must become more sophisticated. Children must also begin to transfer their emotional display rules from their family setting into the classroom, onto the ball field, into the synagogue or church, and so on. In these new settings, they will experiment with speech to learn which emotions can be verbalized in which social settings.

As I list in previous chapters, the three main functions of emotions throughout each developmental phase are to assist in 1) energy mobilization, 2) self-regulation, and 3) social adaptation. In reference to social adaptation, 6- to 11-year-old children's emotions are crucial psychological stimuli through which they learn social responses and construct their social identity by continuing to learn how to perceive and react to emotional information emanating from their parents and others. They are constantly learning how words and feelings communicate more than just words or actions. In becoming better able to perceive emotions in others, they become more adept at guiding their behaviors to adapt their wishes and needs to those of another. Izard (1977) stated that the principal functions of emotions are to motivate adaptive cognition and action and to facilitate social communications.

Beginning at ages 6–7 years and continuing throughout latency, children are also becoming more aware of their anxious emotions or developmental anxieties. They gradually learn to use developmental anxiety as an internal signal that warns them to become vigilant about an external threat (e.g., a physically dangerous person) or an internal threat (e.g., their own building rage toward their little sister who has just destroyed their new video game but whom they are forbidden to physically strike). They become more proficient at using these internal developmental anxiety signals because of the following developmental accomplishments:

1. During infancy, having parents who kept them from experiencing too many distressingly overstimulating (panic inducing) or understimulating (boring) experiences and who responded to their external signals of distress with soothing responses in a timely and consistent manner.

2. During toddlerhood, having parents who gradually delayed responding to their external signals of distress. In being allowed to experience a delay, they could begin to learn that they were capable of soothing themselves. During these delays in their parents' response, they also gradually became aware of their feelings—specifically, their internal anxiety feelings—that motivated them to send external signals of distress. By age 3 years, they began to become consciously aware of their own internal signal of distress (i.e., their anxiety), being able to say, "Mom, I'm afraid!"

3. During early childhood, developing the ability to call on their positive representational images of their parents to help them tolerate any anxiety consciously and to delay immediately sending an external signal of distress or engaging in a fight-flight behavioral response. Also important was their having learned that they could act, talk, engage in fantasy play, write a story, or engage in other similar behaviors when they experienced anxiety.

A child's ever-developing self is the main scanner, organizer, and director of all of that child's mental activities and surface behaviors. Although a child's self operates unconsciously, that child's self-representation allows him or her to be consciously aware of his or her inner mental world. As the representation of their autonomy, assertion, separateness, gender identity, and other parts of their identity, children's self-representation integrates all representational structures to allow them to achieve an awareness of their own self-initiative versus their self-inhibition and self-reflection. This self-representation is supraordinate to the other complex mental structures of the id, ego, and superego. Whereas the ego generates emotions, it is the self-representation that allows children to be aware of the products of their ego (e.g., anxiety). Thus, when children become aware of their anxiety in response to a current perception, they are revealing an aspect of their self-representation.

It is a child's self-representation that monitors an internal anxiety signal and then initiates a delay in activating a behavior to give the child time to think and internally perceive his or her feelings and memories. After such a delay, the child's self-representation activates an action or surface behavior, initiates speaking, or initiates a delay and speaking while the child consciously contemplates a fantasy, belief, or feeling. If the level of the anxiety signal reaches or exceeds the child's unique threshold for stimulation, the anxiety will be highly displeasurable. Then, as Yorke and Wiseberg (1976) stated, "signal anxiety gets no chance to function" (p. 131), meaning that the emotion of anxiety is too painful to tolerate. In that situation, the child's self-representation will automatically—and hence unconsciously—direct the ego to either 1) enact a behavior or series of behaviors in an automatic fight-flight type of response, 2) activate one or more mental mechanisms of defense, or 3) activate the defense mechanism of somatization. Children who can use defense mechanisms in an adaptive manner (i.e., transiently and sparingly) are invariably those who are growing up in a family where the emotional display rules permit verbalization of feelings and those who have not been exposed to too many traumatic life events (e.g., serious accidents, physical abuse).

By age 6 or 7 years, therefore, normally developing, nontraumatized children have, through their interactions with their parents and others, consciously experienced the following developmental anxieties (in contrast to children growing up with rules that restrict their verbalization of feelings or those growing up exposed to multiple traumas that cause them to avoid consciously experiencing these developmental anxieties):

1. Stranger anxiety in recognizing that a person is unfamiliar (first emerges at about age 6 months)
2. Separation anxiety about losing their parents' love and protection (first emerges at about ages 8–10 months)
3. Disintegration anxiety or fear of a total absence of parental attributions of value (first emerges at about age 18 months)
4. Body damage anxiety about the possible occurrence of bodily injury, sickness, or death (first emerges at about age 3 years)

5. Superego anxiety about the possible disapproval of their super-ego (first emerges at about ages 4–5 years)

In addition, from ages 6 to 7 years to about age 12 years, through their socializing interactions with their parents, siblings, and others, children growing up in a family where a goodness of fit has been maintained continue to acquire the knowledge that

1. These developmental anxieties do not indicate an impending inevitable calamity.
2. Defense mechanisms can help them deal with current anxieties but can be given up in time.
3. They will survive and master future experiences that stimulate developmentally normal anxieties.
4. Action (particularly locomotion), speech (i.e., words of distress), and solitary, sibling, and peer play (i.e., symbolic play using compensatory fantasies) can all be used to control and eventually master an event that may generate one or more of these anxieties.

In summary, throughout late childhood, children increasingly acquire knowledge of different developmental anxieties that can be generated by their own wishes, beliefs, fantasies, and feelings and by their not living up to the standards contained within their own superego and those of their parents, teachers, and others. From the first through the sixth grades (between ages 6 and 11 years), they increasingly learn to tolerate these developmental anxieties as internal signals of possible calamity if they delay action and think about what they are doing, think about what others are doing to them, or both. They come to understand that they are able to alleviate proactively their developmental anxieties; this knowledge increases their confidence in their ability to regulate their own emotions.

For example, during her first few days of grade school, a 6½-year-old girl encounters the following new situations:

- She sits in her classroom seat and is greeted by her new teacher (a stranger).
- She sees her parents leave (separation).

- She is told by the teacher that she likes to teach new children (an attribution of value for children).
- She notices at lunch time that some children seem to threaten and bully others (a body damage issue).
- She is told repeatedly about the rules and regulations she must follow in school (a challenge to obey standards).

In response, she generates several types of developmental anxiety, but she does not raise her hand and say to her teacher,

Look, I'm leaving. You are a stranger whom I'm expected to trust but I don't. My mother is at home, but is she really? Maybe she went somewhere and I won't find her if I suddenly need her. So I don't trust her either. You say you like me for being here but I think you will only like me if I produce all the time, if I am real smart and almost perfect. And a few more things. This school is dangerous. You have kids here who hit and look like they can hurt you. So forget about the whole thing. I'm going home. Life is too scary! And all these rules. I know I'll break some sooner or later. And if I do, I'll feel real guilty and everyone at school will say that I did wrong and I'll feel real ashamed. So forget about the whole thing. I'll have all these bad feelings and I won't be able to control them or do anything to make myself feel better. I'm going home because starting school is too scary!

Instead, she finds all these developmental anxieties manageable. She stays in her seat at school, albeit with mild trepidation, and calms and soothes herself; thereupon, she is able to begin to perceive all sorts of novel and interesting new events as she begins her grade school career.

Maturation and Development of Verbal Language Abilities
Progression From Speech Dominance to Thought Dominance

In late childhood, verbal language comes close to its adult functioning. It serves children in 1) maintaining their emotional self-regulation, 2) maintaining their emotionally close attachment relationships with their parents, siblings, and other close individuals while they continue to develop their autonomous self, 3) acting as a principal source of performance and establishing relationships in the world of peers, and 4) assisting them in progressing from action dominance to speech dominance to thinking dominance. This latter function is illustrated in the following example:

> A 7-year-old boy was angry at another boy. He delayed acting while he worried about what would happen to him if he hit the other boy. He told his teacher what he was angry about and that he wanted to hit the other boy. His teacher said he shouldn't hit, but perhaps he could wait until recess and if he still was very angry at the other boy then she would stage a running race between him and the other boy. He told his teacher he did not want a race but wanted a boxing match instead. In talking to his teacher about his feelings and wishes, he instituted a delay in his wish to act. He consequently had time to think things over. By the afternoon, he had decided on a running race with the other boy instead of a boxing match.

The following is an example about how children begin to use speech to better identify and understand the motivation of their feelings:

> A 7-year-old girl sat alone at a picnic. Her mother sensed her sadness and encouraged her to talk about her feelings. The girl stated, "I'm sad because I want to play with my friends and Dad said this morning that this is a new big park, and I had to watch and take care of you at the picnic." Mom smiled inwardly and then explained that Dad was only telling her to be a big girl, and that Mom would be okay by herself. The girl then look relieved, smiled, and went to play with her friends.

Verbal language development in late childhood also assists children in beginning the transition from speech dominance to more thought dominance. They now begin to think more before they speak, and in the process develop their ability to delay gratification.

During this phase of childhood, psychologically aware parents empathically sense that they need to support their children's need to develop their ability to form secrets. However, parents also need to make clear that verbal communication is necessary for any group of people (e.g., a family, a class of children, a peer group) to function in a socially acceptable way. In supporting the use of speech to enhance group cooperation and conflict resolution, parents—especially those with 6- to 11-year-old children—must schedule time to talk with their children. This could be at breakfast, at dinner, on the way to soccer practice, or during any regular activity in which a parent and child are together and also when the entire family is together. If not, children at this age lose this important life experience of taking part in daily family events during which people talk to each other.

In expressing an interest in speaking to their children, parents' facial expressions, body language, and willingness to give children their total attention will often communicate more to their children than their words of interest. Older children, especially those ages 9–10 years, are quite adept at sensing the emotions of others and reading facial and body language. For example, a parent's words can be heard as untruths by a child if the parent's facial expression and body language give another message. When this repeatedly occurs, the child begins to equate words with denying or covering up true feelings and wishes. If the child then identifies with this parental defensive use of words, then he or she may avoid speaking to the parents, thinking, "Why should I? My parents talk but they don't really care about talking to me." The child may even adopt the same behavior; he or she may tell a parent, "Everything is just fine," while keeping his or her worries and anxieties secret.

In order for fantasies to be used by children to solve internal conflicts (i.e., those between their wishes and conscience) and external conflicts (i.e., those between their wishes and the prohibitions of their parents and others), they must involve language. When a private fantasy is used as the only means of gratifying a child's wishes or feelings, it can become a maladaptive defense mechanism that enables the child to avoid interactions with others. Consequently, that child's development of a peer and social identity is greatly inhibited.

Even though, by age 8 years, the content of children's verbalized fantasies being used as an adaptive defense begins to become more disguised, the children's parents must continue to emphasize that speech is crucial for interpersonal adaptation. Although they teach their children that thinking should come before speech, they should not allow their 8- to 11-year-old child to think only and not speak. It is possible for a manifest fantasy to become an "action" within an 8- to 11-year-old child's mind that gratifies a forbidden wish or feeling in symbolic thinking rather than in action or speech, as in the following example:

> A 9-year-old boy was angry at his father when his father deducted 2 days' worth of his weekly allowance because the son did not clean the family backyard as he had agreed to do each week. The boy was afraid to verbalize his anger at his father and instead wrote a story alone in his room about a boy who was a famous bank robber. In his story, the successful thief made the bank president angry, but the president also realized that sometimes he was too hard on people who wanted to save money in his bank.

Obviously, the bank president in the boy's story symbolized his father. This fantasy helped the boy to keep his angry feelings unverbalized as he discharged them in a symbolic fantasy. In rereading his own story, he realized that he was like a thief if he expected money from his father when he did not do his chores.

If this boy did not share some of his ponderings with his father, in time he might begin to construct the belief that, when he had a conflict involving other people, he should go off alone, think it out, and then keep the whole incident private. Such a belief would be incorporated into whatever former emotional control structures he had constructed. In time, he might repress his now pathogenic belief that talking is useless. However, this was not the case in this boy's family, because his father used his paternal empathy to sense that his son had become upset with him, as follows:

> The next evening, before his son initiated speaking to him, the father told his son, "When you're ready to talk, we should talk about what you've thought and felt about my taking your allowance away." His son responded, "I don't want to talk about it." The father, allowing his son an opportunity to think instead of

talk, said, "Okay. But it's important we talk about this." The next morning, after the boy once again pondered his own fantasy-derived discoveries, he initiated talking to his father. In the interchange, he was able to recall and consciously experience his guilt in reference to not cleaning the yard. He told his father that at first he was angry, but then realized he was not meeting his part of the bargain by avoiding his chores and then expecting his full allowance. His father told him he was proud of his response and was glad he had figured so much out on his own. The boy smiled.

If children are to believe in the value of their speech in solving internal and external conflicts, it is crucial for their parents to keep requesting verbal communication from them.

Another important function of speech emerging during late childhood, especially for 6- to 7-year-old children beginning grade school, is the use of verbalization to continue to differentiate between primary process and secondary process thinking. By age 7 years, children begin to notice when they verbalize a magical thought, and begin to treat these verbalizations as slips of the tongue, in much the same way as do adults. In a *slip of the tongue,* some unconscious thought, not always primary process, "slips" out in words; usually children notice they have just said something that did not make logical sense, that they spoke magically, that they have let out a feeling about which they are embarrassed, or something similar. Their recognition of a slip of the tongue indicates their increasing ability to use self-reflection to listen to their own words and use those reflections in deciding whether their words are helping them communicate their thoughts and feelings or hide them. In beginning to reflect on their own words—even before they receive a response from the listener—they become their own source of feedback about the effectiveness of their words in achieving their intended goal for speaking in the first place.

By age 7 years, children demarcate their recalled dreams and conscious daydreams from their nonpretend thinking. If a mother tries to pretend her 7- to 8-year-old child's dream is real, her child will often respond with, "Oh, Mom. It's not real. You're pretending my dream is real." Children are thus using speech to differentiate primary from secondary process thinking.

As an aspect of their normal living experiences, 6- to 11-year-old children will periodically experience highly displeasurable or distressful events. When highly distressed, 6- to 7-year-old children begin to call on their ever-developing capacity to form fantasies, which function as a temporary escape (i.e., an internal flight) when an external flight response (e.g., leaving the house, leaving school) or fight response is limited. When children are using fantasy formation to deal with such an experience, they need to continue to talk to their parents as a means of staying anchored in reality. Obviously, this helps children when they are not in the midst of a chronic traumatic life situation. When they are faced with an unbearable reality, their use of fantasy, while functioning to keep their consciously unbearable, rageful, frightening feelings repressed within their unconscious, will nevertheless begin to take a great toll on their developmental process, as in the following example:

A 9-year-old girl was sexually stimulated by her father. When her mother was away, her father coerced her to allow him to rub her nipples. She became sexually stimulated despite her high level of anxiety. She asked her father to stop but he ignored her and continued. She then became very passive (a type of behavioral flight), and after several minutes her father stopped, but told her to not tell her mother. Over the next several weeks, she avoided her father, spent more time absorbed in silent fantasy, and began to avoid playing with her school friends, especially boys. For this girl, fantasy was now becoming both an internal flight and a fixed and rigid defensive way of avoiding reality—the real world of men and boys—because reality, as represented by her father, had become too frightening. Tragically, this girl, in addition to having an incestuously driven father, had a mother who viewed her new silence around the family as the appropriate secretiveness of a normal 9-year-old child. As such, she did not seek to break through her daughter's silence. Consequently, the secret of her father's now periodic seductive behavior became both a silent and pathogenic memory and an ongoing fear within this girl's representational world. For this girl, speech was no longer a valued possession to help her adapt to life's challenges. In fact, she believed that, the more she kept silent, the less her father might notice her presence.

Continuing Influence of Preexisting Representational World

Transference Reactions in the Service of Achieving Mastery of Current Experience

By the time children reach age 6 or 7 years, their representational world has become a crucial source of information. They use this information to strike a balance between their internal adaptation to their innate needs and their external adaptation to the demands, guidelines, and developmental taskings of their parents, peers, teachers, and others. In this process, children will call on their preexisting representational world (psychological stimuli) of beliefs, fantasies, emotional control procedures, and other mental contents in an attempt to achieve the following:

1. Use their memories to generate transference predictions about their daily experiences with people.
2. Discover which transference predictions about people do seem to be true and reinforce their prior experiences with people.
3. Discover which of their transference predictions do not seem to be true and thereby challenge their prior experiences with people. This stimulates the accommodation-transformation process, in which they begin to transform prior memories of people into revised and new representations of people.

In normally developing children, their transference reactions are a transfer of positive or negative feelings, thoughts, wishes, and conceptions from a person or experience in the past onto a person or experience in the present. In particular, children will transfer what they believe to be true—whether the truth is emotionally pleasurable or displeasurable—in their attempt to achieve an immediate sense of intellectual mastery. The motivation for 6- to 11-year-old children's positive transference reactions is their continued attempt to prove their existent beliefs as true by attempting to assimilate current experiences into past pleasant and nurturant experiences they recall. Negative transference reactions are motivated by their attempt to avoid experiences in the present that remind them of past highly displeasurable, and even traumatic, experiences. The tendency to repeat prior experiences by attempting to make a new facsimile of an old experience is an unconscious function of a child's ego. The goal is mastery and control of current life experiences with those people who are in a position of authority or a position of providing for the child's needs.

Motivated by their continuing innate need to establish a sense of mastery and control over the outside world, children will unconsciously enact certain behaviors or procedures in an attempt to manipulate the outside world so it matches their inner world of beliefs. In this way, they use their beliefs in an attempt to influence the future, as did the girl in the following example:

> A 9-year-old girl had come to believe that all teachers were always mean. In attempting to maintain this pathogenic belief, she selectively perceived only the mean behaviors in all her new teachers, and did not perceive their kindnesses. Consequently, she then told herself, "I just knew this new teacher was going to be mean, just like all the teachers I have ever had in this school." She was not happy with her "discovery" that her prior pathogenic belief about teachers was true, but she also did not have to experience the emotionally displeasurable state of anxious uncertainty (i.e., cognitive dissonance) that accompanies experiencing a perception (a new teacher's kindness) that did not match what she believed she knew about teachers.

Whether children have more normal or pathogenic beliefs, they will try to receive ongoing validation for their beliefs. Hence, the above girl who believed that all her teachers were mean, and who subsequently "discovered" that her new teacher was also mean, may have unwittingly set it up or manipulated her teacher to bring out her "mean side."

I am not suggesting, however, that normally developing children's experiences with new events and new people—like a new teacher—are completely dictated by their preexistent beliefs. Those beliefs do, however, influence how children initially color their perceptions of current reality. Adults who deal with 6- to 11-year-old children are quite aware of how these children differ in their individual responsiveness to completely new events, new opportunities, and new people. Children's memories and past experiences, captured in their currently held beliefs, are not sufficient to explain how they will react, for example, to a new kind and empathic teacher. A further unique quality that varies quantitatively from child to child must be added to the equation: the overall flexibility or rigidity of those beliefs. Beliefs, as a function of children's cognitive capabilities, are controlled by their ego. Hence, children's egos can be viewed as possessing either more flexibility and malleability or more rigidity. An example from my work as a child psychiatrist graphically illustrates the flexibility versus rigidity in the beliefs of 6- to 11-year-old children.

> A 10-year-old black boy was assigned to me for twice weekly psychotherapy because of his tendency to be belligerent and hostile to his peers and to adults. For several months, whenever we met, he generated an intense negative transference toward me in which he automatically enacted his pathogenic belief that I would physically harm him in an unexpected and intense physical attack. In his use of the unconscious defense mechanism of projective identification, he projected his own rage onto me (for the attack he believed would occur) and then repeatedly attempted to provoke me into becoming rageful enough toward him to attack him. For example, he entered each session verbalizing much profanity, attempted to throw toys at me, spit at me, and exhibit other similar behaviors. He then would state repeatedly, "I know you hate me; white people hate black people." Thus, he was now attempting to get me to accept his projected hatred and act hatefully toward him. If he was even momentarily successful, he could identify—in essence, misidentify—his own projected hatred in me.
>
> At the end of a year of treatment, I and other members of a multidisciplinary treatment team had not seen evidence that this boy was psychotic; however, we were in agreement that I and his teachers, both white and black, had been unable to help this boy relinquish, even partially, his strongly entrenched pathogenic belief and associated internal image of white men as harmful, dangerous, and attacking. This pathogenic belief allowed him to continue to repress his partially remembered rage that he had previously felt in experiences he had had with rather sadistic

white men. This rage was stimulated whenever he was in the presence of a white adult male.

Before his black father had left the family when the boy was age 5 years, the father had been extremely physically abusive of both the boy and his mother. When the father left, his wife's initial rage at her husband caused her to repeatedly talk negatively about him. When the father returned 1 year later, he immediately took his wife on a 1-week vacation to an island resort and lavished her with gifts. The boy stayed with neighbors, and, when his parents returned, he was spanked by his mother for saying he was angry at his father about being left, first at age 5 years and second when his father took his mother away. A few days later, his father left again, but continued to return a few times per year to spend time with his wife, but never with his son.

Now this 10-year-old boy's mother spoke only positively about her husband and forbade her son to talk negatively about him. However, she did repeatedly tell her son that her white male supervisor was mean in not offering his father a job so that the father could come back and live with her and the boy. His mother was using the defense mechanism of displacement by displacing her anger at her own husband onto white men—which added to the angry feelings she already had toward white men because they had slighted, criticized, and discriminated against her in the past—because she could not consciously tolerate her angry feelings toward her husband. Now she had organized whatever disappointment, rage, and depression she had experienced in her life as being caused by white men. She believed white men hated her and would continually cause her harm. Her son, under the continued threat of being abandoned by her, had identified with and taken into his representational world his mother's belief about and rage toward white men. With me, her son was always on the offensive in continually enacting and trying to prove his pathogenic belief; if he could get me to physically attack him or seem to attack him in any way, then he could reaffirm his pathogenic belief through a projective identifying process.

Almost concurrently, I was treating in twice-per-week psychotherapy an 8-year-old black boy whose pathogenic belief was similar to that of the 10-year-old black boy. However, the outcome of the therapy was quite different.

This 8-year-old boy was being treated for severe inhibition of his assertion. He did not manifest a normal degree of curiosity and initiative in any of his relationships. In the interview-playroom, he warily withdrew whenever I attempted to acknowledge that perhaps, in time, we might become friends. For several months he maintained a distant relationship with me. He played alone with blocks or other toys. Gradually his play began to put into action his negative transferentially formed expectation (based on his pathogenic belief) that I might physically attack him. However, unlike the 10-year-old boy, who acted out his fear that I would attack him by trying to provoke such an attack, this 8-year-old boy was able to use speech and fantasy play to reveal his pathogenic belief.

For several weeks he invited me to play cowboys and Indians with him; he played the Indians and assigned me the role of the cowboys. In each play fantasy, the Indians were able to kill all the cowboys quickly before they killed the Indians. One day, he set up the toy cowboys and Indians, assigning himself his usual role as playing the Indians, and assigning me my usual role of playing the cowboys. However, before this day's "war" was to begin, he stated, "The cowboys hate the Indians because they are another color, like white people hate black people. But that's the way I used to feel. You are a good cowboy. Now I know some cowboys wouldn't hurt any of the Indians." An important preexisting pathogenic belief was beginning to be restructured and transformed in this boy.

In separate meetings with his parents, I subsequently learned how highly prejudiced and suspicious they were, although their prejudicial and pathogenic beliefs were mostly unconscious. Consciously, they hoped that their son would not be prejudiced toward white people. However, they both had had miserable childhood experiences in which the white people living in the same small Southern town where they had both been raised expressed much hostility toward them. As adults, they did not realize how much they had taken the prejudicial beliefs of their own parents into their representational worlds. They would periodically communicate in their unconsciously motivated enactments—but not in words—their disapproval of their son's current wishes to develop close friendships with white children and white adults.

A few days after the session in which the boy realized that I was a "good cowboy," he heard his father tell his mother that black people needed to be wary of the intentions of white people. The boy told his father, "You're wrong. Dr. Gemelli is fair. I like him a lot, and he likes me. He'd never hurt me." This statement became a catalyst for his mother and father to discover and acknowledge the presence, within their own unconscious inner worlds, of prejudicial beliefs that originated in their childhood and that were still influencing their adult behaviors. At the end of this boy's treatment, which did ameliorate his inhibitions, his and his parents' representational worlds and associated pathogenic beliefs about white people had been changed.

The 8-year-old boy was able to use a therapy experience with a new person (me) to form new normal beliefs and eventually restructure his prior pathogenic beliefs, something the 10-year-old boy was unable to do. The 8-year-old boy and his parents possessed egos marked by flexibility and malleability, whereas the 10-year-old boy and his mother possessed egos marked by rigidity (Meissner 1992). The case of the 8-year-old boy illustrates the more normal process in which 6- to 11-year-old children use new experiences to restructure preexisting normal and pathogenic beliefs as contained within their long-term memories.

More than ever before in their lives, children ages 6–11 years are increasingly thinking about their past and coming up with new intuitive ideas about their memories. Many of a child's memories from the first 6 years of life undergo reconstructive revision or representational reorganization (Karmiloff-Smith 1979) as the child's conscious and unconscious mind activates and uses the accommodation-transformation and hierarchical-restructuring principles. As a result, older children will restructure and transform prior memories and reprioritize the relative importance they attribute to certain memories as being crucial in shaping their life, or what experiences were most valuable in the past and those that they will seek to repeat in the future.

It is difficult to know how much of what children report happened to them represents actual memories constructed in the past and how much represents a more recent reconstruction and transformation of those memories (M. L. Lewis 1995; Terr 1994). In fact, children's reconstruction of their past is just that: a composite memory comprising an original memory (i.e., the initially constructed memory of an experience) plus one or more reconstructions of that original memory (Perry 1992). Thus, at any point in time, what children remember about their past is what they currently believe about what happened in the past.

The ongoing reconstruction of a child's database of long-term preconsciously and unconsciously stored memories from his or her representational world takes place in varying degrees in every child. The extent to which each child engages in reconstruction of those memories depends on that child's maturing cognitive abilities to better integrate and comprehend both current perceptions and memories. With greater cognitive capacity comes a greater capacity to integrate past and present memories, beliefs, and representations of oneself and others.

Loftus (1993) describe this memory reconstructive process as follows:

> Perhaps we would use a child's analogy and think of memory as a chunk of clay that we hold in our hands, allowing it to warm before we mold it into different shapes. We can't change the clay into a rock or water or cotton, but we can transform it, push it, dent it, bend it, make animals and shapes, faces and forms, designs and textures. When we have finished with our manipulations, we put the molded form into the oven of our minds where it bakes until it is hard and firm. Our distortions have become a hard reality, part fact, part fiction, but in our minds an exact representation of the way things were. (p. 8)

Another factor affecting the extent to which each child engages in reconstruction of memories is the degree to which parents allow, encourage, and support their child's reconsidering old memories and seeking new information to modify them. Psychologically attuned parents allow their children to ask questions such as in the following exchange:

Daughter: Mom, when we went to Grandma's house last summer, why was I so unhappy with [her cousin] Mary? I remember her teasing me a lot and I got mad at her but I didn't tell her

because she was older than me. But this year when we go back
to Grandma's house, I'm not going to let her order me around.

The mother encourages her daughter's reconstructive process and
her use of her increasing cognitive skills to reconsider past behaviors and feelings by responding as follows:

Mother: I remember you avoiding Mary and I'm glad you are
thinking about what happened last summer. Tell me more about
what you remember and what questions you have about Mary.

Development of the Self and Object Relationships

■ Development of a Social Identity in the Context of Continued Development of a Peer Identity

As I note under "Functions of the Social Environment," above, children's attainment of an autonomous and valued identity enables
them to approach grade school with a sense of taking pleasure in
being curious and taking the initiative in approaching the learning
process (Erikson 1963). Between ages 6 and 11 years, children
begin to show "in miniature" an early picture of the personality
they will have as an adult. Longitudinal data reveal that the highest
correlation of childhood behavior predicting future adult behavior
exists for this age period, especially for children between ages
8 and 11 years (Roff and Wirt 1984).

Developmentalists have documented that teachers perceive
children rejected by peers as manifesting disruptive behaviors in
class (i.e., demonstrating a high degree of distractibility, impulsivity,
and motoric hyperactivity) and overaggressiveness in social interactions with peers outside of class (Coie et al. 1990). From age 6 or
7 years onward, children have an active need to interact with and
achieve acceptance into a peer group and produce and perform in
front of their peers. Children are often involved with more than
one peer group. Through each peer group they demonstrate many

of the skills, attitudes, and ethical and moral values they learned prior to entering first grade. Cahan et al. (1993) observed the following:

> School classes, Boy Scout and Girl Scout troops, stamp clubs, athletic teams, and countless other sorts of midrange institutions constitute significant social environments for children. . . . These peer groups provide a socialization setting for the child to learn values and attitudes that may be continuous or discontinuous with the values and attitudes learned in the home world. (p. 199)

Colarusso (1992) noted how children's acceptance or rejection by their peers is an important indication of whether children are developing normally. In my view, this is true only if children are exposed to peers who share many of the same developmental taskings, standards, moral values and behaviors for adapting to conflicts that they learned in their own family. Colarusso described this need for acceptance as follows:

> The latency peer group acts as a cruel but accurate triage group, accepting those children who manifest the ability to psychologically separate from parents and engage the developmental tasks of latency, and rejecting those who are regressed and immature. Consequently, acceptance by the same sex peer group is one of the best gauges of psychological health during latency, and rejection is a frequent indication of pathology and a very common presenting symptom. (p. 84)

The following example illustrates the need for acceptance into a peer group:

> A 9-year-old boy had a birthday party with several male friends. During the party, one of his invited friends—one who had difficulty because he was highly distractible and periodically overly aggressive—was progressively shunned by the other boys. The birthday boy had empathy for his shunned friend and consoled him when the friend isolated himself from the other boys. This friend was facing a developmental conflict: he needed the support of a peer group while his peers were rejecting him.

Such a child needs more than an empathic friend; he needs the help of his parents and perhaps a child psychiatrist.

As children begin to spend less time with their family, their peer group becomes a major source for maintenance of their self-esteem and continued development. The peer group is where they receive important feedback about their attempts at mastery within their classroom and playground environments. This need for peer group support of their self-worth is illustrated in the following example:

> A 9-year-old boy selected the assignment to teach his class about tarantulas as his school science project. He drew a tarantula on a large poster board and listed various facts about its habitat, habits, characteristics, and so on. Although his mother and father both enthusiastically admired his project, he was strongly motivated to present his project to his friends for their reaction. He came home beaming after his classmates complimented his work. (Derek Belaga, personal communication, April 1994)

It is interesting that there tends to be a high correlation between low acceptance by 8- to 10-year-old children's peer groups and those children's behavioral problems in adolescence and tendency to drop out of school (Roff and Wirt 1984). In another study, 8-year-old children were evaluated by measuring peer ratings of their behavior. When these children reached ages 19–21 years (11–13 years later), the highest correlation was found between poor peer ratings in childhood and psychological problems in early adulthood (Cowen et al. 1973). Kupersmidt and Dodge (1990), in reviewing studies of peer social status and child development, observed the following:

> Low peer social status in childhood is predictive of nonspecified mental health problems in adolescence and adulthood. The causal role of social rejection in these problems is not at all clear, nor is the strength of this relation. (p. 283)

■ Continued Development of Gender and Sexual Identities

Development of gender identity. Before approximately age 6 years, children's gender identity is fueled by their identification with both of their parents; this identification also plays a crucial part in their learning what constitutes being a boy or girl. Also, once their oedipal wishes have been partially relinquished after age 6 years, they adopt the new goal of growing up to be like their parents but not replace either one of them. One motivating force that propels 6- to 7-year-old children to identify with their same-gender parent is their need to feel more competent as a boy or girl and to feel a sense of power.

Between ages 6 and 11 years, children learn that there are three types of mechanisms through which to gain power or prestige in their society: first, there is intrinsic power that comes from being loved and valued unconditionally by their parents; second, there is attributed power based on their performance in mastering stimuli presented to them during their first 6 years of life; and third, there is formal or bestowed power, which is power given by some social organization (Horner 1989).

During the first few years of grade school, children construct the new category of "people with power" and then further refine this general category into different types of power. Police officers, ministers, priests, presidents, and so on all have different types of power and manifest their power in different ways. Children feel that they have power through identification with those whom they perceive as being powerful. Thus, a major source of 6- to 8-year-old children's overall feelings of having power is their identification with their parents and other significant people in their life (e.g., an older sibling, a grandparent, an uncle). At the same time, identification with parents becomes the basic template for children's further identifications with peers, teachers, coaches, and so on.

By ages 9–10 years, boys want to be with boys and girls, with girls. This segregation helps older children "put aside" in their mind the issue of sexual object choice and instead do more work on consolidating gender-appropriate identifications and construct more categories of what it means to be their gender. Social pressures help boys and girls learn how their gender should act, with each culture defining age-appropriate behaviors for each gender. Same-gender peers and adults (e.g., teachers, uncles, aunts, athletic coaches) become new identification figures for latency-age children. By ages 10–11 years, children are able to incorporate their gender identity into their other identities: their autonomous, sexual, peer, and social identities. For example, a 10-year-old boy might tell himself, "Boys do different things (e.g., assert their autonomy) than girls."

Development of sexual identity. Children ages 6–11 years continue to develop their sexual identity during an era that has traditionally been called the *latency period.* Although it has been argued that children's sexual feelings rest in a latent state in this phase, sexual self-stimulation and gratification still persist. Elias and Gebhard (1969) reported that 83% of boys ages 4–14 years had masturbated, with more beginning to masturbate between ages 3 and 7 years than after age 7 years. Other developmentalists (Noshpitz and King 1991; P. Tyson and Tyson 1991) have observed that masturbation occurs in most children between ages 6 and 11 years. However, it is not a dominant activity in their life and, when they do masturbate, most children keep it very private.

Sexual identity development in late childhood comes under the sway of society's message about whether children can sexually pursue their object of sexual choice. In general, most civilized societies say no to direct sexual activity between children. Indirect activity does take place. As Rosenfeld and Wasserman (1993) noted,

> During the early school years, both boys and girls normally start to conceal much of their sexual interest, talk and play from adults. With peers, however, children in the early school years talk, fantasize, play and act about sexuality with increasing frequency as they approach puberty. They share these interests in conversations with close friends and weave them into rhymes and coarse jokes that mingle orality, elimination and genital sex. (p. 403)

Although direct heterosexual activities are prohibited between children, the school classroom and playground become the places where children subtly develop their sexual identities and more obviously develop their concurrent peer and social identities.

Despite the segregation that generally takes place between latency-age boys and girls, heterosexual children have a secret interest in the opposite gender; their feelings for each other are not neutral. Sexual undercurrents begin in the first grade and extend through the sixth grade (about ages 11–12 years). Girls ages 6–9 years may speak of their "boyfriend" in their class, but are easily embarrassed when someone reminds them of this stated admission. The same occurs in boys, but boys tend to be much less open about their interest in a "girlfriend." Boys may fantasize about what kissing a girl might be like, but will fight with any friend who teases them about wanting to kiss a girl.

As they continue to develop their autonomous identity, latency-age children use their well-developed fantasy formation and game-playing abilities to indirectly assert their wishes with their parents and others (Noshpitz and King 1991). Beginning around age 6–7 years, they discover that both physical games (e.g., sports) or non-physical games (e.g., board games) can be competitive. They also learn that games have rules. Once they truly understand the concept of games, they begin constructing their own games and set rules that help them gratify a wish through the game that would be more difficult to gratify more directly. For example, a boy may have the wish to defeat his father in a wrestling match. Recognizing that he is outmatched, he sets up a game with his father and makes rules that will give him an unfair advantage. If his father becomes upset in recognizing his son's strong wish to win, and confronts him about his wish to win, the boy would most probably sense his father's displeasure, denying it in saying, "No. I'm just playing a game." Sports and other games bring children face-to-face with their special abilities and talents as well as their intellectual limitations, hand-eye coordination limitations (e.g., they are not good at video games), and physical limitations (e.g., they are not good at soccer).

In addition, children come to acknowledge that their parents do not always succeed, win, or dazzle others. These self-observations and observations by children's parents once again stimulate children to resurrect their idealizing wishes to be perfect and to have parents who are perfect. For example, a normally developing 7-year-old boy with an image of his father as being "the greatest" gradually comes to learn and understand that other men run faster, are smarter, and so on, than his father. This boy needs time to deal with this reality, a reality that involves his slow realization that there are no "superdads" to completely protect a son from life's dangers and disappointments. So this boy begins to collect posters of a favorite sports star and then tells his father he will grow up to be great like the star. His father must respect these grandiose fantasies—and allow his son to hang his posters on his wall—knowing that they will eventually be given up. This will happen when the son realizes that 1) he does not have to be great and that his father and mother do not have to be great in order to be a success, and 2) no one is perfect. These realizations develop slowly; it is not unusual for a "hero" to remain so in children's eyes until well into mid-adolescence (ages 16–17 years).

As children continue to find other people to idealize and then de-idealize and struggle with acknowledging those people's value despite their having imperfections, some will construct the family romance fantasy (S. Freud 1909/1963). This is a grandiose and perfectionistic fantasy in which the children fantasize that they were adopted; hence, they can fantasize having more nearly perfect, loving parents than they have in reality. It is as if this fantasy is an effort by children to wish for an innate or genetic perfection, especially given that they have an increased intellectual understanding that challenges their wishes for a perfect parent or to be perfect themselves.

From ages 9 to 10 years, children will often manifest a period of being quite discouraged when faced with their limitations. The child is now perceiving that he or she does not always get an A on every test, or may not be the best in gymnastics class. And in believing that he or she will never attain perfection, the child gives up and states, "School stinks!" or "I don't care anymore about going to soccer" (Thompson 1996). Once again, psychologically attuned parents—and teachers and coaches—must tolerate children's discouragement while being firm in not allowing children to quit staying engaged in these activities that bring children face to face with their limitations and imperfections.

As children approach ages 10–11 years, compensatory fantasies such as the family romance fantasy and their abject discouragement about not being perfect begin to give way to the development of more realistically attainable ambitions and ideals. Kohut and Wolf

(1978) suggested that children's transformed (through *transmitting internalizations*) ideal self-image eventually becomes, as a new representation within their overall self-representation, their more realistic ambitions, whereas their ideal parent images become their more realistic but still somewhat idealistic goals. For 10- to 11-year-old children to begin to transmute their perfectionistic images of themselves and their parents, they must believe that their parents value them despite their limitations and imperfections. When they believe this, they can use their parents' realistic view of them to begin to transform their perfect self-image and perfect parental images into more realistically attainable ambitions and ideals.

These ambitions and ideals will be further developed in adolescence with periodic regressions of wishing once again for a perfect self and for perfect parents or perfect others to protect them from the risks of failing as they apply their ambitions to attempt to achieve their ideals.

Latency-age children's experiences in constructing their early ambitions and ideals must take place in a family where they are, as I noted above, valued despite having imperfections and limitations and are permitted to verbally express their perfect wishes when they are resurrected. When children's parents, however, have experienced a major life defeat themselves (e.g., if they fail in their occupational or professional pursuits), their children's view of them as wonderfully perfect is too quickly shattered. This will cause children to resurrect a family romance fantasy of once having perfect parents but losing them, or resurrect their fantasy of eventually finding new and perfect parents sometime in the future. However, they may be unable to consider these fantasies when they are confronted by a depressed parent. These grandiose fantasies can then go into repression, where they may remain unmodified into adulthood. One developmental outcome for this scenario might be for a child to develop a narcissistic personality disorder. People with this disorder are constantly seeking a perfect, idealized teacher, school, wife, and so on who will give them constant praise and pronouncements of being perfect coupled with always trying to be perfect themselves. When they fall short of their goal of perfection, they tend to become enraged with themselves and view themselves or others who do not tell them that they are still perfect as totally de-idealized and devalued and a "nothing." This brings on a state of intense depression. When another person they have been idealizing (e.g., a teacher) shows his or her imperfections, they react toward him or her with the same intense criticism, narcissistic rage, and devaluation. The teacher now is a devalued "nothing."

In more normal situations, as 10- to 11-year-old children are able to more acknowledge their parents' failures, they gradually become more tolerant of their own limitations and failures.

Development of the Superego

Superego's Provision of Internal Anxiety Signals as a Source of Self-Control and Self-Esteem

As I note earlier, forerunners to 6- to 7-year-old children's superego are all of the experiences, beginning in infancy, in which they learned about the shoulds and should nots and the rights and wrongs of their behavioral choices. However, constructing a superego and then being able to use it to guide behavior are two different matters altogether.

Before about age 7 years, children have what Stillwell et al. (1991) labeled an *external conscience,* meaning that they know how to label their behaviors as good or bad and how to obey rules. However, they have yet to view the rules as their own. They obey authority and expect others to monitor their behavior, often looking shamefully toward adults to see if there is going to be a reaction to a misdeed (Stillwell et al. 1991). When children ages 3–6 years are asked to draw their conscience, they draw themselves in good actions and bad actions while drawing authority figures as the people with the conscience (i.e., the people who know and reinforce their rules). In Figures 6–2 and 6–3 are depicted the drawings of a 5-year-old child in Stillwell et al.'s (1991) research. Those authors described the two drawings as follows:

In the "good" picture [Figure 6–2, p. 435] he is riding his bicycle along even ground. In the "bad" picture [Figure 6–3, p. 436] he is crashing down a hill into the mud. What is "bad" is that he didn't use his brakes like his cousin told him to do. He fears that his cousin won't take him riding again. The "rights" and "wrongs" of bicycling reside in his cousin.

By ages 6–7 years, as children partially relinquish their oedipal wishes toward their same-gender parent, they both acknowledge their parents' authority and power over them and identify with parental authority (Loewald 1979). In doing the latter, they are literally infusing their superego with authority. They then begin to learn how to listen to the voice of their superego as the authority of their parents. If they have repressed their oedipal wishes only out of fear of parental retaliation, their superego will become an unwelcome internalized parent against which they will begin to rebel. Normally developing 6- to 7-year-old children, however, begin to believe that their superego is an ally—residing within their heart or brain (labeled by Stillwell et al. [1991] as a *brain or heart conscience*)—that begins to perform two basic functions: 1) to regulate and control their behavior relatively independent of external restraints and 2) to become a source of self-esteem that is relatively independent of external feedback.

By age 7 or 8 years, a child's superego sends him or her internal signals of distress—superego anxiety—that warn when a new developmental calamity—the disapproval of one's superego—is imminent if the child says or does what he or she is contemplating to say or do. When this internal scanning, signaling, and listening process works well, it greatly assists children in using their representational world to delay both speech and action in order to think and formulate a new strategy or select a different set of procedures. However, for this process to work well, children must begin to delay speech or action long enough to tolerate their internal superego anxiety signal. Some children have significant trouble tolerating this internal signal mainly because 1) they are still developing their general ability to delay speech or action so that they may think, or 2) they have a superego that is still quite immature in its development.

Stillwell et al. (1991) described normal 7- to 10-year-old children as being

> fascinated by information processing: input, storage and retrieval. [They] are fascinated by how rules move from outside to inside. . . . Even though there are internal rules, children add that it's often a good idea to consult both the brain and the heart and authority figures for certainty. It is obvious they are in the midst of a transition from external to internal understanding. (p. 19)

Children in the early stages of internalizing their conscience and beginning to listen to their internal superego anxiety signals still view rules as coming from external authority. This view is depicted in a 7-year-old girl's drawings of doing something good (Figure 6–4, p. 437), which she defined as playing with her toys on a table, and doing something bad (Figure 6–5, p. 438), which she defined as telling another child she hates her. However, this 7-year-old girl had begun to internalize her own rules: she stated that her knowledge of what was good or bad came from her own brain and within her brain was contained her conscience (Stillwell et al. 1991).

One of the reasons for 6- to 9-year-old children's difficulty in accepting their conscience's rules as their own is the intensity of the guilt that emanates from their conscience or superego. Their superego is rather like a very harsh, strict, uncompromising parent who threatens to punish them quickly with no empathy for their needs or conflicts. Children in the early latency period, therefore, begin to carry on a kind of second rapprochement crisis in their life. At times they are proud to follow their conscience and are proud that they are a big boy or girl who knows how to behave on his or her own; at other times, they feel just as proud in disobeying their conscience. It is as if they are saying to their conscience what they said to their mother at age 2½ years: "Sometimes I like to listen to you. But you can't always be the boss. I won't listen to you when you stop me from doing what I want to do." Thus the goal of 6- to 9-year-old children is to restructure their conscience not into one that enshrines their ideal self-representation and ideal parental representation (i.e., by demanding that they be perfect and by totally devaluing them when they transgress a rule or moral value) but into one that, like their parents, loves and admires them when they behave well and disapproves and demands some type of punishment and reparation from them when they misbehave.

Obviously, children's restructuring of their superego is greatly assisted by authority figures who point out their transgressions with firmness but also with kindness and empathy. Such transactions motivate children to identify with authority figures because the authority figures 1) verbalize their criticism without assassinating children's self-esteem, 2) give punishments that are reasonable, and 3) treat children as valuable, even though they do not always behave perfectly. Thus children produce a superego that contains their parents' esteem for them. Children will receive internal superego admiring signals when they contemplate obeying their parents' rules and standards of behavior that are already internalized within their conscience.

The attainment of reversible thinking also lessens the impact of doing something bad. Children now realize that something bad they have done can be reversed; in essence, the bad behavior can be undone by replacing it with a new, good behavior. Parents help this process when they give their children a task to make up for a wrong.

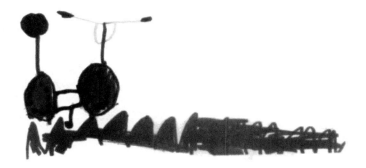

Figure 6–2. A 5-year-old child's drawing of something good.
Source. Stillwell et al. 1991. Used with permission.

Superego development also occurs through children's need to both adhere to and change rules in peer group play. Through peer group games, children practice living with the rules laid down in their conscience—rules dictated by their parents, school, television, and many other sources. Adherence to the rules protects chil-

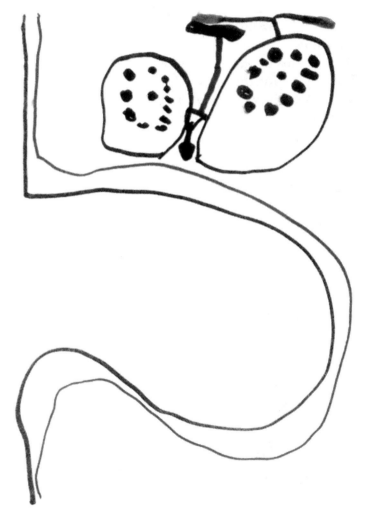

Figure 6–3. A 5-year-old child's drawing of something bad.
Source.   Stillwell et al. 1991. Used with permission.

dren from regressing during play and manifesting less socially acceptable behaviors. For example, one 8-year-old boy in a football game became angry and punched another boy. Because he hit another child, the other boys did not allow him to continue playing the game. This helped this boy develop more self-control with his friends. He returned the next day and chose to play according to the rules and refrained from hitting.

Most children's peer groups are selected by both children and their parents on the basis of their matching the children's standards and values. By ages 7–8 years, a moral code of fairness with a sense of group justice is becoming internalized within children's conscience. Latency-age children are motivated to internalize their peer group's rules and standards of fairness because of their need for peer group approval (Coie 1990) and their fear of peer group rejection (Asher and Coie 1990; Putallaz and Dunn 1990). Hence the

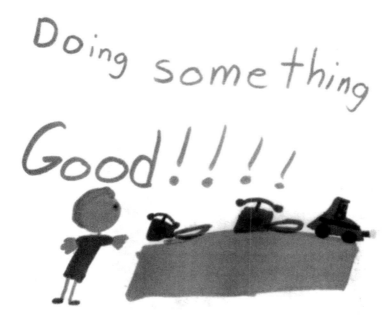

Figure 6–4. A 7-year-old girl's drawing of doing something good. *Source.* Stillwell et al. 1991. Used with permission.

peer group can occasionally override a child's healthy moral internalized rules within his or her conscience. Indeed, some children have succumbed to peer pressure and done something greatly out of character when exposed to a strong peer group collective demand to do a certain asocial act (e.g., take an illicit drug, inflict physical harm on an animal).

During this period of superego development, peer groups also become a source of admiring signals even when children are not obeying all the rules laid down within their conscience. Thus when children break a rule, their sharp pangs of guilt and the impact of the withdrawal of their superego's admiration is lessened when they find friends who tell them that they still like them or that they have recently broken the same rule and also gotten into trouble with their parents.

Sullivan (1953) emphasized that, between ages 8 and 10 years, the role of a close friend helps children further modify their con-

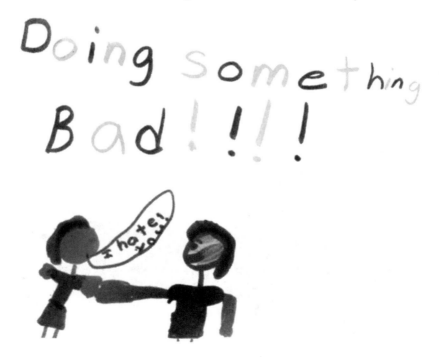

Figure 6–5. A 7-year-old girl's drawing of doing something bad.
Source.   Stillwell et al. 1991. Used with permission.

science. Through this relationship, children have a chance to share their worries about not living up to some of the high demands concerning behavior that have been internalized within their conscience. In this sense, the close friend helps them relinquish their periodically resurrected wishes to be perfect. These wishes for a perfect self are maintained when children are not able to believe that they can admit their worries, fears, and anxieties—that is, their imperfections—to a friend and still be accepted. When they tell their friend about their imperfections, they feel relieved when the friend responds with something like, "Big deal! I'm not perfect either."

Close friend relationships are also children's first real experience with making the problems, worries, and anxieties of a peer their own. In this sense, such relationships are felt by Sullivan (1953) to be a precursor for children's eventual ability to enter into a mature intimate heterosexual loving relationship in young adult life. In an adult intimate relationship, mutual concern for each other, acceptance of each other's imperfections, and willingness to be vulnerable and dependent are all necessary for true love and trust to develop.

By age 11 years, children have done considerable work on developing their superego, not only in being able to listen to its internal signals, but also in accepting it as their own internalized set of rules and ethical and moral values. Figure 6–6 is the drawing of a conscience by an 11-year-old child. It is a brain with rules imprinted on it. This child commented, "A conscience is part of your mind . . . it tells you what to do" (Stillwell et al. 1991, p. 20).

Development of Adaptational Capabilities

Maturation and Development of New Defense Mechanisms

The predominant defense mechanisms used by children in late childhood are fantasy formation, isolation of emotion, sublimation, reaction formation, displacement, and suppression.

Fantasy formation. *Fantasy formation* is used more than ever before as an adaptive defense by children in this age period. Instead of verbally or behaviorally expressing an anxiety-provoking wish or feeling that is associated with a developmental anxiety, children construct an unconscious latent fantasy that expresses the wish or feeling in a way that brings gratification. This latent fantasy stays repressed while a disguised manifest fantasy is experienced in consciousness.

Isolation of emotion. *Isolation of emotion* is an automatic barring from consciousness of an emotion that, if expressed, would produce an intolerable level of one or more developmental anxieties. When this defense is used, there is only the conscious awareness of the thoughts being experienced at the moment, but without the associated feelings connected with those thoughts.

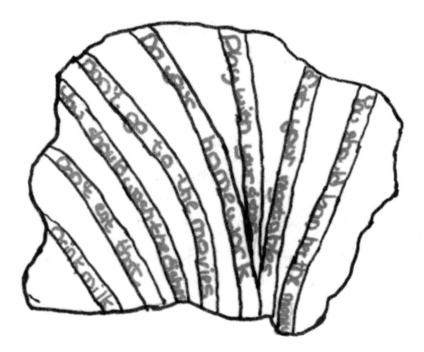

Figure 6–6.   Drawing of a conscience by an 11-year-old child.
Source.   Stillwell et al. 1991. Used with permission.

This process is illustrated in the following example:

> An 8-year-old girl witnessed a boy peer being slapped by a
> teacher for talking angrily. The girl herself had been slapped
> quite often during the first 5 years of her life by her biological
> mother. As a result, she had constructed an emotional procedure
> memory in which she pathogenically believed that she should
> not verbally express angry feelings toward those in authority lest
> she be slapped. By the time she was age 8 years, this pathogenic
> belief had become repressed, along with the anger she felt to-
> ward her biological mother for being repeatedly slapped. Now,
> when this belief was stimulated by seeing children slapped, her
> unconscious mind automatically used the defense of repression
> to keep her anger unconscious.
>
> This girl's father remarried when she was age 6 years, a year
> after her biological mother had abandoned the family. On the day
> when the teacher slapped her friend, she did not even think of
> mentioning the incident to her stepmother. She had repressed
> both her thoughts and anger about the incident. She uncon-
> sciously believed that, if she told her stepmother how angry she
> was at the teacher for slapping her friend, her stepmother would
> slap her. Her repression of the event, however, was interfered
> with by her stepmother's empathy. Her stepmother empathically
> sensed she was upset about something and gently inquired about
> her school day. The girl's repression gave way to some extent. In
> responding to her stepmother's empathy she was able to risk
> revealing part of the school event. She used isolation of emotion
> to allow her to tell her stepmother her thoughts about the boy's
> being slapped without revealing her anger in her voice. Her an-
> ger remained within her unconscious mental domain.

Sublimation. *Sublimation* is an automatic, unconscious process in which the gratification of a wish is achieved by changing the
object or aim of the wish. The aim or object is altered from one
that may have been socially objectionable to one that is socially
acceptable. This process is illustrated in the following example:

> An 11-year-old boy had a wish to impress his female teacher with
> his athletic prowess and physical development. These wishes
> produced excessive body damage and superego anxieties be-

cause they occurred at a time when the boy was close to returning to oedipal wishes, something associated with his early pubertal development (see Chapter 7). Also, his oedipal wishes were causing him anxiety because his mother had been quite seductive toward him over the last 6 months, ever since his father had been leaving on long business trips.

In an unconscious process, he displaced his anxiety-provoking oedipal wishes toward his mother onto his teacher. Then he sublimated his oedipal wishes toward his teacher into a new aim to build architectural models, but was not aware of his motivation for building the models. He found himself wanting to build a model of Pearl Harbor before the Japanese attack. He spent hours building this model. He then built a model of a university he had visited on a class trip. Consequently, he brought both of these models to school to show his teacher and his class. He was not aware that his teacher was interested in both subjects of his models. Several months before he built the models, his teacher had told the class that the brother she admired the most of her three brothers attended this same university, and sometime later showed the class a book she admired greatly, *A Day of Infamy* (Bishop 1955), about the Japanese attack on Pearl Harbor.

Reaction formation. *Reaction formation* is an automatic unconscious process that bars from consciousness an unacceptable wish or feeling and produces in consciousness the opposite wish or feeling. It is a predominant defense mechanism for children ages 3–11 years. As with all defenses, it is adaptive when used for a short period of time. When it is used extensively or too often, it is usually being used to defend against assertive wishes that are causing children internal and possibly external conflict. If their assertiveness is then handled by chronic reaction formation, they may become passive and inhibited and tell people that they like to be nonassertive and watch others take the initiative.

Displacement. *Displacement* is an automatic unconscious mental mechanism that displaces the expression of a wish or feeling from the original person or object that is causing high levels of developmental anxiety to another, less anxiety provoking person or object. For example, a boy will talk about his friend as being hateful, when really it is his father who he believes is being hateful; in this case, he is displacing his feelings onto his friend.

Suppression.   *Suppression* is the conscious and willful attempt to put mental contents out of one's conscious awareness. It is the only specific mechanism of defense that is defined as consciously volitional. Valliant (1977) noted that, with suppression, one says, "I will think about it tomorrow," and the next day remembers to think about it. Thus, when children use suppression, they are deliberating and temporarily postponing—but not deciding to permanently avoid—thinking and eventually talking about conflictual thoughts, wishes, and feelings. Werman (1985) postulated that children appear to possess differences in their ability to suppress thoughts, wishes, and feelings.

Parents can support either an adaptive or a maladaptive use of suppression. They can remind their children that something that was suppressed was not supposed to be suppressed forever. On the other hand, in supporting the maladaptive use of suppression, they can encourage their children to suppress something and then never remind them to talk about the suppressed issue.

Chapter 7

Adolescent Phase of Mental Development
Age 12 Years to Age 19 Years

Biopsychosocial Stimuli Involved in the Structural Organization of Mental Development

Adolescence as a developmental period, and adolescents as members of society, have both been the subject of considerable interest, speculation, and, regrettably, bad press. In most societies, it is during adolescence that young individuals truly begin to assert their own views and preferences as separate from those of their parents and teachers; accordingly, it is during adolescence that they begin to make their presence known as future adults who will eventually take a place within society. As Esman (1990) noted,

> Probably the outstanding fact about contemporary adolescents is their visibility. Never before in history have young people, at least in the industrialized world, been so blatantly *present* in their

445

modes of dress, their hairstyles, their musical tastes. (p. 3; italics in original)

This entry process from late childhood into adolescence is not without its "sparks" and developmental anxieties, for both adolescents and their parents and other adult members of society (McCarthy 1995). Just as adults throughout antiquity tended to project onto infants those aspects of their human selves that they wanted to deny and be rid of, a similar collective projective process tends to occur with regard to adolescents. Feinstein (1987) expressed this tendency as follows:

> More than those of any other stage of development, adolescents seem to serve as a repository for the conflicts of the culture and as a bearer of its mythic projections. The more complex society becomes, the more perplexing, troubling, and problematic their role appears to be, at least to those adults who require an external focus for their own sense of anomie [i.e., their own tendencies to deviate from the common rule]. (p. 3)

The biopsychosocial stimuli of adolescence can be understood as follows. The biological changes that take place at the onset of adolescence—which is called *puberty*—are quite striking, and in many families become more of a triggering stimulus than the biological changes associated with prior developmental phases. Adolescents also enter puberty with a much more complex representational world. This world is a source of psychological stimuli with which adolescents can engender quite elaborate internal responses—beliefs, fantasies, feelings, and memories—to their own biological, pubertal changes. A society's developmental taskings for its adolescents will profoundly influence the further development of the adolescents' sexual identity and the consolidation of the various aspects of their overall identity (i.e., their autonomous, gender, sexual, peer, and social identities) into an emancipated identity. All in all, each adolescent will emerge from this phase at about age 18 or 19 years with an emancipated identity that is defined by the way in which he or she has cognitively processed the transactions between these biological, psychological, and social stimuli.

For purposes of this discussion, I split adolescence into two periods: *early adolescence* (from puberty [about age 12 years] to age 15 years) and *late adolescence* (from age 16 years to age 19 years). Early adolescence is a period of great change. It can be viewed as the time in which the individual is preparing for "emancipation." The stimulation of adolescents' innate need for sensual-sexual stimulation and gratification restimulates the return of their oedipal wishes, which were partially relinquished around age 6 years. Also, pubertal development fuels a new surge toward adolescents' developing greater independence from their parents. All this results in early adolescents' gradual decreasing involvement with their parents and increasing involvement with their peer group. Close friendships with same-gender peers are particularly important.

Early adolescents also begin to reevaluate their beliefs, standards, values, and ways of behaving, which, in great part, were all derived from the various identifications they made in the first 12 years of life. These identifications led to the construction of representations within their pubertal self- and object representations. A reevaluation of these representations leads to the object relations conflicts that begin to consume early adolescents' attention (see below). The peer group becomes an important sounding board for them (e.g., complaining to one another about how out of style or old fashioned their parents are).

Late adolescents have lessened considerably their childhood dependencies on their parents. They are developing a sense of being separate individuals with their own opinions and perspectives. They realize now more than ever that they possess views about life that do not always agree with those of their parents. However, at times this newly emerging individuality in thinking leads them to feel isolated and misunderstood. This is the time when the peer group and the special same-gender friend become allies. Adolescents take refuge in believing they are joined by other adolescents in their struggle to achieve emancipation from their childhood dependencies.

Major Developmental Tasks of Adolescence

Construction of an Emancipated Identity, Realistic Ambitions, and Reasonable Ideals, and the Further Development of Sexual and Social Identities

Construction of an emancipated identity.   With the advent of the cognitive maturational advances that emerge at about age 12 years, adolescents become more capable of slowly integrating the various aspects of their subidentities (i.e., their autonomous, gender, sexual, peer, and social identities) into one overall identity. This integrated knowledge of themselves—as contained within their self-representation—eventually becomes a new mental structure called an *emancipated identity.* This emancipated identity allows them to demonstrate all components of their subidentities while functioning autonomously within their society and concurrently maintaining important transactional relationships with their parents and others.

Construction of realistic ambitions and reasonable ideals. This task is achieved through adolescents' relinquishing their periodically resurrected wishes for an ideal self as well as for ideal parents, people in authority, educational institutions, forms of government, and so on. Relinquishing ideal wishes also involves adolescents' coming to terms with earlier traumatic events that may have occurred in their life. Adolescents eventually master such traumas, at least for the most part, instead of denying their occurrence and resurrecting a belief in being an ideal self or an ideal object.

Further development of a sexual identity.   This task is achieved through adolescents' embarking on and continuing to develop direct experiences involving their sexual object choice (P. Tyson and Tyson 1991). Inherent in the development of sexual identity during adolescence is the attainment of *genital primacy.* This entails adolescents' focusing on their genitals as the primary mode of gratification of their need for sensual-sexual pleasure.

Further development of a social identity.   This task is achieved through adolescents' coming to understand that choices they make in life often lead to irreversible actions, commitments, and consequences in the context of their being a member of their society. In the further development of their social identity, adolescents accept certain social, ethical, moral, and legal responsibilities as they demonstrate their right to assert their emerging emancipated identity. With the establishment of a more developed social identity, they attain a new understanding of the relative influence of their past life in shaping their current wishes and wishes for the future.

Maturation and Development of Innate Needs

Further Maturation and Development of the Innate Need for Sensual-Sexual Pleasurable Gratification

Of the five innate needs possessed by adolescents, the need for sensual-sexual pleasurable gratification undergoes the most visible phase-specific maturational changes (S. Freud 1905/1963). These changes coincide with the observable bodily changes that accompany adolescents' entrance into puberty.

The "surgent" maturation at puberty of 11- to 13-year-old boys' innate need for sensual-sexual pleasurable gratification causes them to experience genital body sensations that are physically quite compelling. Boys awaken most mornings and notice that they have an erection. Likewise, 11- to 13-year-old girls have their first episode of menstruation. They wake up many mornings with obvious genital sensations that coincide with the fact that their breasts are de-

450 NORMAL CHILD AND ADOLESCENT DEVELOPMENT

veloping and their pubic hair is beginning to show. They may avoid processing these new body perceptions or not even notice some of the subtle bodily changes that accompany these sexual sensations. But those in their social environment will not. Noshpitz and King (1991) gave a good example of this process:

> Two boys in sixth grade watch a girl walk past. They have known her for years through earlier grades, but now one of them pokes the other and says, "Hey look. She's walking with a wiggle." And indeed she is. Her pelvis has broadened, her trochanters have changed their angle, and her gait has altered accordingly. The metamorphosis has been a completely silent one; she has no awareness of any of this until her classmates call the wiggle to her attention. Once alerted, however, she must make some decisions. She can decide to ignore the whole thing; she can anxiously try to suppress the wiggle; or she might find it interesting to exaggerate this novel development. But in one way or another she has this to take into her future calculations; she is different now and must adapt to the new reality.

Early adolescents are given two rather new signals concerning their sexual identity: one signal is from their maturationally intensified innate need for sensual-sexual gratification, which manifests itself in an increased genital sensitivity and reactivity; the other is from their society that now tells them that it is normal and permissible for boys and girls to begin to pursue each other as boyfriends and girlfriends and, eventually, as sexual partners and lovers. Thus, the societal prohibition regarding sensual-sexual activity that was operative during all of childhood is now lifted, although with restrictions. In effect, society tells the young adolescent,

> There are limits on your need-driven interest in sexual stimulation and pleasure. Be careful of AIDS (the acquired immunodeficiency syndrome), other sexually transmitted diseases, and pregnancy, and don't let sexual activity interfere with other developmental tasks (i.e., to establish an emancipated identity such as arriving at realistic ambitions as to how you will support yourself in the future, to decide which relationships you will maintain and develop, and to become a productive and contributing member of society outside of your family).

This societal message is not an easy one for all early adolescents to acknowledge. For some it creates too much anxiety about failing to attain the developmental tasks contained within the message. This anxiety can then suddenly propel them to become engaged in heterosexual activity or possibly illicit drug use as a way of avoiding their adolescent development. Such behavior will disguise the real source of their difficulty: truly negotiating the developmental tasks of adolescence, and particularly beginning to develop an emancipated identity.

Each person's gender identity undergoes progressive development after its initial formation at about age 2½ years. During latency, children have many experiences through which they consolidate their gender identity. Some abnormally developing children, however, experience some confusion during latency in understanding what it means to place themselves in the category of "heterosexual male," "heterosexual female," "homosexual male," or "homosexual female." When these children reach puberty, there may be some confusion about their sexual object choice (Green 1985). In early adolescence, they may then manifest a bisexual object choice, which propels them to seek sexual gratification from both sexes. This, however, is not the experience for most developing pubertal adolescents. And this variant of development should not be confused with the heterosexual pubertal child's periodic preoccupation with trying to understand the criteria for inclusion into the categories of homosexual male and homosexual female, and the homosexual pubertal child's periodic preoccupation with trying to understand the criteria for inclusion into the categories of heterosexual male and heterosexual female. These usual preoccupations in heterosexual and homosexual adolescents can lead to some transient experimentation with homosexual and heterosexual activity, respectively. But this experimentation is in the service of acquiring new knowledge through having direct experience with homosexual and heterosexual activity. It also is in the service of adolescents' coming to terms with their ideal self-representation and object representations. In reference to the latter, in later adolescence, a 16- to 19-year-old heterosexual male (or female) may seek a homosexual experience with another adolescent in the process of loving himself or herself through loving someone of the same gender. This

homosexual activity is often motivated by heterosexual adolescents' concern that no one of the opposite gender will love them
because of their faults and imperfections. (I further discuss
this point in "Development of the Self-Representation and Object
Representations," below).

Maturation and Development of Physical Capabilities

Secondary Sexual Characteristics

Puberty is defined as the phase in the life cycle when the external
bodily changes, defined as *secondary sexual characteristics,* make
their appearance. These characteristics are induced by sex hormones (estrogen or androgen) (Frank and Cohen 1979; Sugar
1993). Secondary sexual characteristics differ from primary sexual
characteristics in that the latter encompass changes that create the
capacity for procreation (Bloch 1995). The entrance into adolescence, in most cultures, is signified by the external physical
changes that occur at the onset of puberty, rather than the new
internal physical and physiological changes that make procreation
possible.

Primary sexual characteristics in boys are their testes, epi-
didymis, seminal vesicles, prostate gland, penis, and urethra; in
girls, they are their uterus and ovaries. *Secondary sexual characteristics* in boys include an increase in the size of the genitals; the
appearance of pubic, axillary, and facial hair; the deepening of the
voice; and bone and muscle growth. In girls, secondary sexual characteristics include breast growth, pelvic and hip changes, appearance of pubic and axillary hair, and the onset of menses (Tanner
1970).

The rate at which boys' and girls' primary and secondary sexual
characteristics mature differs (Khatchadourian 1977). At age
13 years, overall physical and secondary sexual development in
girls is often thought to be 1½–2 years ahead of that in boys. How-

ever, this is incorrect, because pubertal primary and secondary sexual maturational changes emerge only about 6 months earlier than in boys (Meyer-Bahlburg 1983). Meyer-Bahlburg (1983) noted,

> The general impression of an overall, considerably earlier maturation of girls is largely due to the fact that the growth spurt [i.e., in body height, bone and muscle diameter and muscle strength] is placed earlier in the sequence of pubertal changes in girls than in boys; the average boy has his growth peak 2 years later than the average girl. (p. 63)

This 1½- to 2-year difference in the overall growth rate between boys and girls remains a relative biological constant throughout adolescence (between ages 12 year and 19 years) (Bloch 1995). By age 13 years, some girls will have completed their entire adolescent physical development, whereas others will not have even begun to mature physically. Girls show a height spurt somewhere around age 11 or 12 years, and usually reach their maximum physical growth by age 16 years. Boys' physical growth and the growth of their secondary sexual characteristics begin when they are age 12 or 13 years; boys do not reach their maximal growth until about age 17 or even 18 years.

The age at onset of menstruation in girls has been decreasing throughout time. Around 1880, the age of onset was age 15 or 16 years; in 1925, age 13 or 14 years; and in 1985, age 12 years (Kestenbaum 1979). Once a pubertal girl begins to menstruate, she will usually manifest irregular periods of menstruation for anywhere from 1 year to 18 months. These ovulatory cycles—as well as boys' nocturnal emissions and penile erections during sleep and upon awakening—are manifestations of activation of hypothalamic functions. Shapiro and Hertzig (1988) described these changes as follows:

> In both sexes these primary and secondary sexual changes correspond to activation of hypothalamic functions, which in turn stimulate the gonadotropic hormones of the pituitary, stimulating both estrogen and luteinizing hormones at the periphery as well as testosterone especially in boys. These changes are

thought to be coordinated with maturation of the hypothalamic cells. They become less sensitive to the feedback dampening effect of circulating sex hormones. In males nocturnal emissions are observed to occur about a year after the secondary sexual characteristics develop and mark the beginning of capacity to procreate. (p. 112)

Pregnancy becomes possible in girls by age 14 or 15 years; mature sperm are in evidence in boys by age 15 or 16 years (Khatchadourian 1977). Thus procreation is possible by about midadolescence (Tanner 1978).

Both sexes experience a spurt in general body growth and increases in body strength, muscle tone, and general body coordination during puberty (Beiser 1991). Despite these maturational advances, adolescents ages 12–15 years can appear awkward and uncoordinated in body management. Beiser, however, noted that this apparent awkwardness and uncoordination does not match the physical evidence; she explained this awkwardness as follows:

It may be that increased hormones are responsible for an observed restlessness in both sexes, but it is harder to explain the impression of awkwardness and uncoordination on this basis, as formal tests actually show an increase in strength and skill during this period. It may well be that psychological changes have an effect on body movements. In other words, awareness of bodily changes, especially changes in height, make children of this age unsure of their physical boundaries. (p. 101)

Indeed, pubertal bodily changes compel adolescents to look at their body. This increased body awareness becomes an important biological triggering stimulus that causes adolescents to have many internal responses (psychological stimuli) and to encounter many external responses (social stimuli) to their changing body appearance. Adolescents' mental processing of these biopsychosocial transactions will lead to new developmental changes in their body image. What developmental changes take place in adolescents' body image become a crucial aspect of what they believe about themselves as valued, as well as sexually attractive, individuals.

Maturation and Development of Cognitive Capabilities

Emergence of Hypothetical Thinking and Constructing the Concept of an Unconscious Mental Domain

What Piaget termed the *formal cognitive phase,* during which *formal thinking* emerges, begins at about age 11 or 12 years, and it is not fully developed until about age 16 years. Overton et al. (1992) defined formal thinking as

> a particular type of thinking, namely, logical thought or logical reasoning. Specifically, this is the type of thought usually understood as rational thought, thought whose main hallmarks are its coherence, its consistency, its precision, and its lack of contradictions. (p. 503)

However, the formal phase of cognitive maturation and development many not ever be fully achieved by all adolescents or adults (Blackburn and Papalia 1992). Also, the attainment of formal operational cognitive capabilities appears to be more dependent on environmental experiences than on the attainment of Piaget's prior cognitive phases (Blackburn 1984; Flavell 1971; Sabatini 1979). Finally, the rate of progression through Piaget's phases of cognitive development tends to differ depending on the individual's culture (Blackburn and Papalia 1992; Dasen 1977; Neimark 1979).

■ Emergence of Hypothetical Thinking

A basic characteristic of formal thinking is the capacity to begin to isolate the elements of a problem and explore all possible hypotheses and solutions. Assisting in this process is the young adolescent's new capacity "to examine the logic and consistency of his existing beliefs" (Bloch 1995, p. 34). This review of existing beliefs also contributes to the adolescent's interest in developing his or her own moral and ethical values (Kagan 1971b; see "Development of the Superego," below). Formal thinking processes—that is, systematic, abstract, rational, and logical thinking—emerge from the further development of secondary process thinking. Latency-age children, particularly between ages 8 and 11 years, engage in a mental operation to solve a presented problem (e.g., an arithmetic problem); however, they have little, if any, cognitive ability to mentally evoke a previously stored problem solution and apply it to the current problem. They cannot internally integrate their intelligence the way they can beginning at about age 12 years. As Kaplan (1991) noted:

> From age 12 on, the child no longer depends on perceived data. Freed from the here and now, he deals with timeless, spaceless information. He can think of the possible, the potential, and is ready to reform data. . . . This developmental advance in thinking between 12 and 16 is from the more concrete, present-oriented, simplistic right-good vs. wrong-bad to the general, formal, logical and abstract. (p. 207)

Pubertal cognitive advances associated with formal thinking operations include the following:

1. *The ability to be able to reason on a hypothesis based on verbal propositions.* At age 12 years, adolescents can begin to understand the idea or concept inherent in a hypothesis without having to see physical proof in order to achieve this understanding. They can, therefore, understand either-or and if-then statements.
2. *The ability to combine propositions and isolate variables to test a hypothesis.* For example, a task may involve being presented with five colorless jars of liquid labeled A, B, C, D, and E. Adolescents are given an unlimited number of jars of each label. They are then asked, "Which particular combination of jars will produce a yellow color and what functions do jars B and D possess?" Before age 12 years, they would combine the jars in two-jar sequences, then all the jars together to solve the problem. By age 12 or 13 years, however, adolescents would proceed methodically, testing all combinations of two-, three-, and four-jar sequences. They would then determine, for exam-

ple, that A, C, and E produce a yellow liquid and that B and D have no relationship to the yellow color. This new increase in their cognitive ability to analytically solve problems leads adolescents to construct executive control structures that are much more complex than before. This type of thinking is the deductive reasoning of the scientist.

Adolescents also increasingly organize their mental operations into ways of finding abstract rules by which they can both solve the problem at hand and extend this new problem-solving information to a host of similar problems. In a sense, formal thought is a generalized orientation toward one kind of problem solving.

3. *The ability to use thoughts and increasingly believe in the power of thoughts in planning for the future* (Overton et al. 1992). Latency-age children tend to be preoccupied with the present, whereas adolescents in the formal operational phase become concerned with hypothetical, remote, and future concerns. Early adolescents begin to develop the ability to integrate past, present, and future when thinking about an issue or a problem. Overton et al. (1992) observed that, with the new capacity for formal thinking, adolescents now possess and begin to develop a "generalized system of logic" (p. 506) that enables them to reflect in a new way on their current and past fantasies, beliefs, and memories. This new way entails their generating many new possibilities in thinking about their immediate present life circumstances and formulating plans for the future.

4. *The ability to classify objects and people based on propositional or hypothetical reasoning.* Prior to age 12 years, children use their cognitive abilities to construct and reconstruct numerous categories that they have stored as memories within their representational world. By age 12 or 13 years, adolescents are capable of thinking about the similarities between categories based not only on concrete evidence they can see but also on mental propositions they can form. Bidell and Fischer (1992) expressed this capacity as their being able to understand that, if A belongs to subclass B1, then A must belong to the class of B, of which B1 is a subclass. This ability to classify

objects based on propositions explaining relationships that are not concretely obvious also helps young adolescents to begin to appreciate fully the meaning of proverbs (Kaplan 1991). In this way, they learn much more about how their society engages in many forms of subtle communication (e.g., irony, hypocrisy, humor).

5. *The ability to be increasingly creative in thinking and more sophisticated in the use of symbolic thinking.* Adolescents begin to become aware that they formulate ideas that are uniquely their own (Noy 1979). Their ability to arrive at creative ideas to aid them in reevaluating previous behavioral patterns helps them to "resolve internal conflicts by utilizing new ways of understanding and coping" (Schneider 1992, p. 414). Langer (1962) noted how adolescents begin to experiment with much more sophisticated symbols. For example, they recognize that if they paint a house a dark color, they are symbolically communicating that the house is causing them to feel sad or even depressed.

6. *The ability to form personal opinions and to construct individual standards and moral values along with an increase in the capability to separate what is theoretically possible from what is realistically possible.* P. Tyson and Tyson (1991) remarked on adolescents' development of a *cognitive egocentrism.* In so doing, they were addressing adolescents' resurrection of their wish for an ideal self (i.e., to be a grandiosely wise person) whose creative ideas (e.g., about government, the meaning of life, poverty) should be listened to as important contributions to the world scene. If parents respectfully tolerate these ideas and offer their own ideas without criticizing those of their adolescent, they (and others) become an audience on whom adolescents can test ideas and thus continue to develop their overall identity. In this way, parents continue in their function of providing acceptance and positive, but not grandiose, mirroring (i.e., they do not tell their adolescent that his or her ideas are the only ones worth listening to). When parents do accept their adolescents' pronouncements—both those that are reality based and those that are grandiose—adolescents will perceive that it is permissible to evaluate

critically those standards, morals, and ethical values that are internalized within their preadolescent superego.

Adolescents also construct an imaginary audience composed of their preexistent object representations. In seeing themselves as they imagine others see them, a new level of cognitive awareness is reached in reference to their own representational world. This self-aware and self-reflective capacity is more expansive in scope and more detailed than was possible before. In becoming more aware of their inner thoughts, feelings, and memories, adolescents begin, according to Selman (1980), to understand

> that there are certain aspects of the self's behavior of which the self is *not in control* and that the self is able to examine its own motivations and behaviors. By putting together these concepts, the subject moves . . . to construct a new psychological process, the *unconscious,* to explain the observation that persons are not always aware of their behavior, that even introspection may not yield the psychological causes which best explain behavior, and that external causes cannot explain all of the self's behavior either. (p. 135; italics in original)

■ Construction of Concept of an Unconscious Mental Domain

Adolescents' eventual discovery that they possess an unconscious mental domain is a slowly evolving process that begins during adolescence and is achieved by most adolescents by age 16 or 17 years. Once achieved, the recognition that not every action, belief, or opinion can be so readily explained through one's conscious mental activity assists adolescents in modifying their demand that their beliefs and opinions be easily supported by the facts as they consciously know them. Adolescents now can consider that an impassioned opinion may be based on unconscious factors of which they are not presently aware.

During adolescence, the 12- to 13-year-old egocentric, hypothesizing adolescents progress to being 18- to 19-year-old young adults who can relinquish their wish for cognitive omnipotence. This process helps adolescents further separate what they think and create in fantasy from what they eventually must accept as actually possible as they consolidate an emancipated identity (Anthony 1982).

Maturation and Development of Emotions
Development of Emotional Self-Awareness

Emotions continue to serve adolescents in 1) energy mobilization, 2) self-regulation, and 3) social adaptation.

■ Emotions as Energy Mobilizers

Adolescence has been designated by many as the time in which emotions are numerous and intensely felt (Blos 1962; Hauser and Smith 1991; Noshpitz and King 1991). As energy mobilizers, adolescents' emotions propel them to seek to repeat remembered activities and initiate new activities. One such emotion is the pleasurable feeling associated with attaining orgasm. Now masturbation takes place more frequently and the orgasmic feelings are more intense. This is one example of how an emotion acts as an energizer. Another emotion is the loving feelings experienced for the first time toward a sexually attractive person.

Adolescents experience a new emotion in adolescence—*cognitive dissonance*—as they reexamine and reflect on their beliefs and standards. For example, an adolescent girl will scan her beliefs and standards for logical consistency and,

> if she detects inconsistency, she automatically tries to rearrange or alter them to attain coherence among her beliefs, and between her beliefs and behaviors. Failure to do so results in a special feeling state we might call *cognitive dissonance*, which is not identical to guilt (which follows recognition that one's voluntary actions deviate form a standard). (Kagan 1984, p. 179)

As an emotion, this cognitive dissonance might be named *cognitive confusion* or even *cognitively generated ambivalent feelings*. Adolescents experience ambivalent feelings: one feeling is the competency pleasure in discovering the cognitive dissonance, and another is frustration and even anger that such dissonance exists. Cognitive dissonance acts as an energy mobilizer in motivating adolescents to reflect on the logical inconsistency between a belief or standard they possess and information being attained from new experiences.

The advances in their formal thinking operations enable adolescents to become aware of much more complex emotions within themselves and others. Hauser and Smith (1991) viewed emotional behavior as

> in part a learned "skill." Fischer et al. (1990) note that adolescents have entered a "new developmental tier," characterized by cognitive advances in abstract thinking. The expression and appreciation of affect begins to take on a more complex meaning. Beyond the basic emotions of anger, sadness, fear, joy and love, for example, adolescents can appreciate more complex, adult like "scripts" for emotions, such as jealousy and resentment as well as the concept of deeply hidden or repressed emotions. (pp. 136–137)

In reference to adolescents' ability to understand the concept of deeply hidden or repressed emotions, Selman (1980) wrote:

> The powerful idea that the mind, the conscience, or the "little person inside" can organize the self's inner psychological life leaves no room for psychological phenomena unavailable to [the young adolescent's] roving eye. . . . [The young adolescent] attains the belief that it is possible to fool the self, but only in the sense that the mind makes a *special effort* to trick itself, that is, fooling oneself is understood to be possible only if one *wills* it; and even then, once one pays attention to the concern, one can no longer truly fool the self. (p. 134; italics in original)

Young adolescents, therefore, are able to understand how they can fool themselves into believing that at the moment they do not possess a particular emotion. In essence, this understanding further assists their becoming aware of their mind's possession of an unconscious mental domain; that is, they begin to recognize when they can consciously suppress or unconsciously repress an emotion and then recall the emotion at a later time.

Lane and Schwartz (1987) hypothesized that adolescents' emotional awareness shows progressive maturational growth that enables them to achieve a more differentiated awareness of their and others' emotional states. They can now view others—and themselves—as having mixed thoughts, feelings, or motives toward one object (Selman 1980). Children ages 6–11 years could be swayed or perceptually dominated by any one strong emotion regarding an individual; their subsequent object representations of that individual would be significantly colored by that one dominant emotion. In contrast, young adolescents begin to inwardly perceive subtleties in emotions and construct emotional experiences from blending various emotions. This new ability assists them in viewing people—including their parents and siblings—more realistically; these people are not loved or hated completely, and they are not viewed as totally perfect or imperfect. With this new ability, adolescents can eventually give up their wishes to achieve an ideal self and find an ideal person within their parents or another person.

Adolescents do at times feel somewhat overwhelmed by their emotions and often experience an overall emotional state of feeling bewildered and even angry that their representational world and the outside world are too complicated to be explained logically or categorized into neat black-and-white categories. They will periodically rebel against acknowledging the "grays" of life. At times, however, they seem to be propelled to act or not act based entirely on their emotions. It is as if they have replaced speech and thought dominance with emotional dominance—in essence, seeming to have abandoned all thinking. Developmentalists have speculated differently about the source of this periodically increased emotionality. Some, like P. Tyson and Tyson (1991), stated that adolescents simply have unpredictable and uncontrollable mood swings that lead them from elation to depression, whereas others, like Offer and Schonert-Reichl (1992), have emphasized that this periodically increased emotionality has led to the myth that adolescents are always in a state of increased emotionality. I agree with Offer in that, although adolescents do seem to be more emotionally energized than latency-age children, they are not always bombarded with intensely generated emotions. Strong emotions are generated periodically, and more so in adolescence than in latency. Another ponderable regarding adolescents' periodically increased emotionality is whether the cause could be some maturational change in innate emotions or whether it could be simply adolescents' increased cognitive awareness of their emotional responses.

■ Emotions as a Means of Self-Regulation

By age 12 years, adolescents have already been using their internal anxiety signals to assist them in guiding their actions in order to remain within their optimal stimulation range. Their new awareness of emotional blends upsets their ability to use their emotions as signals of distress. For some time during adolescence, therefore, adolescents find that their emotional signals are difficult to decipher.

To help them maintain self-regulation, young adolescents slowly develop the ability to use reversible mental operations. They begin to become aware that hating a person does not negate their affectionate feelings toward that person. In other words, they learn that their hatred is not an irreversible feeling (Hauser and Smith 1991). For example, instead of an adolescent girl's becoming anxious when she realizes she hates her father for something, she can now calm herself in recognizing that she also has preserved her loving feelings toward her father. These loving feelings will help her tolerate her hatred without her becoming too anxious. This reversibility of feelings greatly assists her in maintaining her overall feelings within a regulated and pleasurable range, which in turn gives her a sense of being in control of her emotions. However, Hauser and Smith (1991) remarked that

> we have little understanding of how certain situations in adolescence (for example, new heterosexual relationships or intensified same sex relationships) may impinge on emotional development in adolescence with respect to stability of affects, reversibility and other possible emergent features. (p. 139; parentheses in original)

Those authors noted the need for new empirical studies of children's and adolescents' understanding of their and others' affective experiences. In no other area is this more pertinent than in achieving a better understanding of how emotional self-regulation develops throughout adolescence.

■ Emotions as an Aid in Achieving Social Adaptation

More than ever before in their life, adolescents are able to use the emotional communications of others to guide their actions. This is attributed to their growing ability to manifest true empathy in relation to another person. They can use empathy and intuitive thinking to view an interpersonal situation involving themselves by seeing themselves through the eyes of another (Lane and Schwartz 1987).

Young adolescents' advanced empathic ability, mediated by the cognitive advance to generate different hypotheses in planning their future, enables them to anticipate the feelings they assume will accompany each of their possible future choices. The 13- to 14-year-old boy, for example, begins to become more interested than ever before in his grandmother's previously told story about her son (the boy's uncle) and how unhappy the uncle had become when he did not follow through with his goal to be a lawyer. The boy imagines how achieving his goals—or not achieving them—will make him feel in the future.

In sensing and empathizing with the feelings of others, adolescents enhance their ability to achieve internal adaptation to their innate needs and external adaptation to the needs and tasks of others. They express their empathic observations to others through the use of verbal language (see next section).

Maturation and Development of Verbal Language Abilities

Facilitating the Verbalization of Adolescent Emotions

In the psychologically aware family, parents begin to allow their young adolescents a new "language space" in which they permit them to verbalize their thoughts and emotions within the family without always encouraging them to think before they speak. It is as if parents encourage them to move back to the speech dominance of early childhood and away from the thought dominance of late childhood. However, in encouraging speech as the vehicle for the expression of their emotions, parents are helping adolescents slowly restructure their emotional control structures through experimenting with when it is useful to verbalize certain emotions and when it is better to leave them unexpressed until they are privately evaluated. The context of a situation becomes quite important for adolescents because of the tenuousness of their newly acquired cognitive capacity for abstraction (Hauser and Smith 1991). Young adolescents (ages 12–15 years), in particular, are not confident in using their abstract thinking in deciding which of their thoughts and emotions should be verbalized in interpersonal situations. They experiment and reveal their abstract ideas, hypotheses, and empathic hunches about other people's thoughts and emotions; however, they are perhaps most sensitive to revealing their and others' inner emotional states. Psychologically attuned parents detect this sensitivity and function as admiring and encouraging selfobjects in communicating a certain degree of pleasure in hearing their adolescents reveal their emotional hypotheses and discoveries in certain contexts. The following example from a conversation I had with a father illustrates this:

> The father of a 14-year-old boy listened as his son told him, "You know, I think that inside, you don't like being so conservative all the time. In fact, I have this feeling that you hate being a lawyer because you have to be so straight and have to look so neat like 'Mr. Clean.'" Although the father did not agree with his son's assessment of his inner feelings about being a lawyer and dressing conservatively, the father told me, "I wanted to smile as he spoke because I was happy he was trying to figure me out. But I gave him my serious attention and told him that these were interesting ideas."
>
> This father wanted to hear his son's feelings, empathic statements, and abstract ideas, even when he did not agree. However, he did hear his son's comment as complimentary in the sense

that the father believed his son was telling him that his conservative outside hid more liberal qualities inside.

When parents encourage their adolescents' emotional statements—about both the adolescents' feelings and their empathic hunches about the parents' feelings—they can follow their adolescents' slow progression during adolescence from being somewhat anxious about the value of verbalizing their emotions to believing in the utility of their emotional verbal expression in maintaining developing enhancing interactions with their parents and others.

When a family does not want to hear an adolescent's emotions, it is often because the family does not want the adolescent to be introspective about family relationships. The adolescents may be discovering a *family myth,* which is a certain belief that all family members avoid mentioning and covertly reinforce (Viorst 1986), as illustrated in the following example:

> A 14-year-old girl who was not doing well in school told me, "In our family these days, I'm not allowed to think about what's going on with my dad. It's like there is this rule—it's not good to ever ask how dad is feeling. But I know he's depressed. My parents already came to see you and I know they didn't tell you what's happened at home. [Her parents had told me that everything was fine within the family.] Since my father did not get promoted to being a captain [in the Navy], he sits and doesn't want to do anything with anybody. He has really changed since this happened. Now I don't like to be around him, because I can't say how I feel."
>
> In time, this girl might have established an emotional display rule that speaking with emotion is not permitted in her family, particularly if emotions involve her father. If this did occur, she would begin to automatically repress her feelings within the family and manifest an overall identity that was true only to her thinking self, while her emotional self would remain within her unconscious. This would lead to her isolation from her family and a state of inner loneliness.

Development of the Self-Representation and Object Representations

■ Construction of an Emancipated Identity While Maintaining Transactional Relationships With Important Others

The attainment of an emancipated identity is the major developmental task of adolescence; as such, it is not fully attained until well into the completion of adolescence at age 18 or 19 years. Before I delineate the steps that lead to the construction of an emancipated identity, I will describe some of its characteristics.

An older adolescent's identity reaches a degree of emancipation in the sense that, by age 18 or 19 years, that adolescent's self-representation and object representations have reached such an advanced degree of development that they enable the adolescent to function more fully as an autonomous individual. Toward the end of adolescence, the person begins to function as an adult—that is, he or she can exist and make autonomous decisions about his or her life without believing that his or her parents or any other adult basically knows what he or she should do. However, this emancipated or fully autonomous identity is not of a person who is an island unto himself or herself. In older adolescents' developed representational world, the important people in their life have become represented within their object representations. These object representations—in addition to ongoing relationships with parents, siblings, teachers, and others—are necessary for late adolescents to maintain self-autonomy or self-emancipation. This is because late adolescents will use the external voices and many of the internalized voices of their parents, teachers, coaches, religious leaders, relatives, siblings, and peer friends both to guide their behaviors and to maintain an internal source of positive acceptance and admiration. They do not normally reject their object representations in favor of resurrecting childhood-derived ideal self-representation or object representations. If they did, they would leave adolescence telling themselves that they did not need anyone's support or guidance (the ideal self) or that they needed to find an external source of power, protection, and admiration (the ideal object representation) in another person, institution, or peer group.

Adolescents' eventual attainment of self-autonomy is obviously the product of many developmental achievements since they first constructed their sense of being an autonomous individual, somewhere around age 18 months. As I note in previous chapters, children slowly construct a series of subidentities (i.e., autonomous, gender, sexual, peer, and social identities). Erikson (1963) described an ongoing process of identity building, extending from infancy through adolescence, that culminates in a person's achieving an identity that must override or counteract the development of identity (or role) confusion. Although Erikson did not use the term *emancipated,* his definition of identity in adolescence is the same as the following definition I offer: late adolescents' emancipated identity is an aspect of their self-representation that defines the self as

1. Being separate and autonomous from their parents and significant others—especially their parents—while maintaining supportive transactional relationships with the parents and important others.
2. Believing in their self-value while possessing individual and different points of view, ideals, and values from those of respected parents, teachers, coaches, and so on.
3. Possessing sex-role behaviors in congruence with their sexual object choice in demonstrating heterosexuality or homosexuality.
4. Possessing social behaviors and beliefs that enable older adolescents to be comfortable in adopting a social role. This social role gives late adolescents a continued sense of trust in entering their society and committing to a particular lifestyle (e.g., as a college student, as someone who is gainfully employed, as someone providing community service).

5. Attaining an appreciation of the progressive continuity in their life between their past, their present, and their fantasies and ambitions for their future. This progressive continuity is facilitated by cognitive advances that enable late adolescents to understand what they conceive themselves to have become during childhood and what they conceive will happen to them in an anticipated future.

In the above definition of an emancipated identity, the first component is the main organizer of adolescents' achieving a sense of true emancipation. Achieving a belief in being truly separate and autonomous speaks to the issue of which mental structure activates and organizes adolescents' self-autonomy. Meissner (1986) discussed self-autonomy as follows:

> [Self-autonomy] involves complex issues of personal freedom, responsibility, moral decision making, a capacity for independence and self-determination, the presentation of a cohesive self in the face of instinctual, interpersonal, environmental, social, and cultural pressures for submission, conformity, dependence and self-evocation. The organization of self-autonomy, then, requires an integration of elements derived from the id, ego, and superego. The acquisition of personal freedom, for example, cannot be realized without the attainment of ego autonomy along with a significant degree of superego autonomy. The theoretical option here rests on the question of whether an adequate account of self autonomy is provided by a mere catalogue of contributions from the tripartite entities, or whether the autonomy of the self involves more than merely the sum of the parts. I would assert the later perspective. (p. 392)

I agree with Meissner in viewing the achievement of self-autonomy as the product of a new integration in late adolescence of the various structures that make up adolescents' representational world. I would add, however, that the development of self-autonomy takes place in the context of, as Miller (1991) wrote, "developing all of one's self in increasingly complex ways, in increasingly complex relationships" (p. 45).

Early adolescents embark on this process of establishing an emancipated identity when they begin to question many of the beliefs, standards, and values that they have previously internalized as long-term memory structures within their representational world. This reevaluation or reassessment of prior knowledge is necessary if they are to become adults who truly believe they possess certain beliefs, goals, ambitions, standards, and values, versus adults who are always trying to agree with or rebel against either their real parents or the internalized representation of their parents.

Blos (1985) viewed adolescents as eventually achieving an emancipated identity through engaging in the "second individuation process of adolescence." The first individuation process began in toddlerhood (see Chapter 3 on the separation-individuation process) where there was more of a need to establish "a relative independence from external objects, while the second, the adolescent step of individuation, aims at the independence from internalized, infantile objects" (p. 145). These internalized infantile objects (here infantile refers to prepubertal) are the positive object constancy that normally developing pubertal adolescents bring to their adolescent state of development. These infantile object representations enabled the infant, toddler, and grade school child to explore autonomously and with industry away from his or her parents. Now in adolescence these object representations must be restructured, not relinquished or replaced. The process during which this occurs in great part involves transferring object relations conflicts into structural conflicts, which I describe in the next section.

Object relations conflicts and structural conflicts.
Dorpat (1976) observed the difference between object relations conflicts and structural conflicts. Adults who possess internal object relations conflicts are those who have an identity that either is forever attempting to please its object representations or rebels against pleasing its object representations, as did the following man:

> A boy grew up with a mother who taught him that weekly church attendance and religious worship were important aspects of life. Now, as an adult, he neither lived with his mother nor was ever

asked by her if he practiced any religion. When he was asked if he believed in religion, he responded, "I go to church to please my mother, but I often hate to go. But if she asked if I go to church and I said no, she'd get upset. I don't know what I believe about religion." During his adolescence, this man did not reevaluate his mother's belief that religious worship was important. He had taken his mother's belief into his object representation of her. Throughout his adolescence, he held the following object relations unit within his inner world: "I go to church because my mother loves me and wants me to go."

This man had never reconstructed this object relations unit about going to church by 1) changing its content or 2) transforming it into an object relations unit that would support an emancipated self. Such an emancipated unit would be something like,

I go to church because it is important to me. Religion is an important part of my life. My mother taught me about religion and wanted me to go as a child. Now I basically believe the way she does, but not on every religious issue. My religion is part of my own identity.

Once such an internal object representation is constructed, the individual is capable of experiencing a true (internal) *structural conflict,* one that would take place between one or more of his or her wishes versus what he or she believes. On a Sunday morning, for example, this man would experience superego anxiety (as an internal distress signal of impending guilt) if he contemplated not going to church. This would be quite different from his experiencing anger at his internalized mother for making him go to church.

Dorpat (1976) noted that emancipated internal object relations units contribute to the development of the mature superego or conscience. Thus truly emancipated individuals have attained self-autonomy in that they are able to use their id, ego, superego, and self in arriving at personal decisions, in contrast to believing that they must rebel against their own superego—which in essence is more their parents' superego than their own—in order to assert their true self. The failure of an early adolescent to begin to work on object relations conflicts leads to his or her eventual failure in establishing an emancipated identity.

In the process of early adolescents' reevaluating and reassessing their representational world and their current relationships with their parents and siblings, internal object relations conflicts are inevitable. These conflicts must be externalized by adolescents, tolerated by their parents and significant others, and worked on by adolescents for adolescents to mature to being adults who experience primarily structural conflicts as opposed to adults who continue to experience object relations conflicts.

Generational conflicts. The transformation of internal object relations conflicts into structural conflicts is, in essence, the psychological work of adolescence (Dahl 1995). Internal object relations conflicts also contribute to the emergence of generational conflicts—that is, conflicts between early adolescents' current and prior, internalized views of their parents (contained within their object representations of them) and their current needs and wishes. Blos (1979) explained this type of conflict as follows:

> The formation of a conflict between generations and its subsequent resolution is the normative task of adolescence. Its importance for cultural continuity is evident. Without this conflict no adolescent psychic restructuring would occur. . . . Generational conflict is essential for the growth of the [emancipated] self and of civilization . . . [and] is aroused by the emotional disengagement from the old and by beckoning of the new that can only be reached via the gradual elaboration of compromise and transformation [of structures within adolescents' representational world]. (pp. 11, 14)

Generational conflicts inevitably are expressed through a certain degree of normal rebellion. Rebellion in adolescents has been romanticized by some adults and overemphasized by some psychiatrists and psychologists who see only a selected population of emotionally disturbed adolescents (Offer and Schonert-Reichl 1992). Generational conflicts are a normal part of the adolescent's developmental process. They are often composed of both an internal object relations conflict that has been externalized onto the original object and a current external conflict between the adolescent's own view and those of his or her parents', as in the following example:

> A 14-year-old boy began to argue quite often with his father. He accused his father of being arrogant and dogmatic, even though the father had not displayed these traits for many years. The father had been quite dogmatic when his son was in grade school, but had become more tolerant of his son's and other people's views since he retired from a quite demanding and high-stress occupation. However, he had regressed to his old arrogance during a recent conversation with his son. The 14-year-old boy was attempting to emancipate himself not only from his [internal] object representation of his father—one that still retained a view of his father as dogmatic and arrogant—but also from current episodes of his father's arrogance.

In the son's externalizing his earlier object representation of his father onto his current view of his father—in part precipitated by his father's recent episode of arrogance—the son was manifesting a negative transference toward his father; that is, he was transferring his old image and relationship with his father onto his current image and relationship with his father. In so doing, he felt compelled to be rebellious lest his father's recent arrogance lead the father to assert his authority dogmatically and arrogantly tell his son that his son's views were entirely wrong.

The externalization of an internalized object relations conflict may or may not generate new external conflicts or aggravate ongoing conflicts with parents (Dahl 1995). In the above example, the father had changed—despite the father's momentarily regressive episode of arrogance—and he and his son had been relating quite well prior to the son's negative transference reaction to the father. However, another father who had not changed might have reacted to his son's normal degree of rebelliousness as a personal attack; his current relationship with his son would then have become mutually rebellious.

In the more psychologically aware family, parents take some measure of pride in their early adolescent's rebellion against their beliefs, opinions, and attitudes. As one father of a 16-year-old girl told me,

> She is really becoming quite an independent-thinking young woman. She used to be a Republican like me, but now she is taking me to task for all the positions I take that she believes are wrong. I'm glad I didn't raise her to be my clone.

Sensitively aware parents, therefore, recognize that early adolescents are in the process of emancipating themselves from the generation that reared them. This process assists early adolescents in negotiating a new social identity that will enable them to take their place within their generation and replace adults. Negotiating generational conflicts entails adolescents' tolerating the emotions that these conflicts generate (e.g., sadness, anxiety, cognitive dissonance, anger, disappointment—particularly the disappointment in recognizing that their parents are not perfect). These conflicts also generate guilt in adolescents about breaking the emotional and physical dependencies on their parents. Restructuring their inner world leads to adolescents' growing emancipation.

Generational conflicts may also be viewed as a social phenomenon. In this view, parents prepare their children to live in a society that no longer exists from the parents' viewpoint. The "generation gap" is not simply a problem of communication, but is a result of the wisdom of past generations that is passed from parents to their adolescents. The majority of adolescents eventually come to value and incorporate the wisdom of their parents in separating from their parents and establishing an emancipated identity. This latter point was illustrated by Offer and Offer (1975). In a worldwide study of approximately 20,000 middle-class teenagers living primarily in urban environments, the authors found that the majority of the teenagers were not in the throes of turmoil. The vast majority functioned well, enjoyed good relationships with their families and friends, and accepted the values of the larger society in which they lived. Offer and Offer characterized these teenagers as follows:

- Most (98%) were task oriented and felt good when they received feedback for a job well done.

- Most (90%) felt a job was waiting for them in their society and felt that they would do well economically.
- Most did not feel overly rebellious or unloved (but 50% reported anxiety as being a regular everyday feeling).
- Most felt that no generation gap existed in their family, and on 18 of 19 questionnaire items reported good feelings toward their parents.
- Most (90%) got into the college of their choice, showing realistic goal setting and good appreciation of their overall ability.

Esman (1990), in reviewing the studies by Offer and Offer (1975), Douvan and Adelson (1966), and Keniston (1968, 1971) wrote,

> The weight of evidence, therefore, seems to argue against the existence of a true "generation gap." . . . Most adolescents in most cultures conform rather quietly to the expectations of their elders. . . . From the previously mentioned normal population studies one gains a picture of general compliance and identification with adult standards with, perhaps, brief and sporadic flurries of rebelliousness around nonessential issues. Indeed, the logic of cultural continuity demands that this be so, were each generation truly to reject or rebel against the values and ideologies of its parents, only chaos could result. (p. 30)

Those teenagers, on the other hand, engaged in generational conflict avoidance (Blos 1979) are unable to tolerate and work through their normative generational conflicts because of various acute and chronic risk factors. Acute familial and nonfamilial risk factors that make it difficult for adolescents to work on their internal object relations conflicts and associated generational conflicts are the highly stressful events that occur during adolescence. These include

- Experiencing a parental divorce
- Becoming a victim of violence
- Suddenly losing a parent's involvement because of the parent's depression

- Experiencing a physical illness that causes one to leave school and one's peer group for an extended period of time
- A sudden relocation of the family into a new environment, which entails losing one's peer group

Coping with these stressful events and having to adapt to a new unexpected set of challenges interferes with the work of achieving an emancipated identity. Those adolescents possessing internal protective factors—such as high adaptability, transient use of defense mechanisms, and an ability to seek help from others—will tend to master acute traumatic experiences and go on to achieve an emancipated self (Offer 1989). Offer described a group of such male adolescents:

> [These adolescents] progressed through adolescence and young manhood with a smoothness of purpose and a self-assurance of their progress towards a meaningful and fulfilling adult life. . . . The subjects were able to cope with external trauma, usually through an adaptive active-orientation. When difficulties arose, they used the defenses of denial and isolation [of emotion] to protect their ego from being bombarded with affect. . . . They did not experience sustained periods of anxiety or depression. (pp. 184–186)

Adolescents who have been exposed to a cumulatively traumatic family environment that operated as a chronic familial risk factor often manifest significant generational conflict avoidance. In the face of such chronic and cumulative trauma, even the possession of protective factors is often not sufficient to protect adolescents' development. Offer (1989) described adolescents within this group as follows:

> These adolescents have been observed to have recurrent self-doubts (often unsuccessfully masked by braggadocio), escalating conflicts with their parents, and debilitating inhibitions. . . . Some of the parents in this group had marital conflicts, and others had a history of mental illness in the family. . . . [These adolescents] experienced more major psychological traumas. The difficulties in their life situations were greater than their satisfactions, and defenses were not well developed for handling emo-

tionally trying situations. . . . Wide mood swings indicated a search for who they were as separate individuals and concern about whether their activities were worthwhile. Feelings of mistrust about the adult world were often expressed in this group. (pp. 189–190; parentheses in original)

Because they are unable to work gradually on achieving an emancipated self, these adolescents seek rebellion—often at school—as a way of avoiding their confusion about what their role will be in their society.

Adoption of a false identity. Earlier in this chapter, I note that Erikson delineated the overall psychosocial conflict that is inevitable during adolescence as one between the establishment of an emancipated identity versus a succumbing to identity or role confusion. Significant role confusion leads adolescents to adopt a false identity that has been attained through some combination of internal rebellion—against unloving and critically harsh parental representations contained within their superegos—and external rebellion—against current unloving and critically harsh voices emanating from others (e.g., parents, siblings, teachers).

A false identity is established in abnormally developing adolescents when they are unable to integrate the many diverse social, peer, gender, and sexual roles that individuals experience at one time or another throughout their adolescence. This can occur in adolescents who have never attained positive self-constancy and object constancy (normally first attained at about age 3 years), and hence are very mistrustful of assuming any socially acceptable role because they believe that people will abandon or hurt them in some way. These adolescents will then often manifest an external rebellion: they search for a new person, group, cult, or organization through which they can discard their previously internalized negative self-constancy and object constancy and associated overly critical standards, values, and so on. The new person or group provides these adolescents with an identity that helps them repress their sense of role confusion and even identity diffusion (Erikson 1968). These adolescents resurrect the generational gap as an impasse and a life preoccupation; they also resurrect—as a permanent solution for their conflicts—their childhood-derived ideal self-representation and ideal parent representations. Blos described this type of adolescent as follows:

> The subjective feeling of the gap lies in its use as a distancing device in which spatial and ideological separations are substituted for inner [object relations] conflicts and emotional disengagement. . . . [T]he generation-gap-minded youth attaches himself to these broader social issues and thus imbues his sense of personal separation and cultural discontinuity with a viable ideology and an emotional referent. (pp. 15, 18)

For their own reasons, there will always be adults who will idealize rebellious generation gap–preoccupied teenagers. For example, Dubois (1965), a biologist, stated, "As long as there are adolescent rebels in our midst, there is reason to hope that societies can be saved" (p. 85).

Some adults subtly encourage adolescents to rebel against parental and societal values. For example, adults who want to rebel themselves know how to attract those adolescents who are looking for an ideal world or a perfect parent substitute to protect them from life's problems. Often these teenagers have experienced acute and possibly chronic traumatic experiences that they cannot tolerate. Consequently, their ideal self-image and object images become their defenses against an intolerable, traumatic reality.

A false identity—or false self—is also established in adolescents who have grown up in a family in which they continually adapted to their parents' needs and expectations at the expense of their own innate needs. Instead of an emancipated identity, such adolescents may construct a *negative identity,* which is an identity almost entirely defined by their parents, peer group, or an institution. In his novel *Beneath the Wheel,* Herman Hesse (1930/1972) described the slow and emotionally painful "death" of the inner vitality of a pubertal adolescent who was unable to stand up to his father's hostile attacks on his attempts to establish an emancipated self.

Adolescents who resort to establishing a false self to avoid the intense anxiety generated by their conscious awareness of their identity confusion—the confusion resulting from attaining a true identity and being compelled to attain a false identity—are unable to do the work of achieving psychological emancipation; they are unable to work on internal object relations conflicts or the external manifestation of these in the observed generational conflicts between adolescents and their parents and society.

■ Parents' Role in Facilitating Formation of Emancipated Identity

Parents need to empathize with their adolescent's need to confront parental values, standards, and beliefs in order to support their adolescent's verbalization and resolution of conflict. Parents must permit and be tolerant of their early adolescent's confrontation of the many values, standards, and beliefs that he or she most likely held to be true during his or her latency years. In order to maintain a developmentally enhancing goodness of fit between their adolescent and themselves, parents must use their empathy in identifying in the teenager the same emancipation currents the parents experienced during their adolescence.

An adolescent's age-appropriate wish may go something like the following: "Look, Dad, I want to argue about some of the things I always accepted. I don't believe everything you believe in." How the parents' parents handled this developmental age-appropriate wish (e.g., whether they rejected and criticized it or supported it) when they expressed it will affect how they handle their own adolescent's wish. In facing this wish, parents may remember their own displeasurable experiences when, for example, their own parents responded to this same wish with some measure of disdain. If they call on and maintain an identification with their disdainful and rejecting parent (thus identifying with the aggressor), they will do the same thing to their teenager that was done to them. However, if they can tolerate their painful memories and give to their teenager what was not given to them by their own parents, the teenager's normal wish to reevaluate his or her own early adolescent beliefs will help the parents reevaluate some of their adult beliefs that were constructed in their developmentally inhibiting adolescent years.

When parents are able to express their views, they encourage their teenager to do the same. When there is disagreement, the parents model for their teenager an important socially adaptive behavior: constructive arguing and conflict resolution. Collins and Laursen, citing Shantz (1987), defined conflicts as being precipitated when "behavior [including speech] by one member of a dyad is incongruent with the goals, expectations, or desires of the other member, resulting in *mutual opposition.* In addressing both the experience of conflict and conflict resolution during adolescence, Collins and Laursen (1992) made the following points:

1. *Conflicts emerge in interpersonal relationships that are closer rather than more distant or superficial.* Collins and Laursen (1992) wrote,

   > Adaptive, well-functioning relationships are marked not by the absence of conflicts, but by responsive engagement in resolving them (Grotevant and Cooper 1985; Kelley et al. 1983). . . . When conflicts occur in close relationships, adolescents have the opportunity to learn about the dynamics of relationships as they assume new roles within them. Perceptions of mutuality and reciprocity in conversations increase during adolescent years. (pp. 226, 235)

2. *The interdependencies between adolescents and their parents—developed before the onset of adolescence—inevitably lead to generational conflict.* Again, returning to Collins and Laursen (1992):

   > During adolescence, rapid and extensive physical, cognitive and social changes necessitate interpersonal adjustments in order to maintain these functional interdependencies, and conflicts often occur in this realignment process. . . . Conflicts are presumed to be more common in relationships with family members, especially parents, on the premise that autonomy issues are central to individual development during this period, and these must be dealt with primarily in parent-adolescent relations (Hill 1987; Steinberg 1991).

> . . . Conflicts become increasingly likely as adolescents de-
> velop cognitive competencies that permit them to recog-
> nize inconsistencies and imperfections in others (e.g.,
> Elkind 1967) and to view many issues as matters of personal
> concern, rather than legitimate areas of parental authority.
> (pp. 218, 220)

3. *The verbalization of conflicts can be developmentally enhancing or developmentally inhibiting in relation to adolescents'
   construction and development of an emancipated identity.*
   Verbalization of conflicts is more developmentally enhancing
   when parents gradually use less of their authoritative power to
   resolve conflicts with their adolescent and instead begin to
   solve conflicts by working out compromises, instituting "time-
   outs" to allow each to reformulate his or her opinion, and ne-
   gotiations. As Collins and Laursen (1992) wrote,

> Abilities for resolving conflicts are believed to be based in
> capacities for reasoning and [emotional] self-regulation. . . .
> [The child's] knowledge of appropriate skills and strategies
> for negotiated resolutions increases linearly from middle
> childhood to late adolescence, on the assumption that logi-
> cal competence, including understanding of interpersonal
> relationships, is more advanced among older individuals
> than younger ones. . . . Parent-adolescent relationships in
> which interactions are marked by responsiveness to adoles-
> cents' expressions of discrepant opinions are associated
> with sense of *identity* among the adolescents, as well as
> social perceptions skills. (pp. 217, 231)

It would appear, therefore, that parents who encourage and
assist their adolescent to engage in verbal conflict expression and
eventual resolution 1) decrease their adolescent's need to act out
their conflicts through rebellious behavior, and 2) assist their adolescent's integration of his or her various subidentities into an eventual emancipated identity.

**Parents need to be consistent in expressing their values
and standards.** Parents must be relatively consistent in expressing their values, attitudes, ideals, and points of view to pro-

vide their adolescents with a frame of reference to test out their views, ideals, and beliefs by entering into verbal conflict with their parents. Parents must appreciate that their teenager will often fluctuate between wanting to agree and wanting to disagree with them.

For adolescents to struggle with those beliefs and values from their childhood that they want to retain as their own, they need their parents to be consistent in manifesting their more stable emancipated identities. For example, it is very difficult for an adolescent girl to argue with her physician mother about the merits of pursuing medical school when her mother one week tells her that being a physician is a worthwhile profession but the next week tells her that being a physician is a terrible profession.

Parents need to encourage their adolescents' continued involvement with their peer group and not be overly competitive with the peer group. Parents need to encourage their adolescents to continue to pursue peer relationships that began in late childhood. Parents who appreciate the crucial role of the peer group in facilitating their adolescent's development of an emancipated identity do not set up a competition between themselves and the peer groups' attitudes, values, and so on. The majority of normally developing adolescents do not join peer groups whose values, attitudes, and rules of behavior differ greatly from those of their parents.

Adolescents' greater interest in developing close ties with peers is fueled by their need for independence. This need propels them to identify with certain aspects of the peer group in order to establish their own views of life. The views adolescents develop before they reach adulthood will be a composite of their own views, their parents' views, other adults' views, and their peers' views.

Despite the increasing importance of the peer group, adolescents will still remain highly dependent on their parents and other adults, but they will be less willing to admit it. Peer groups often assist adolescents in working on internal object relations conflicts and current external conflicts with their parents. For example, an adolescent girl tells her peers about one of her father's edicts that she has long believed to be true. Now she is questioning this edict. Her peers may give her the support she needs to feel confident enough to enter into a conflict discussion with her father about this very edict.

By midadolescence, peers are vitally important. As Rakoff (1992) wrote,

> In middle and late adolescence, an alternate and transitional family develops. . . . A society of friendly brothers or sisters emerges that will facilitate the essential move away from family into the society at large. In that society, the individual moves almost as if without parents. The adolescent must, in a sense, become an orphan in order to become an adult. If he is fortunate, the cohort of friends in which he has to establish his new self, a self that will continue for the rest of his life, will permit a secure sense of community in the nonfamilial world. . . . Such a family provides security, a sense of personal value, without it having to be constantly earned and justified. (p. 110)

However, as the majority of mid- to late adolescents restructure their positive self-constancy and object constancy by working on their internal object relations conflicts through adaptive confrontation and conflict negotiation with their parents, many of the basic moral and ethical values of their parents will remain within these representations. Adolescents will now make these moral and ethical values more their own, mostly as internalizations within their more developed conscience, as well as in various restructured and new identifications with the views and behaviors of their parents and significant others (e.g., teachers, political and cultural figures, coaches). By the end of adolescence, the processes of conflict negotiation and adaptive confrontation lead adolescents to arrive at a set of beliefs and values that define their emancipated self.

■ Further Development of Sexual and Social Identities

The first and perhaps most significant catalyst that sets into operation the process of establishing an emancipated self is puberty. This is the first step in adolescents' constructing a sexual identity. Having attained a solid gender identity (i.e., a basic sense of maleness or femaleness with associated identifications with gender role behaviors) and sexual identity (in which they make their sexual object choice), adolescents begin to discover and consider embarking on new behaviors as they enter the world of sexual activity. Blos (1979), in writing about puberty, stated,

> While pubertal maturation remains the biological initiation of adolescence, the advanced state of personality formation allows all kinds of transformatory influences to be brought to bear on the sexual drive. . . . Adolescence is the sum of the total of accommodations to the condition of puberty. (p. 105)

Blos's "accommodations to puberty" refer to adolescents' experiences of the many social reactions to their pubertal changes, which then lead to their construction of conceptions of these experiences. These conceptions further develop their social identity. In Chapter 2, I describe two 12-year-old boys' experiences with the emergence of their masculine secondary sexual characteristics; the difference between their experiences was based primarily on their fathers' responses to their changes. For the first boy, puberty triggered and facilitated his further healthy maturation and development; for the second boy, puberty further triggered a developmentally inhibiting relationship with his father. Therefore, in the first boy, puberty enhanced the development of his social identity, whereas in the second boy, puberty inhibited the development of his social identity by causing him to avoid interacting with men in authority.

Puberty becomes a major sexual and social event for both adolescents and their parents. Parents now have an emerging sexually active person living within their family. When they become unduly anxious in seeing their pubertal boy or girl exhibit the pubertal bodily changes, they and other adults, as Bayrakal (1987) noted, may

> deal with these uncomfortable feelings by shaming, reproaching, and provoking youth. . . . Jealousy in adults and a resurgence of their own unresolved adolescent conflicts can find solution in the projection to the negative aspects of the current culture onto youth. (p. 113)

It is not only 12- to 13-year-old adolescents' perceptions of their own pubertal body changes that trigger the development of their sexual identity, but also their family's, their peer group's and other people's responses to these body changes that determine to a large degree what conception of a sexual identity adolescents will begin to construct within their self-representation. Young adolescents react to their secondary sexual characteristics as new discoveries about themselves and experience a wish to exhibit these discoveries within social contexts and have them admired and valued. However, there is always some anxiety.

Young adolescents experience a new variant of the developmental anxiety I discuss in earlier chapters as disintegration anxiety (i.e., the anxiety that is associated with not receiving positive mirroring and admiration for one's characteristics or performances). They feel anxious that their bodily changes will not be accepted by their parents, teachers, and peers. Throughout their development, their body has been, and still is, an important source of positive or negative self-esteem. This form of disintegration anxiety can be thought of as body reflection anxiety about not being viewed as a potentially sexually attractive individual. No heterosexual adolescent wants to be told or believe that he or she has no sexual appeal or attractiveness to those of the opposite gender, just as no homosexual adolescent wants to be told or believe that he or she has no sexual appeal or attractiveness to those of the same gender.

Pubertal changes. Important rite of passage events for 12- to 13-year-old boys are buying their first underarm deodorant and their first athletic supporter. Some boys are also anxious about being told they must wear gym shorts because they do not have any hair on their legs or their legs are underdeveloped.

Both pubertal boys and girls have some anxiety about having to take a shower in public locker rooms (e.g., at school, at a health club). Girls worry about their breast size (that they are either too big or too small) and the presence or absence of axillary and pubic hair (Bloch 1995). Boys worry about their axillary, chest, and pubic hair growth. All boys are aware of penis size (Sugar 1993) and may avoid taking a locker next to a boy in the class who is taller than they because they believe that the taller boy will have a bigger penis.

Girls age 11 or 12 years approach buying their first brassiere as a rite of passage into adolescence. When doing so, they experience some anxiety about not being developed enough or being too developed. Again, their anxiety is primarily what they see reflected in the eyes of others in reference to their new sexual bodily appearance. Pubertal girls will want to go to the store with their mothers, who are more psychologically attuned to this experience, and will avoid going with their fathers.

Both pubertal boys and girls become preoccupied with how to dress their sexually maturing bodies. They now embark on the important personal task of shopping for and selecting their own clothes (Rizzuto 1992). In working on eventual self-emancipation, early adolescents assert their separation from their parents by shopping with peers and in the process communicate to their parents that their adolescent body no longer belongs to the parents (Rizzuto 1992).

As a triggering biological stimulus, menarche propels adolescent girls to begin to more seriously contemplate a feminine sexual identity (Ritvo 1976). Its emergence will either enhance or inhibit their development based on 1) how it emerges (i.e., whether it unfolds smoothly with regular periods and is not associated with any severe abdominal cramping or pain or unfolds erratically and is associated with painful cramping) (biological stimuli), 2) how their parents' and others' respond to it (social stimuli), and 3) what their own perceptions, emotions, memories, and new conceptions are about it (psychological stimuli). A normally developing adolescent girl eventually processes the transactions between these biopsychosocial stimuli and constructs a developmentally enhancing conceptual belief about what having menstrual periods means to her. Each girl's unique normal belief will then begin to influence her developing sexual identity. A normal belief would be something along the lines of "I believe having periods is a sign that I'm healthy, that I can have babies someday, that I'm becoming a woman, and that my parents are proud of my new feminine body changes."

P. Tyson and Tyson (1991) emphasized the importance of menarche as a potent conceptual organizer of the pubertal girl's image of her female body. Her new conceptualization of what it means to be having regular periods enables her to place herself into the category of "women who can produce babies," which fuels her identifications with her mother. She then is motivated to tell her father, "Someday I'll be a mother and have babies." The psychologically attuned and empathic father compliments his daughter for her wish to have babies, which helps the daughter believe that becoming a mother can enhance her self-esteem.

Puberty is a time when adolescent girls identify strongly with the feminine aspects of their mother. Indeed, as Dahl (1995) observed,

> Normative research suggests that during adolescence the relationship of the daughter to her mother is best characterized as one of strong attachment rather than of conflict and rejection. (Apter 1990)

Around the time of the expected onset of menarche, the sensitively aware mother initiates an interest in discussing her daughter's use of tampons and the body events associated with having a period. The mother will attempt to find out what her daughter knows about menarche and what fantasies and possible worries she is currently having about beginning her periods. In these discussions, the mother communicates to her daughter that she wants her daughter to understand and respect her body (Kestenberg 1968). This strengthens her daughter's gender identity, consolidating her identification with females. And, as Dahl (1995) further observed, "Through the experience of her mother's bodily care, the girl's relationship to her own body is established" (pp. 201–202).

In asserting her new femininity, an adolescent girl is taught by her parents and others that asserting her sexual identity has limits. For example, as a model for femininity, her mother—who respects and takes care of her own body—communicates to her daughter that a sexually developing feminine body is a possession to be valued, not used or abused by others.

Thus, as the adolescent girl begins to become more interested in the idea of eventually engaging in sexual activity with males, she seeks more information about protected sex and sexually transmitted diseases, particularly how one contracts the human immunodeficiency virus (HIV), and becomes more interested in becoming aware of how to protect herself from such crimes as rape and sexual abuse.

This new interest in acquiring knowledge about sexual activity does not propel the pubertal girl to engage in sexual activity in the first few years after menarche. Her acquisition of the shoulds and should nots of becoming sexually active prepare her for the actual sexual activity that will often begin in late adolescence (i.e., between ages 16 and 19 years) (Wyatt 1990). Sometimes the new sexual knowledge acquired by younger adolescent girls (i.e., those between ages 12 and 15 years) creates significant anxiety. One reason for this anxiety may be the current emergence of an incestuous or potential incestuous situation between the heterosexual girl and her father, uncle, or brother, or between the homosexual girl and her mother or another woman. (I discuss this below in the context of adolescents' dealing with reawakened oedipal wishes.) Another reason for a young adolescent girl's anxiety is her becoming aware of the past occurrence of a sexually traumatic event that took place in her childhood. Her new focus on her genital anatomy can stimulate her recall of such a sexually traumatic event in her childhood. At the time of the event, it may not have been experienced as traumatic, both because of her lack of understanding as a child and because of one or both parents' denying the significance of the traumatic event in accordance with their own need. In adolescence, however, the remembered past event will become traumatic as the girl is able to understand it with a new awareness of its consequences on her development at the time and in the ensuing years. This traumatic awareness occurred in the girl in the following example:

> A 15-year-old heterosexual girl had become very depressed after she attended a child and adolescent sexual abuse consciousness-raising lecture at school. She had just experienced her first menstrual period. One week after the lecture, I was asked by her principal (with her mother's permission) to interview her. Early in the interview she began to cry while she told me the following:
> "I grew up on a farm. We never saw a lot of people. When I was 7, my [maternal] uncle did things to me around my private

area, and I remember telling my mother, who told me that she would talk to my uncle so that he wouldn't do it again. But for about a month it hurt to go to the bathroom. My mother took me to the doctor, but she told me on the way that what my uncle did was no big thing and not to tell the doctor. I didn't say anything to the doctor and he just said I had an infection. I remember then taking pills for a while and I got better. I don't think I ever thought about what happened with my uncle until the lady giving the talk at school started to tell us what incest was, and how bad it was, and how the infection you could get from incest could mean that a girl might never have babies."

I then asked if she had begun to have periods, and she responded, "Yes. And maybe that's another reason why I was interested in this sex abuse talk today. I feel so dirty and like I'm a terrible person. And I am even starting to believe that my mother didn't really love me. I've even been imagining what would my uncle do if I killed myself? Would he then confess and get punished for what he did to me?"

She suddenly understood that she had been sexually abused, that her mother had protected her uncle more than she had protected her, that the doctor had also protected her uncle, and that her mother had never allowed her to talk about her intense anxiety and rage about what her uncle had done to her. These discoveries caused her to consciously experience the sudden loss she had repressed as a child: the loss of a mother who was an advocate in protecting her developing feminine body. This sudden conscious experience of her childhood loss was causing her current tearful depression, a depression that hid her still-repressed rage at her mother and uncle. Her construction of her new belief that she was defective and damaged was necessitated by her inability to tolerate her rage. In assessing her own self as dirty and terrible, she was using the defense of turning aggression upon herself which, in part, enabled her to achieve some sense of control in the face of a sense of being dirty.

This girl entered into adolescent psychotherapy, which entailed her mother meeting separately with the psychotherapist. In these parent sessions, the mother was helped to tolerate her own guilt about not protecting her daughter. She was then able to recognize that her daughter needed to verbalize her rage at her, and eventually began to believe that this rage would not destroy their relationship. She was advised by the psychotherapist that she could help her daughter to express her rage if she could have the courage to begin to respond in a rather normal way to her daughter's menarche (the mother had never prepared her daughter for its onset).

As the mother began to ask her daughter about how she was feeling about her monthly periods, this new maternal interest became the trigger for a new rapprochement between the girl and her mother. Eventually, the girl told her mother about her rage. The mother was able to listen to her daughter's rage without criticizing or withdrawing from her daughter. The mother then told her daughter that she had been wrong in not helping her understand what had happened and in not exposing the uncle. Over a period of 6 months, as mother and daughter continued to talk, the girl began to understand her mother's motivations for reacting to the abuse the way she did and forgave her for her mistake.

This girl's menarche and subsequent new awareness of what had happened to her as a child thus had become the catalysts for a new, developmentally enhancing goodness of fit between a mother and daughter who had previously had a distant and lonely relationship.

Reemergence of the oedipal phase. As I discuss at length in Chapter 5, in partially resolving their oedipal wishes, heterosexual children relinquish their wish to have an exclusive sensual-sexual relationship with their opposite-gender parent and begin to identify with their same-gender parent. This turning away from their competitive and envious wishes toward their same-gender parent enables them not only to put to rest their oedipal conflict between wishing to compete with, conquer, and replace their same-gender parent while at the same time physically fearing that parent's retaliation, but also to avoid the guilt feelings that threatened them should they try to rid themselves and the family of their same-gender parent. This oedipal conflict is traditionally called the *positive oedipal conflict.* During early adolescence, the reawakening of adolescents' sexual drives restimulates their previous oedipal wishes. In a psychologically attuned family, the onset of puberty, with its associated physical and sexual development, can upset the equilibrium that had been present in the family since early childhood.

In addition, however, a negative oedipal conflict exists for heterosexual adolescents with their same-gender parent (Blos 1985). Girls' *negative oedipal wishes* involve their wanting to identify with their mother, the love they experience for their mother, and their wish to be dependent on and taken care of by their mother. These wishes evolve from girls' infant and childhood attachment relationship with their mother. In essence, throughout development, much of a mother's role as an empathically attuned admiring object for her daughter (or an admiring selfobject) is subsumed in this concept of the negative oedipal conflict. The *negative oedipal conflict* for the heterosexual girl is one in which she experiences all those feelings listed above, but, at the same time, begins to fear that these feelings indicate that she may be drifting from her previous heterosexual object choice to a homosexual object choice. The negative oedipal conflict becomes stimulated in early adolescence because of the concurrent stimulation and return of the positive oedipal conflict.

At around age 12 years, the physical, sexual changes that boys experience propel them to a new realization that they are becoming a man. This brings their attention to the developmental task of putting more energy into developing their sexual identity. A boy's innate assertiveness in desiring to manifest his innate need for sensual-sexual gratification is supported not only by what his parents, siblings, relatives, teachers, ministers, and coaches tell him, but also by what movies, television, and classic and contemporary works of literature tell him about what constitutes a normal heterosexual sexual identity. More often than not in contemporary American society, the early adolescent heterosexual boy learns that the male who is assertive in seeking and winning the girl is demonstrating a healthy heterosexual sexual identity (a derivative of his positive oedipal complex), and the boy who wants his father or another man to take care of him or find him a girlfriend is demonstrating a diminished or even "wimpy" heterosexual sexual identity (a derivative of his negative oedipal conflict). As one grandmother often told her grandson when he asked advice about how boys were supposed to find girls to date, "Men are hunters" (M. Avallone, personal communication, August 1960).

In his book *Iron John: A Book About Men,* Bly (1990) lamented the dilemma of single mothers who are trying to instill masculine and heterosexual identities in their heterosexual adolescent sons. Bly recognized their difficulties, stating his belief that

> only men can initiate men, as only women can initiate women. Women can change the embryo to a boy, but only men can change the boy to a man. Initiators say that boys need a second birth, this time birth from men. (p. 16)

Bly also empathized with the dilemma in which both parents or a single father is raising an adolescent son:

> We know that today many fathers now work 30 to 50 miles from the house, and by the time they return at night the children are often in bed, and they themselves are too tired to do active fathering. (p. 19)

With the absence of a father's presence in the life of an adolescent son, Bly noted that the father and mother must pay close attention to encouraging their son—especially when he reaches puberty—to spend some separate time with his father. Otherwise, the pubertal adolescent male will find it more difficult to resist or fight his own temptation to become physically close to his mother—a temptation stimulated by the return of his oedipal wishes as a result of entering puberty.

Early adolescents' positive oedipal wishes cause them to experience various anxieties: body damage anxiety (i.e., at the hands of their same-gender parent), superego anxiety for contemplating a wish to dispose of the symbol of family authority, and a certain degree of disintegration anxiety in reference to possibly losing their same-gender parent as a mirroring source of admiration (i.e., as an admiring selfobject). So what do pubertal adolescents do? Katan (1951) noted that they must engage in a mental process of *object removal.* This process entails more than just their displacing their sexual desires toward their same-gender parent onto new sexual objects outside of the family. It is an adaptive defense mechanism that involves the unconscious transfer of a highly displeasurable wish or feeling from one person or situation onto another person or situation that is associated with less emotional displeasure. Displacement is adaptive, however, only when it is used transiently and the adolescent reverses the displacement in time when he or she is better able to deal with the displeasure associated with the original person or situation. The normal pubertal adolescent's object removal is not reversible. As Katan (1951) explained,

> The process of displacement per se does not imply a specific, preordained direction in which it is bound to occur. . . . In the case of the defense mechanism of puberty, however, we are dealing with an irreversible process of displacement in a specific direction, namely, away from the incestuous object on to other, innocuous [nonincestuous] persons. (p. 42)

For example, a boy will remove his mother from his "list" of possible sexual love objects and begin to look for an appropriate nonincestuous love object. If he does not engage in incestuous object removal, he is left with two other developmentally inhibiting options: 1) he can fight his positive oedipal wishes by regressing to prepubertal behaviors and avoiding any contact with girls his age and socializing with prepubertal boys, or 2) he can fight experiencing sexual sensations by fighting his body (e.g., he may overeat and become grossly overweight in an unconscious attempt to avoid developing any degree of sexual attractiveness in body appearance). Parents do not have to look too hard to notice their pubertal boy's desire to distance himself from physically close encounters with his mother.

Occasionally, however, even in a reasonably psychologically attuned family, a son and mother may have developed too close an attachment relationship during the boy's latency period. This can happen when, during the boy's latency years, the father is regularly and periodically away from the family on business trips or military duty or has been too little involved with his son. The boy, during his father's absence, acts as the man in the house and enjoys the closeness this brings with his mother. When such a boy reaches puberty, this overly close bond with his mother does not create the normal degree of oedipally stimulated anxiety, because his father has not been an authoritative presence in the family. The psychologically attuned—and not incestuously driven—mother in this situation will recognize her son's entrance into puberty as a triggering stimulus for her to reassess her overly close latency-age attachment bond with her son.

Heterosexual pubertal boys' need to avoid close physical contact with their mother is motivated by the societal rule prohibiting incest. It may also be motivated by boys' healthy prepubertal attachment relationship to their mother, which, as I note in Chapter 5, Erickson (1993) hypothesized serves as a protective factor against the threat or risk of incest. Bly (1990) furnished a dramatic example of the young adolescent's innate need to maintain a nonincestuous attachment to his mother by strenuously avoiding any possible sensual-sexual stimulation attendant with physical contact with her. He described the following family in which a mother was the single parent for her son and two daughters:

> The girls were doing well but the boy was not. At 14 the boy went to live with his father, but he stayed only a month or so and then came back. When he returned, the mother realized that three women in the house amounted to an overbalance of feminine energy for the son, but what could she do? A week or two went by. One night she said to her son, "John, it's time to come to dinner." She touched him on the arm and he exploded and she flew against the wall. . . . [There was] no intent of abuse . . . and no evidence that the event was repeated. . . . The psyche or body knew what the mind didn't. When the mother picked herself off the floor, she said, "It's time for you to go back to your father," and the boy said, "You're right." (pp. 18–19)

The normal heterosexual adolescent does not usually have to engage in such explosive avoidant behaviors in reference to his or her opposite-gender parent. The normally developing pubertal boy will tend to avoid his mother and spend more time with his father and other men. As his relationship with his father becomes stronger, he begins to relinquish his positive oedipal wishes for the second time in his life, and as he becomes more aware of his emotional closeness with his father, he begins to deal with the issue of asserting his heterosexuality and further putting himself in the category of "heterosexual men." This categorization inevitably includes his learning more about the category of "homosexual men." When he is physically close with his father and other men and male peers, he may become a bit anxious: too much physical and emotional closeness concerns him that he may be drifting toward homosexuality. His negative oedipal wishes toward his father will, throughout his adolescence, cause him some measure of anxiety.

Similar dynamics exist for the heterosexual girl. She too experiences a return to positive oedipal wishes toward her same-gender parent. She pulls away from her father and becomes closer to her mother. Like boys, she begins to fear her emotional and physical closeness with her mother (her negative oedipal wishes) will cause her to drift toward a homosexual object choice. Although her fear of closeness with her mother is stronger than the boy's fear of closeness with his father (something I discuss below), the girl still has considerable fear of engaging in physically close encounters with her father.

Both the young adolescent boys and girls are assisted by their peer groups in their attempts at object removal. In early adolescent boys, there is a tendency to turn away from girls, with some need to depreciate femininity. Boys ages 12–14 years will boast, "Who needs or wants a girlfriend!" However, when a boy turns too strongly away from girls, it may indicate his intense body damage anxiety about developing a heterosexual sexual identity. This boy inevitably may have had problems identifying with his heterosexual father (e.g., the father has often pushed his son away or has been hostile or too critical). Alternatively, the boy's childhood relationship with his mother may have been too close, and the boy may have had and still have strong resentment about his father's asserting his authority in maintaining his special marital relationship with the mother. This boy has not relinquished his positive oedipal wishes. Accordingly, his intense body damage anxiety around girls may be caused by either 1) his projecting his own anger at his father onto his father for possessing his mother and then fearing that his father would be angry at him for pursuing a girl of his choice, 2) his father's hostile and threatening responses to the boy's healthy assertive expression of his heterosexual sexual identity, or 3) both of these. Both the first and second causes will make it difficult for an adolescent boy to identify with his father. Without such heterosexual identification, the boy may begin to identify more with a kindly and admiring homosexual male or with his mother and drift toward making his sexual object choice a male, which can lead to homosexuality. Alternatively, the boy may continue to develop his heterosexual sexual identity while beginning to avoid his father because of his expectation that his father will criticize his heterosexual behaviors. In the latter case, he may seek a new heterosexual male figure as the model for his developing heterosexuality, a behavior that could be viewed as being a protective factor for the boy in that it would counteract the negative effects of the father's criticism, criticism that could put the boy's developing heterosexuality at risk.

The normal developing early adolescent male (ages 12–15 years) who is on his way toward establishing a heterosexual identity struggles with holding onto his heterosexual identifications and tends to stay away from excessive involvement with girls, because acting sexual around girls is still a new behavior for him. For many boys, their wish to be involved in sex-role behaviors with girls creates a conflict: they want to try to assert their heterosexuality in front of girls and yet fear they will not behave in a way that girls will admire. Because of this fear, they may transiently attempt to rid themselves of this conflict by regressing to an anal phase of development (e.g., telling toilet jokes and making anal noises, using profanity, manifesting crude eating habits, suddenly maintaining a very sloppy bedroom). As girls between ages 12 and 15 years turn away from their father, there is a general reaction against their regressing to a more emotionally close and dependent relationship with their mother. The early adolescent girl becomes anxious about wanting and needing her mother to help her develop her sexual identity. This anxiety is related to the girl's worry that she will become too dependent on her mother, thereby losing her "hard-won activity" (Dahl 1995) and burgeoning self-emancipation. As a result, early adolescent girls have a period in which they turn away from involvement with their mothers and often develop a close relationship with a particular same-age peer, who then becomes their best friend. Now the girl and her friend shop for clothes together as their mothers are excluded. Concurrently, the early adolescent girl turns toward the opposite gender. Boys are often the topic of discussion at gatherings of girls. During this age, a normally developing heterosexual girl may become overly competitive with boys. This behavior is propelled, in part, by her identification with an assertive mother who is able to compete with men when necessary. Adolescent girls' developmental need to establish an emancipated self may lead them to manifest a short-lived tomboy reaction. This tomboyishness represents their sudden urge to disavow their feminine identifications with their mother. In time, they become less anxious about their closeness with their mother. They then return to developing their heterosexual identity as they begin to reidentify with their heterosexual mother. Both girls' and their mothers' goal is for the girls to emerge from adolescence as assertive, competitive, and feminine women and still maintain a good relationship with their mother.

Masturbatory behaviors. In early adolescence (ages 12–15 years), as heterosexual teenagers are attempting to establish a heterosexual identity and construct a set of standards about sexual behavior, they are assisted in this process by being able to masturbate. Masturbation now leads to orgasm and ejaculation in the boy and orgasm in the girl. The first ejaculation for a boy is a statement of his emerging heterosexuality, further defining his thoughts and fantasies of what heterosexual activity will eventually entail. Sarnoff (1987) described the importance of this sexual behavior:

> Erection, orgasm, and ejaculation provide the child with a means of articulating the drives with reality objects. . . . Erections have always been present, so they cannot be used by a pubescent youngster as a sign of sexual maturity and readiness for object-directed sexuality. The ability to ejaculate alone carries the impact of a capacity to communicate, procreate and involve oneself in reality. . . . With the onset of the first ejaculation, a discharge pathway involving reality becomes available. At that point, fantasy is opened to reality influences. . . . Should the fantasies accompanying the first ejaculation be comfortable for the child— either because they themselves or sexuality is acceptable to him—the maturational step is taken in stride. (p. 155)

Masturbation for 12- to 15-year-old adolescents serves multiple functions (Laufer and Laufer 1984). First, it becomes a means of discharging sexual tension. In early adolescence, masturbatory fantasies express wishes that were subjected to repression during the latency years—namely, positive oedipal wishes. A teenage boy, through his masturbatory fantasies, "can express the latent fantasy more directly, release it from repression, and decide whether or not he wishes to keep it (Sarnoff 1987, p. 160).

Similarly to how children had to learn to use speech as a trial action to delay immediate action and think about different behaviors, including speech, early adolescent masturbation becomes "a trial action experienced within one's own thought and a way of testing which sexual thoughts, feelings, or gratifications are acceptable to the superego" (Kaplan 1991, p. 222).

When adolescents discover in their masturbatory fantasies a wish (i.e., an incestuous wish) that they feel is wrong or forbidden—either externally by society or internally by their superego—they can gradually begin to relinquish the wish. Adolescents' healthy need to emancipate themselves from the family—which involves removing their family members from their list of eligible sexual objects—will assist them in relinquishing their forbidden incestuous wish. They will gradually replace these wishes in their masturbatory fantasies with more nonincestuous wishes, which in their content begin to become a rehearsal for later interpersonal sexual activity with the appropriate gender person.

Masturbation can also become an adaptive defense mechanism when the wish to engage in heterosexual activity causes undue anxiety. It is a developmentally enhancing adaptive defense when it is transient and functions in the service of slowly resolving either a current external conflict with parents, an internal object relations conflict with one or both parents, or both, as is illustrated in the following example:

> A 14-year-old boy wanted to ask a girl to his first school dance. He fantasized that he would be alone with her on his first date. He was quite physically attracted to the girl, and yet, whenever she called him or he called her and his mother walked into the room, he became uneasy and expected to hear his mother's criti-

cism of his interest in the girl. He began to fantasize about the girl after these episodes involving his mother, and, for a while, he masturbated and thought about the girl, but stayed away from her. One night, he awoke from an anxiety-provoking dream with an erection. Now awake, he masturbated thinking about his dream: in his dream he was watching his mother undress. Over the next few days, he noticed that he was attracted to his mother's figure and how she looked, the perfume she wore, and other physical attributes. He also knew that he was quite anxious about these attractions. He continued to masturbate but now began to enjoy, more than he had in the past, his images of the girl he wanted to take to his first dance. He had now discovered his incestuously derived wish toward his mother and decided that it was time to give it up and move on to new, nonincestuous feminine objects. He had solved an object relations conflict involving his mother through his use of masturbation as an adaptive defense mechanism.

Positive oedipal wishes are never truly destroyed (Loewald 1979), but only wane significantly; they must be repeatedly addressed throughout life. The need to compete with the authority of the same-gender parent must be reconciled within each person with his or her love and respect for this parent.

As dating begins, teenagers want their parents, particularly their opposite-gender parent, to acknowledge them as a sexually attractive person. For example, a 16-year-old boy's mother told him before he left for a date, "You are becoming quite handsome; I'm really proud of you." Adolescents' internalization of a belief in having a competent and attractive heterosexual identity initially begins to be developed in the admiring visual gazes of the opposite-gender parent.

Initiation of sexual activity. The age of initiation of heterosexual activity in adolescents is quite variable. Most current studies reveal that, by age 18 years, 45%–55% of teenagers have experienced intercourse (Hofferth et al. 1987; Wyatt 1990; Zelnik and Shah 1983). However, a study by Offer and Offer (1975) of gifted, highly academically oriented teenagers (having an IQ of 140 or higher) revealed that, as a group, they were uninvolved sexually, were rather puritanical, and had little knowledge of sexual practices. A possible explanation for these findings could be these teenagers' sublimation of their normal heterosexual desires into a strong wish to learn and be creative.

Sublimation used in this way would be an adaptive defense mechanism. At other times, however, sublimation of heterosexual desires can function as a maladaptive defense mechanism. This happens when the teenager's own wishes, or the wishes of another, make the teenager's original wish fraught with excessive anxiety. For example, in her desire to gratify her normal heterosexual needs, a teenage girl wishes to date and spend time with boys, but her mother demands that she study all the time and punishes her when she does date. Consequently, her sexual wishes are sublimated into wishes to study all the time. She might be viewed as having a love affair with her books.

The issue of when the loss of virginity is normally supposed to take place is a problematical one. Virginity lasting up until age 25–30 years or older may indicate not abnormal heterosexual or homosexual development, but moral and value choice in a person who has achieved self-emancipation. Adolescents need to be helped in not being exposed to too much sexual stimulation, especially because each adolescent has his or her own "clock" concerning sexual activity.

In late adolescence, the body's physical sexuality has bloomed. Sexual interests and activities now assume an importance that they never have before in an adolescent's life. Normal rites of passage that 16- to 17-year-old teenagers see as necessary to feel self-confident and in step with their peers include experiencing at least the first official date and first kiss, but possibly also sexual body explorations and oral and genital intercourse. For adolescents who so choose, their first experience with sexual activity can be quite self-centered. They are initially focused on their own sexual performance rather than on caring and concern for their partner's feelings. They seek admiring feedback about how they have performed.

Sexuality will become more of a preoccupation in late adolescence (ages 16–19 years). Esman (1990) noted the following three characteristics about current adolescent sexual behaviors:

1) A "new morality" developed in the adult world in the decades of the sixties and seventies, one that sanctions, if it does not encourage, a free sexuality among adolescents. 2) The predominant shift underlying the "new morality" has been in the values and behaviors of adolescent girls, who now feel permitted to do what had earlier been forbidden them. . . . 3) The characteristic pattern of "new sexual behavior" is that of "serial monogamy." Promiscuity is not the rule and, indeed, appears to be found only among the more disturbed members of the youth population. (p. 70)

The "serial monogamy" to which Esman referred was defined by Sorensen (1973) as

a close sexual relationship of uncertain duration between two unmarried adolescents from which either party may depart when he or she desires, often to participate in another relationship. (p. 219)

Testing of heterosexual and homosexual sexuality still involves heterosexual and homosexual fantasies during masturbation. This masturbation, if the teenager believes it is not harmful or sinful, continues to assist the teenager in developing his or her fantasies in how to achieve pleasure with a heterosexual and homosexual dating partner. Some adolescents may masturbate to totally avoid heterosexual or homosexual activity because of their concern about loss of virginity, pregnancy, or contracting HIV or other sexually transmitted diseases (STDs). In reference to HIV and STDs, Esman (1990) observed that little research has been done on the effect of these diseases, especially HIV, on adolescent sexual behavior. Furthermore, despite the current effort to educate teenagers better about STDs, a 1989 study by the Carnegie Council reported the following:

Fully one-fourth of all sexually active adolescents will become infected with a sexually transmitted disease before graduating from high school, a grave situation that makes AIDS [acquired immunodeficiency syndrome] a potential time bomb for millions of American youth. (p. 25)

Esman (1990), in reviewing the Carnegie Council data and how those data indicate that the AIDS epidemic has had a minimal effect on adolescent sexual behavior, wrote,

> It seems likely that cognitive awareness [in teenagers] may be outdone by the pressure of [sexual] impulse, coupled with the adolescent's characteristic of omnipotence and invulnerability ("It can't happen to me"). It may be that more time, more profound penetration of new social constraints and less ambiguity in transmitted information will be needed before a substantial change occurs in the sexual mores of American adolescents. (p. 80; parentheses in the original)

Development of the Superego

Facilitating the Construction of Realistic Ambitions and Reasonable Ideals

Reconstruction of standards and beliefs. Normally developing adolescents begin to attain self-emancipation when they begin to accept their wish to take authority for directing their life from their parents. Adolescents' wish to compete and win the battle of becoming an emancipated self generates guilt (Loewald 1979); the guilt comes from their viewing their wish to sever the relationship of parent and child as a sin that demands atonement. This guilt is alleviated when late adolescents (ages 16–19 years) reconstruct their superego to become truly their own ethical and normal standards and beliefs. Loewald (1979) described this process as follows:

> Responsibility to oneself within the context of authoritative norms [or standards] consciously and unconsciously accepted or assimilated from parental and societal sources is the essence of superego as an internal agency. . . . It involves appropriating or owning up to one's needs and impulses [or wishes] as one's own, impulses and desires we appear to have been born with or that seem to have taken shape in interaction with parents during

infancy. . . . Such appropriation, in the course of which we begin
to develop a sense of self-identity, means to experience ourselves
as agents. . . . The self, in its autonomy, is an atonement [for
the sin of severance], and, as such, a supreme achievement.
(pp. 760–763)

Before the emancipated self emerges, changes must occur in adolescents' conscience, as well as concurrent changes in their long-standing childhood wishes to be perfect and to have perfect parents.

Throughout adolescence, the conscience becomes more and more internalized. Consequently, conscience slowly becomes better able to achieve its main two functions:

1. To regulate and control behavior relatively independently of external restraints
2. To become a source of self-esteem that is relatively independent of others' evaluations of the person's worth and value

Throughout adolescence, teenagers evaluate the moral rules and values defined by peers, teachers, and other adults; some are internalized and become further building blocks of conscience development (Sugar 1992).

Stillwell et al. (1991) described a sequence in conscience development from early to late adolescence. Young adolescents symbolize their conscience as existing somewhere within the body (usually heart or mind) or as humanlike figures emerging from the self (as depicted in the drawing of by 12-year-old boy in Figure 7–1.) Stillwell et al. viewed this drawing as this boy's symbolic depiction of his heart-mind or personified conscience. The boy described this as a picture of his conscience, which is

a blob with eyes. A blob is an abstract shape to represent my abstract thinking. The eyes watch over me. No mouth . . . it doesn't say anything, but makes me think. (Stillwell et al. 1991)

Figure 7–2 is another drawing by a 12-year-old adolescent, this time a girl who illustrates her heart-mind or personified conscience.

She symbolically views her conscience as a tape recorder with lips that talks to her. She explained her tape recorder conscience as something that

> records what you're saying and doing, . . . comes back, processes what you've said, . . . decides what is the output. . . . [It is] not really like a machine . . . because it changes. You could rewind it if you wanted to . . . when you're sleeping, it stops unless you're having a dream. The process . . . takes in information, analyzes it, decides whether [it is] good or bad. You can't turn it down, but you can push it to the back of your mind and try to think of other things. (Stillwell et al. 1991)

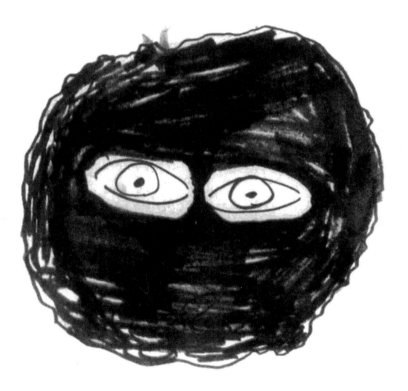

Figure 7–1.   Drawing of a conscience by a 12-year-old boy.
Source.   Stillwell et al. 1991. Used with permission.

Early adolescents engage in conversations with their parents about what they perceive about their conscience. In the process, their internal object relations conflicts are externalized onto the parents. Psychologically aware parents encourage these conflictual conversations and help their young adolescent realize when he or she has set unattainable standards of behavior for himself or herself. When parents themselves have set unattainable standards of behavior and rigid moral values for their adolescent throughout his or her childhood, the adolescent may be prone to overthrow such a rigid conscience and be too ready to accept the standards of behavior and moral values of a peer group, religious sect, or other group. For example, a young adult who, as a child, developed a conscience with unattainable, perfectionistic standards of behavior

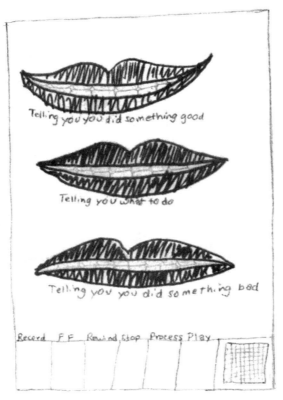

Figure 7–2. Drawing of a conscience by a 12-year-old girl.
Source. Stillwell et al. 1991. Used with permission.

and rigid, unyielding moral values, and did not modify these during adolescence, is a young adult who is overly critical of himself or herself and others and is prone to becoming depressed when he or she fails to achieve the unattainable perfect goals demanded by his or her conscience. Psychologically attuned parents begin to recognize when their teenager is struggling with his or her own wish to find rules about life by which the teenager can live.

A "confused conscience." Stillwell et al. (1991) described the next sequence in the development of adolescents' conscience, occurring at about age 15 years, as the possession of a confused conscience. This conscience is characterized by

> confusion, indecisiveness, and struggles with the intermediate "gray" zones of good and evil. The confusion occurs in behalf of moral growth. As the teenager's moral world expands to include the challenges of their peer culture and the popular culture, the conscience is pressured to reorganize its concepts as well as its dynamic power. The competition between adult authority and peer authority stresses it. The typical issues of distress are time away from the home environment, reputation with peers, alcohol and drugs, sexuality, and the use of vehicles. . . . The younger teenager in the midst of moral growth seems very inconsistent, as though talking out of both sides of the mouth at once. Behavior and emotional responses are likewise unstable. This becomes a time of great parental and societal anxiety as young people appear to have lost sight of their earlier training. Impulsiveness may reemerge, forcing elders to exert more external control. Parents should have faith that the struggles of this period lead to a more integrated conscience ahead. (p. 20)

Figure 7–3 is a drawing of a conscience done by a 15-year-old boy. He described his drawing as follows:

> It's just thoughts and feelings . . . all jumbled up. . . . I don't think about it much . . . it just all comes out at once. (Stillwell et al. 1991)

Figure 7–4 is the response of a 15-year-old girl when she was asked to draw her conscience. She explained her drawing as follows:

The bad part . . . I didn't care what I drew . . . lots of sharpness and points . . . like the rough times. Some of them may be in the future. Hot dazzling colors . . . kind of blah. All messed up. In between . . . it's a confused state . . . it's not too sure of which side to take. Doesn't know . . . maybe should go to one side or another. The bad there is interfering with the good. (Stillwell et al. 1991)

Much of the confusion associated with the struggles in midadolescence with conscience is related to the concurrent struggle—begun in early adolescence—between establishing realistic ambitions and maintaining ideals. In puberty, adolescents begin to work not only on developing their sexual identity but also on developing new views of themselves and their parents. Their old childhood and latency-stage views no longer work. They can no longer see themselves as simply someone who goes to school, obeys the

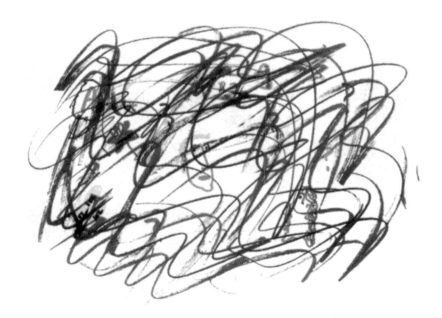

Figure 7–3.   Drawing of a conscience by a 15-year-old boy.
Source.   Stillwell et al. 1991. Used with permission.

family's and school's rules, does schoolwork, and has fun playing sports and pursuing hobbies. They no longer have an unquestioned dependence on their parents. Now, in adolescence, they hear a repetitive message not only from their parents but also from various voices in school, on television, and in the movies: "Now that you're an adolescent, it's time to think about becoming independent and think about your future."

Adolescents do not accept this message without a fight. Just as they did at ages 3–4 years and again at ages 9–10 years when they fought accepting that themselves and their parents were not omnipotent—which gave birth to their ideal self and ideal object wishful representations (see Chapter 5)—they now resurrect these ideal representations to fight accepting their new, anxiety-provoking feelings as they become disillusioned with their parents' not being able to protect them from all the pressures that the challenges of emancipation brings. In so doing, they once again become quite

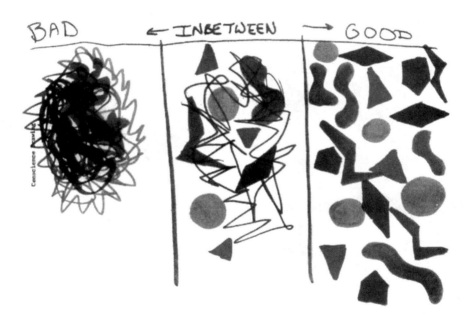

Figure 7–4. Drawing of a conscience by a 15-year-old girl.
Source.   Stillwell et al. 1991. Used with permission.

ambivalent in their feelings toward their parents, first idealizing them and then criticizing them for not living up to those ideal images. As I note earlier, Blos (1967) described this ambivalence as being precipitated by adolescents' second individuation from their parents. The first individualization took place between ages 18 months and 3 years, culminating in the rapprochement crisis at about age 2½ years. At this age, young children were quite ambivalent toward their parents as they became more aware of 1) the limitations their parents put on their assertive will, and 2) the fact that both they and their parents were not perfect and that their parents were not omnipotently able to protect them from experiencing separation anxiety.

This process of idealizing and de-idealizing parents goes on for much of mid- to late adolescence. Consequently, parents must tolerate behaviors in their teenagers that remind them of when they were younger: their tendency to become upset, angry, and even depressed when faced with their own imperfections, alternating with their tendency to become equally upset in viewing their parents' imperfections. This process becomes most prominent in 16- to 19-year-old adolescents when their positive oedipal wishes begin to wane and the relationship and identification with the same-gender parent becomes stronger. A process of de-idealization of both parents now begins in which they ultimately give up any residual wishes to have perfect and all-powerful parents to protect them from life's challenges.

The recrudescence of adolescents' childhood-derived wishes to be perfect and to have perfect parents is primarily caused by their turning toward the same-gender parent as an admirer and protector. For a while, adolescents will wish that this parent be able to provide total protection and perfection. This parent inevitably fails them, and adolescents are unwilling to seek the closeness and admiration from the opposite-gender parent. Thus, for a period of time, both parents are viewed as rather limited and imperfect.

Once again, the peer group rescues teenagers from feeling too disappointed and anxious about becoming emancipated, and they can eventually relinquish their view of their parents as all-protecting and all-admiring. In so doing, teenagers feel, for a while, a sense of loss in losing their parents as a source of admiration and positive self-esteem. Also, their parents' standards about sexual behavior (which teenagers have now internalized in their conscience) become somewhat less of an influence as the peer group assumes the increasing role of facilitating independence from the parents and providing a source of admiring feedback and self-esteem. This process of a gradual (but not total) devaluation of parental standards results in teenagers' conscience becoming less of a source of self-control, from whence comes the confused conscience of the 15- to 16-year-old adolescent.

A transient period develops where there is a turning inward and looking toward the peer group and occasionally other adults to assist adolescents in controlling their behavior; for example, peer group rules and attitudes about dating become very important. A narcissistic stage occurs when adolescents alternate between overly admiring themselves and being overly critical of their imperfections and of their not possessing abilities and attributes they admire in other adolescents. They may now develop a close friendship with a same-gender peer whom they admire; this peer may have qualities and abilities that they feel are lacking in themselves. It is as if adolescents, in losing their parents as a source of admiring feedback in supporting their wished-for perfection and in not quite being able to achieve perfection through self-admiration, attempt to make up for their imperfections by filling them in with a friend who possesses what they do not. For example, the shy teenager may have a best friend who is uninhibited, outgoing, and somewhat of a daredevil.

This close friendship (occurring about ages 12–16 years) may lead to some transient and experimental homosexual activity in the heterosexual adolescent. In fact, much of the homosexual type of activity in heterosexual young adolescents is in the interest of sexual experimentation (e.g., mutual masturbation). In addition, homosexual activity affords an outlet for sexual tension in heterosexual adolescents that allows them to avoid the anxiety attendant with performing sexually with the opposite gender, or the guilt associated with such sexual behavior because of the return of positive oedipal wishes during adolescence. Sarnoff (1987) gives an example:

An 11-year-old girl came into her [psychotherapy] session a little late. "I think you'll like the story I have to tell you," she said. "I was on top of my girlfriend. We were making believe we were having sex. She got a little frightened and asked if what we were doing was wrong. I told her, think how wrong it would be if I were a boy!"

Eventually, in late adolescence, teenagers begin to relinquish their wish to be perfect or have their parents be perfect. Their ideal images of their same-gender parent had stimulated their negative oedipal wishes toward this parent. In eventually relinquishing this wish as being realistically unattainable, adolescents will construct realistic (i.e., de-idealized) ambitions and reasonable ideals for themselves. P. Tyson and Tyson (1991) described this process as follows:

To the extent that the adolescent is able to differentiate the omnipotent, idealized object representations of his infancy from parents of his current life, he will be able to establish "friendly," respectful relationships with his parents and still feel himself to be independent (i.e., emancipated) of them. (p. 115)

Attainment of an integrated conscience. The more highly developed superego now enables late adolescents to experience true structural conflicts. It becomes a more realistic and friendlier internal guide for behavioral choice and an internal source of admiration when late adolescents attain more realistic ambitions. Stillwell et al. (1991) labeled this more developed superego in late adolescence as the *integrated conscience*. Stillwell et al. (1991) described a 17-year-old boy's drawing of his conscience as follows (see Figure 7–5):

The angel with the crooked halo and the broken string is an excellent representation of the concept "good within evil, evil within good" that comes with mastery of the *confused conscience* with its transformation into an *integrated conscience*. This angel represents the imperfections of conscience functioning. This 17-year-old boy explained that because he thinks killing animals is basically wrong, he only lets himself hunt with a bow and arrow, never a gun. It is his compromise with good and evil.

Stillwell et al. (1991) also noted that, in the integrated conscience, good dominates evil. One example of this is shown in Figure 7–6, drawn by a 17-year-old girl. Stillwell et al. delineated the characteristics of the integrated conscience as follows:

> The Integrated Conscience (model age 17) conceptualization is characterized by flexibility, choices among more than two options, and the understanding of the overlap of good and evil. With the evolution of this harmony and balance, there is a return of confidence regarding moral issues, increased modulation of

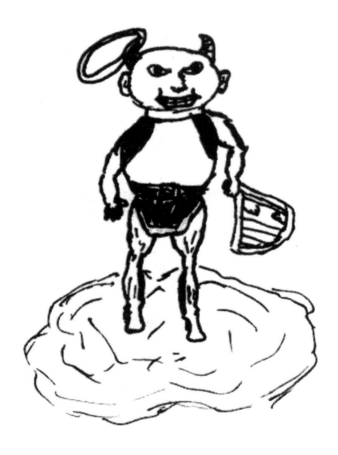

Figure 7–5.   Drawing of a conscience by a 17-year-old boy.
Source.   Stillwell et al. 1991. Used with permission.

moral emotions, and tolerance for the coexistence of good and evil within the self as well as in the environment. With the Integrated Conscience comes understanding, benevolence, optimism and a desire to reach to the unknown. The older teenager can comprehend both the possibilities and the difficulties of dealing with changes within the self. S/he can actively choose courses for moral action that include partial if not total goodness. The ability to deal with grayness and partial success argues against harshness and rigidity and for flexibility and forgiveness. (p. 20)

The integrated conscience of the 17- to 18-year-old adolescent eventually becomes the more developed conscience of the 18- to 19-year-old young adult who has attained an emancipated identity. Without such a conscience, true emancipated functioning is not possible.

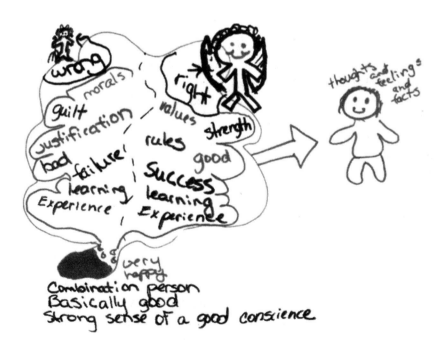

Figure 7–6. Drawing of a conscience by a 17-year-old girl.
Source. Stillwell et al. 1991. Used with permission.

Development of Adaptational Capabilities

Emergence of More Socially Mature Mechanisms of Defense

Psychologically aware parents, despite how annoying some of their adolescent's current confrontations may be, know that an avoidant, nontalking teenager is using too many defense mechanisms to avoid working on his or her internal object relations conflicts and current external conflicts with parents, siblings, teachers, peers, and others. Parents, therefore, must work at 1) creating a communication space within their home and 2) being models of how to socially communicate. This first requirement involves figuring out ways to help teenagers keep a certain amount of communication going between themselves and their parents. This involves not allowing too much time to go by during which their teenager is silent around the family. The second requirement involves the parents' modeling how teenagers should verbalize their feelings and conflicts and what are socially acceptable defense mechanisms.

Defense mechanisms have been shown to be associated with healthy adult functioning (Valliant 1971, 1974), particularly in adults who have a good capacity to adapt to different social, educational, and professional situations. These mechanisms include the following:

1. *Intellectualization*—This is an automatic process in which thoughts about a topic that is causing emotional displeasure remain within adolescents' consciousness while the emotionally displeasurable feelings are relegated to their unconscious mental domain. Intellectualization is a derivative of the defense mechanism of isolation of emotion. It is useful to think of intellectualization as a prominent adolescent defense mechanism, because adolescents are quite adept at using their new formal thinking capacities to suppress or to repress displeasur-

able feelings. This process is illustrated in the following example:

> A 16-year-old boy was asked by his parents if he had com- pleted his application to take the Scholastic Aptitude Test (SAT; an achievement test used for entrance into university- level education). The teenager had been avoiding filling out his application because of his high degree of separation anxiety associated with the possibility of his eventually leav- ing home to go to college. So he answered, "That's an inter- esting question. The whole idea of what this test really measures is never discussed at school. Some students think it is a realistic measure of college potential, and others don't. . . . "

2. *Humor*—Humor is used as a defense mechanism throughout adolescence, especially in late adolescence. Humor, according to Valliant (1987), is the

> overt expression of feelings and thoughts without discom- fort or immobilization and without unpleasant effects on others. The forbidden wish is expressed but not acted on. Humor that affects others unpleasantly, such as satire and practical jokes, can often be thought of as displacement or passive aggression. (p. 120)

For example, a 17-year-old girl, anxious about telling her first boyfriend that she wants to date other boys, consciously decides to suppress the whole issue of her independence. They were then out on a date, and an elderly couple walked by. The elderly couple was holding hands. The girl suddenly says, "He looks like he can't let her go." They both laughed, but the humorous comment enabled her to express something of her own uncomfortable dilemma.

3. *Anticipation*—This is the automatic delay of action accompa- nied by consciously experiencing the thoughts and feelings of a future event or an encounter with a person. Anticipation sig- nifies the development of adolescents' progression from ac- tion to speech to thought dominance in directing their life. In anticipating a future, adolescents are able to tolerate many cur-

rent displeasurable feelings associated with achieving certain developmental tasks. For example, anticipation helps teenagers tolerate deprivation associated with studying for an entire week for final examinations.

Progress in the Transition From Adolescence to Young Adulthood
One Set of Criteria

The word *adolescence* literally means "becoming an adult." Hence, when adolescence ends, it is usually defined by what society associates with adult behavior and adult psychological maturity. This is quite difficult to clearly define. As Blos (1979) noted,

> Behavior alone never renders a reliable assessment of an individual's developmental status, nor does it reveal the working of his motivational system. (p. 85)

The following are criteria that can be used to define the end of adolescence and collaboratively lead the late adolescent into the beginning of adult functioning (Blos 1979). Most of these are the psychological tasks outlined above for the entire period of adolescence. They criteria are developmental achievements emerging at around age 18 or 19 years. In each of the criteria below, the attainment of the task is relative—that is, in order for development into adulthood to be smooth and nonconflictual, there must be more rather than less of an attainment of these criteria. All four tasks below lead to new possessions within the late adolescent's self-representation. This self-representation defines the emancipated self.

Establishment of autonomy from parents (self-autonomy). This addresses late adolescents' belief in being able to assert control over their life. This does not mean that their relationships with others are less important. Self-autonomy occurs in the context of being comfortable with needing to be in emotionally intimate relationships with others (J. B. Miller 1991).

Parents have been, for the most part, de-idealized and have come to be viewed more as advisers, guides, and friends. Parents are no longer viewed as having all the answers and being all wonderful, nor are they viewed as being completely uninformed, old-fashioned, and "out of it." Superego anxiety (signal of impending guilt) is used to guide behavior and make thoughtful and appropriate moral and value choices.

Establishment of realistic goals (realistic self-image). There has been a progressive relinquishment of wishes for perfection, signified by the ability to set reasonable goals and tolerate the realization that every goal will not be achieved. Imperfections, setbacks, or faults do not greatly inhibit adolescents from using the abilities they possess. Adolescents no longer primarily blame parents, authority figures, and institutions for their own limitations. Late adolescents who have experienced traumatic events in childhood come to terms with those events and, in so doing, give up holding a grudge and forever blaming their parents (or others) for these events. For example, an 18-year-old boy, disappointed with and angry at his mother ever since his father left when he was age 13 years, was now able to understand his mother's predicament at the time. He stopped blaming his mother for his father's leaving and stopped feeling sorry for himself.

There also is the attainment of the ability to direct the effects of a childhood trauma into a commitment to a socially acceptable goal—that is, turn a childhood trauma into a success. For example, a college student had been bitter throughout her adolescence after having been raped at age 13 years. However, at age 20 years, she began to do volunteer work at the college on a rape hotline. This eventually led to an interest in helping people with childhood traumas, and she later became an adult and child psychiatrist.

Establishment of a stable sexual identity. This addresses the growing capacity to make a mutually caring choice of a heterosexual or a homosexual partner and to treat the partner's body with kindness and respect. Sexual activity is separated from wishes to dominate and control the person of one's sexual object choice through sexual performance. This occurs as a direct result of late adolescents' ability to relinquish their wishes to be perfect and find someone (e.g., a sexual partner) to mirror this perfection or to worship this sexual partner as being perfect. Relinquishment of perfectionistic wishes can take place only when late adolescents have begun to develop enough healthy self-esteem that is based on their true sexual and other capacities and is not unduly rejecting of their limitations. Through the sexually intimate relationship that emerges for some in late adolescence and for others in young adulthood, they gain more experience in relating to another with equality and reciprocity and further relinquish the need for one or both partners to be perfect.

Establishment of a sense of continuity between past life experiences and present motivations and beliefs. Late adolescents gain a new understanding of the relative influence of their past experiences on their present wishes, motivational goals, and beliefs. This understanding often entails seeking out the life histories of family members to help understand present problems, as is illustrated in the following example:

> A 19-year-old man started college and fell madly in love with a 19-year-old woman. She was not attending college, and she began pressuring him to abandon college and get married. He sought out the advice of an uncle, who many years before had left college in his freshman year to get married. This uncle had been a role model for this 19-year-old man during his childhood.
>
> As his uncle talked about his own struggles and the positive and negative aspects of leaving college, this 19-year-old young man began to realize how he had modeled himself after his uncle in this respect: like his uncle, he was quite worried about being rejected by a woman if he did not do what she wanted him to do. He became aware of how much separation anxiety he was experiencing in thinking about telling his girlfriend that he did not want to leave college and worrying that she would react by leaving him.
>
> Over the next several weeks, he more fully realized that his separation anxiety was fueled by a long-standing identification with his uncle: he, like his uncle, believed that a woman would not love him if he manifested his true wishes and feelings. He

ultimately decided to stay in college and tolerate the anxiety that was stimulated when he told the 19-year-old woman of his decision. Surprisingly, after she voiced some of her anger, she continued their relationship and in time became quite supportive of his need to stay in college.

Epilogue

In Chapter 1, I note how some developmentalists believe that an integrated theoretical model of the mind's maturation and development is not currently possible. This means that the medical student, psychology graduate student, and residents in psychiatry, pediatrics, and family practice are on their own in coming up with any degree of integration of human development. Thus the adult psychiatry resident may ask, "What should I believe about what should occur in each phase of development, if I want to establish my own beliefs about what is normal and what is abnormal in the different phases of the life cycle?" In this book, I have attempted to answer that question by presenting one possible integrated view of development. I believe that the multiplicity of variables involved in the genesis of all mental activity and surface behavior in the developing child can be organized and integrated by the use of the biopsychosocial model. My hope is that individuals will be able to use the sequential and integrated developmental concepts presented in this book in 1) understanding normal infants, children, and adolescents, and 2) assessing the presence of psychopathology in those infants, children, and adolescents with signs of abnormal development (Gabbard 1992).

In studying the human developmental process, to dismiss the formation and subsequent influence of the representational world constructed by the child seems analogous to going back to the situation present from antiquity to early modern times that children's internal, representational world, and the influence of that world on their behavior as future adults, was considered to be

1) inconsequential, 2) uninteresting, and 3) not worthy of the true attention of the great thinkers and scientists of the time. Let us not repeat the past.

References

Abrams S: Is memory not the trusted archivist? The American Psychoanalyst 29:31, 1995

Ainsworth MD: Patterns of attachment behavior shown by the infant in interaction with his mother. Merrill-Palmer Quarterly 10:51–58, 1964

Ainsworth MD, Belehar M, Waters E, et al: Patterns of Attachment: A Psychological Study of the Strange Situation. Hillsdale, NJ, Lawrence Erlbaum, 1978

Aires P: Centuries of Childhood. New York, Random House Vintage Books, 1962

Alexander F: Fundamentals of Psychoanalysis. New York, Norton, 1948

Ames LB, Ilg FL: Your Three-Year Old. New York, Dell Publishing, 1976a

Ames LB, Ilg FL: Your Four-Year Old. New York, Dell Publishing, 1976b

Ames LB, Ilg FL: Your Five-Year Old. New York, Dell Publishing, 1976c

Ames LB, Ilg FL: Your Six-Year Old. New York, Dell Publishing, 1979

Anastasi A: Psychological Testing, 6th edition. New York, Macmillan, 1988

Andrews G, Harris M: The syndrome of stuttering. Clinics in Developmental Medicine 17:19–45, 1964

Anthony EJ: Normal adolescent development from a cognitive viewpoint. J Am Acad Child Adolesc Psychiatry 21:318–327, 1982

Anthony EJ: Studies of risk, vulnerability and resilience in children, in Psychiatry: The State of the Art, Vol 5. Edited by Michels R. New York, Plenum, 1985, pp 7–10

Appelbaum MI, McCall RB: Design and analysis in developmental psychology, in Handbook of Child Psychology, Vol 1: History, Theory and Methods. Edited by Kessen W. Series edited by Mussen PH. New York, Wiley, 1983, pp 242–289

Applegarth A: On structures. J Am Psychoanal Assoc 37:1097–1107, 1989

Apter T: Altered Loves: Mothers and Daughters During Adolescence. Columbine, NY, Fawcett, 1990

Arlow J: Summary comments: panels on psychic structure. J Am Psychoanal Assoc 36 (suppl):283–295, 1988

Asher SR, Coie JD: Peer Rejection in Childhood. New York, Cambridge
University Press, 1990

Baker H, Baker M: Heinz Kohut's self psychology: an overview. Am J Psychiatry 144:1–9, 1987

Baldwin JD, Baldwin JI: Open peer commentary: the stage question in
cognitive-developmental theory. The Behavioral and Brain Sciences
2:182–183, 1978

Baldwin JM: The Development of the Child and of the Race. New York,
Macmillan, 1894

Bandura A: Self-efficacy: toward a unifying theory of behavioral change.
Psychol Rev 84:191–215, 1974

Bayrakal S: Sociocultural matrix of adolescent psychopathology, in Adolescent Psychiatry, Vol 14. Edited by Feinstein S. Chicago, IL, University of Chicago Press, 1987, pp 112–118

Beal CR, Flavell JH: Development of the ability to distinguish communicative
intention and literal message meaning. Child Dev 55:920–928, 1984

Beebe B, Sloate P: Assessment and treatment difficulties in mother-infant
attunement in the first three years of life: a case history. Psychoanalytic Inquiry 1:601–624, 1982

Beiser HR: Ages eleven to fourteen, in The Course of Life, Vol 4: Adolescence. Edited by Greenspan SI, Pollock GH. Madison, CT, International Universities Press, 1991, pp 99–118

Berg C: Perspectives for viewing intellectual development throughout
the life course, in Intellectual Development. Edited by Sternberg J,
Berg C. New York, Cambridge University Press, 1992, pp 1–16

Berk LE: Why children talk to themselves. Sci Am 271:5, 1994

Bettleheim B: The Uses of Enchantment: The Meaning and Importance
of Fairy Tales. New York, AA Knopf, 1985

Bever J: Regression in the service of development, in Regressions in Mental Development: Basic Phenomena and Theories. Edited by Bever
TG. Hillsdale, NJ, Lawrence Erlbaum, 1982

Bezirganian S, Cohen P: Sex differences in the interaction between temperament and parenting. J Am Acad Child Adolesc Psychiatry 31:790–
802, 1992

Bidell TR, Fischer KW: Beyond the stage debate: action, structure, and
variability in Piagetian theory and research, in Intellectual Development. Edited by Sternberg R, Berg C. New York, Cambridge University Press, 1992, pp 100–141

Binet A, Simon T: Méthodes nouvelles pour le diagnostic du niveau intellectue des anormaux. Année Psychologique 11:191–244, 1905

Bishop J: A Day of Infamy. New York, Bantam Books, 1955

Blackburn JA: The influence of personality, curriculum, and memory correlates on formal reasoning in young adults and elderly persons. J Gerontol 39:207–209, 1984

Blackburn JA, Papalia DE: The study of adult cognition from the Piagetian perspective, in Intellectual Development. Edited by Sternberg R, Berg C. New York, Cambridge University Press, 1992, pp 141–160

Bloch HS: Adolescent Development, Psychopathology, and Treatment. New York, International Universities Press, 1995

Blos P: On Adolescence. New York, Free Press, 1962

Blos P: The second individuation process of adolescence. Psychoanal Study Child 22:162–186, 1967

Blos P: The Adolescent Passage: Developmental Issues. New York, International Universities Press, 1979

Blos P: Son and Father, Before and After the Oedipus Complex. New York, Free Press, 1985

Blum HP: Superego formation, adolescent transformation, and the adult neurosis. J Am Psychoanal Assoc 33:887–909, 1985

Bly R: Iron John. New York, Wesley Publishing, 1990

Boesky D: The concept of psychic structure. J Am Psychoanal Assoc 36 (suppl):113–137, 1988

Boswell J: The Kindness of Strangers. New York, Pantheon Books, 1988

Bowlby J: The nature of the child's tie to his mother. Int J Psychoanal 39:350–373, 1958

Bowlby J: Attachment and Loss, Vol 1: Attachment. New York, Basic Books, 1969

Bowlby J: Attachment and Loss, Vol 2: Separation, Anger and Anxiety. New York, Basic Books, 1973

Bowlby J: Attachment and Loss, Vol 3: Loss, Sadness and Depression. New York, Basic Books, 1980

Bowlby J: Developmental psychiatry comes of age. Am J Psychiatry 145:1–10, 1988

Brainerd C: The stage question in cognitive-developmental theory. The Behavioral and Brain Sciences 2:173–213, 1978

Brazelton TB: Neonatal Assessment, in The Course of Life, Vol 1: Infancy. Edited by Greenspan S, Pollack G. Madison, CT, International Universities Press, 1989, pp 415–417

Brenneis CB: Memories of childhood sexual abuse. J Am Psychoanal Assoc 42:1027–1055, 1994

Brenner C: An Elementary Textbook of Psychoanalysis. New York, International Universities Press, 1965

Brenner C: The components of psychic conflict and its consequences in mental life. Psychoanal Q 48:547–567, 1979

Bringuier JC: Conversations Libres Avec Jean Piaget. Paris, France, Editions Robert Laffont, 1977 (Conversations With Jean Piaget. Translated by Laffont R. Chicago, IL, University of Chicago Press, 1980)

Brodal A: Neurological Anatomy. London, Oxford University Press, 1969

Brody S: Psychoanalytic theories of infant development and its disturbances: a critical evaluation. Psychoanal Q 51:526–597, 1982

Brothers L: A biological perspective on empathy. Am J Psychiatry 146:10–19, 1989

Bruner J: Child's Talk. New York, WW Norton, 1983

Buchsbaum HK, Emde RN: Play narratives in thirty-six-month-old children: early moral development and family relationships. Psychoanal Study Child 45:129–155, 1990

Buss A, Plomin R: A Temperamental Theory of Personality Development. New York, Wiley, 1975

Buxbaum E: Between the Oedipus complex and adolescence: the "quiet" time, in The Course of Life, Vol 3: Middle and Late Childhood. Edited by Greenspan S, Pollack G. Madison, CT, International Universities Press, 1991, pp 333–355

Cahan E, Mechling J, Sutton-Smith B, et al: The elusive historical child: ways of knowing the child of history and psychology, in Children in Time and Place. Edited by Elder GH Jr, Modell J, Parke RD. New York, Cambridge University Press, 1993

Campos J, Barrett KC, Lamb ME, et al: Socio-emotional development, in Handbook of Child Psychology, 4th Ed, Vol 2: Infant Development. Edited by Haith M, Campos J. New York, Wiley, 1983, pp 785–915

Carey W: Temperament and pediatric practice, in Temperament in Clinical Practice. Edited by Chess S, Thomas A. New York, Guilford, 1986, pp 210–235

Carnegie Council: Turning Points: Preparing American Youth for the 21st Century. New York, Carnegie Council of New York, 1989

Case R: Neo-Piagetian theories of child development, in Intellectual Development. Edited by Sternberg RJ, Berg CA. New York, Cambridge University Press, 1992, pp 161–197

Case R, Hurst P, Hayward S, et al: Toward a neo-piagetian theory of cognitive and emotional development. Developmental Review 8:1–51, 1988

Chandler M, Fritz A, Hales S: Small scale deceit: deception as a marker of two-, three- and four-year olds': early theories of mind. Child Dev 60:1263–1277, 1989

Chess S, Thomas A: Temperament in Clinical Practice. New York, Guilford, 1986

Chess S, Thomas A: Temperament and its functional significance, in The Course of Life, Vol 2: Early Childhood. Edited by Greenspan SI, Pollock GH. Madison, CT, International Universities Press, 1989, pp 163–227

Chomsky N: Syntactic Structures. The Hague, Mouton, 1957

Chused JF: Consequences of parental nurturing. Psychoanal Study Child 41:419–438, 1986

Cicchetti D, Schneider-Rosen K: An organizational approach to childhood depression, in Childhood Depression. Edited by Rutter M, Izard C, Reed P. New York, Guilford, 1986, pp 71–135

Clower VL: Theoretical implications in current views of masturbation in latency girls. J Amer Psychoanal Assoc 24 (suppl):109–125, 1976

Clyman R: The procedural organization of emotions: a contribution from cognitive science to the psychoanalytic theory of therapeutic action. J Am Psychoanal Assoc 39:349–383, 1991

Coen S: Notes on the concepts of self object and preoedipal object. J Am Psychoanal Assoc 29:395–411, 1981

Cohn JF, Tronick EZ: Three-month old reactions to simulated maternal depression. Child Dev 54:185–193, 1983

Coie JD: Toward a theory of peer rejection, in Peer Rejection in Childhood. Edited by Asher SR, Coie JD. New York, Cambridge University Press, 1990, pp 365–403

Coie JD, Dodge KDA, Kupersmidt JB: Peer group behavior and social status, in Peer Rejection in Childhood. Edited by Asher SR, Coie JD. New York, Cambridge University Press, 1990, pp 3–14

Colarusso CA: Child and Adult Development. New York, Plenum, 1992

Collins W, Laursen B: Conflicts and relationships during adolescence, in Conflict in Child and Adolescent Development. Edited by Shantz CU, Hartup WW. New York, Cambridge University Press, 1992, pp 216–242

Compton A: On the psychoanalytic theory of instinctual drives, part IV: instinctual drives and the id-ego-superego model. Psychoanal Q 28:739–774, 1981

Condon W, Sander L: Neonate movement is synchronized with adult speech: interactional participation and language acquisition. Science 183:99–101, 1974

Cowen EL, Pederson A, Bebigan H, et al: Long-term follow-up of early detected vulnerable children. J Consult Clin Psychol 41:438–446, 1973

Crockenberg S: Predictors and correlates of anger toward and punitive control of toddlers by adolescent mothers. Child Dev 58:964–975, 1987

Dahl EK: Daughters and mothers. Psychoanal Study Child 50:187–204, 1995

Damon W: The Moral Child. New York, Free Press, 1988

Darwin CA: A biographical sketch of an infant mind. Mind 2:285–294, 1877

Dasen PR: Piagetian Psychology: Cross-Cultural Contributions. New York, Wiley, 1977

DeCasper AJ, Fifer W: On human bonding: newborns prefer their mothers' voices. Science 208:1174–1176, 1980

DeLoache JS: Rapid change in the symbolic function of very young children. Science 238:1536–1557, 1987

Demos EV: Affect in early infancy: physiology or psychology? Psychoanalytic Inquiry 1:533–574, 1981

Demos EV: Facial expressions of infants and toddlers: a descriptive analysis, in Emotion and Early Interaction. Edited by Field T, Fogel E. Hillsdale, NJ, Lawrence Erlbaum, 1982, pp 118–129

Diaz M, Berk LE (eds): Private Speech: From Social Interaction to Self-Regulation. Hillsdale, NJ, Lawrence Erlbaum, 1992

Dorpat T: Structural conflict and object relations conflict. J Am Psychoanal Assoc 24:855–873, 1976

Douvan E, Adelson J: The Adolescent Experience. New York, Wiley, 1966

Dowling S: Abstract report from the literature on neonatology. Psychoanal Q 50:290–296, 1981

Dowling S, Rothstein A (eds): The Significance of Infant Observational Research for Clinical Work With Children, Adolescents and Adults. Madison, CT, International Universities Press, 1989

Dubois R: So Human and Animal. New Haven, CT, Yale University Press, 1965

Dunn J: Individual differences in temperament, in Scientific Foundations of Developmental Psychiatry. Edited by Rutter M. Baltimore, MD, University Park Press, 1981, pp 8–15

Edgecumbe RM, Burgner M: The phallic narcissistic phase: a differentiation between preoedipal and oedipal aspects of phallic development. Psychoanal Study Child 30:161–180, 1975

Eisenberg L: Mindlessness and brainlessness in psychiatry. Br J Psychiatry 148:497–508, 1986

Eisenberg N, Mussen PH: The Roots of Prosocial Behavior in Children. New York, Cambridge University Press, 1989

Eisendrath S: The Mind and somatic illness: psychologic factors affecting physical illness, in Review of General Psychiatry. Edited by Goldman H. Norwalk, CT, Appleton & Lange, 1988, pp 126–155

Ekstein R: Children of Time and Space and Action and Impulse. New York, Appleton-Century-Crofts, 1966

Elias J, Gebhard P: Sexuality and sexual learning in children, Phi Delta Kappa 50:401–405, 1969

Elkind D: Discrimination, seriation, and numeration of size and dimensional differences in young children: Piaget reproduction study VII. J Genet Psychol 104:275–296, 1964

Elkind D: Egocentrism in adolescence. Child Dev 38:1025–1034, 1967

Ellenberger HT: The Discovery of the Unconscious. New York, Basic Books, 1970

Emde RN: The prerepresentational self and its affective core. Psychoanal Study Child 38:165–192, 1983

Emde RN: The affective self: continuities and transformations from infancy, in Frontiers of Infant Psychiatry, Vol 2. Edited by Call JD, Galenson E, Tyson RL. New York, Basic Books, 1984, pp 38–54

Emde RN: Risk, intervention and meaning. Psychiatry 51:254–260, 1988

Emde RN: Positive emotions for psychoanalytic theory: surprises from infancy research and new directions. J Am Psychoanal Assoc 39 (suppl):5–44, 1991

Emde RN, Buchsbaum HK: A psychoanalytic theory of affect, III: emotional development and signaling in infancy, in The Course of Life, Vol 1: Infancy. Edited by Greenspan SI, Pollock GH. Madison, CT, International Universities Press, 1989, pp 193–227

Emde RN, Harmon RJ: Continuities and Discontinuities in Development. New York, Plenum, 1984

Emde RN, Metcalf D: An electro-encephalographic study of behavioral rapid eye movement states in the human newborn. J Nerv Ment Dis 150:376–386, 1970

Emde RN, Gaensbauer TJ, Harmon RJ: Emotional Expression in Infancy. New York, International Universities Press, 1979

Emde RN, Biringen Z, Clyman RB, et al: The moral self of infancy: affective core and procedural knowledge. Developmental Review 11:251–290, 1991

Engel GL: The need for a new medical model: a challenge for biomedicine. Science 196:129–136, 1977

Engel GL: Clinical application of the biopsychosocial model. Am J Psychiatry 137:535–544, 1980

Engel S: Learning to reminisce: a developmental study of how young children talk about the past. Unpublished doctoral dissertation, City University of New York, New York, 1986

Erickson MT: Rethinking Oedipus: an evolutionary perspective of incest avoidance. Am J Psychiatry 150:411–415, 1993

Erikson E: Identity and the Life Cycle. New York, Norton, 1959

Erikson E: Childhood and Society, Revised Edition. New York, Norton, 1963

Erikson E: Identity, Youth and Crisis. New York, Norton, 1968

Erikson E: Psychosocial tasks. Paper presented at Symposium on Normal Development. College Park, MD, October 1980

Esman A: Adolescence and Culture. New York, Columbia University Press, 1990

Etchegoyen A: Latency: a reappraisal. Int J Psychoanal 74:347–357, 1993

Fantz RL: The origin of form perception. Scientific American 204:62–72, 1961

Fantz R: Pattern vision in newborn infants. Science 140:296–297, 1963

Farrington DP: Longitudinal research strategies: advantages, problems and prospects. J Am Acad Child Adolesc Psychiatry 30:369–374, 1991

Feinstein SC: Editor's introduction, in Adolescent Psychiatry, Vol 14. Edited by Feinstein SC. Chicago, IL, University of Chicago Press, 1987, pp 3–5

Feldman D: Beyond Universals in Cognitive Development. Norwood, NJ, Ablex, 1980

Ferguson C, Farwell C: Words and sounds in early language acquisition. Language 51:419–439, 1975

Fischer KW: A theory of cognitive development: the control and constriction of hierarchies of skills. Psychol Rev 87:477–531, 1980

Fischer KW, Canfield RL: The ambiguity of stage and structure in behavior: person and environment in the development of psychological structures, in Stage and Structure: Reopening the Debate. Edited by Levin I. New York, Plenum, 1986

Fischer KW, Carnochan P, Shaver PR: How emotions develop and how they organize development. Cognition and Emotion 4:81–121, 1990

Fivush R: Theoretical and methodological issues in memory development research. Paper presented at the annual meeting of the American Academy of Child and Adolescent Psychiatry, San Antonio, TX, October 1993

Flavell JH: The Developmental Psychology of Jean Piaget. Princeton, NJ, Van Nostrand Reinhold, 1963

Flavell JH: Stage-related properties of cognitive development. Cognitive Psychology 2:421–453, 1971

Flavell JH: The development of children's knowledge about the mind: from cognitive connections to mental representations, in Developing Theories of Mind. Edited by Astington JW, Harris PL, Olson DR. New York, Cambridge University Press, 1988, pp 244–267

Fogel A, Melson G: Child Development, Individual, Family and Society. New York, West Publishing, 1987

Fosshage JL: Toward reconceptualizing transference: theoretical and clinical consideration. Int J Psychoanal 75:265–281, 1994

Fraiberg S: Object constancy and mental representation. Psychoanal Study Child 24:9–47, 1969

Fraiberg S: Some characteristics of genital arousal and discharge in latency girls. Psychoanal Study Child 27:439–475, 1972

Fraiberg S: Pathological defenses in infancy. Psychoanal Q 2:635–642, 1982

Fraiberg S, Adelson E, Shapiro V: Ghosts in the nursery: a psychoanalytic approach to the problems of impaired infant-mother relationships. J Am Acad Child Adolesc Psychiatry 14:387–422, 1975

Frank RA, Cohen DJ: Psychosocial concomitants of biological maturation in preadolescence. Am J Psychiatry 136:1516–1524, 1979

Freidrich WN, Gramsch P, Broughton D: Normative sexual behavior in children. Pediatrics 88:456–464, 1991

Freud A: The Ego and the Mechanisms of Defense, Vol 2 (1936), in The Writings of Anna Freud. New York, International Universities Press, 1966

Freud A: Observations on child development. Psychoanal Study Child 18:245–265, 1951

Freud A: The concept of the rejecting mother (1955), in The Writings of Anna Freud, Vol 4, Revised. New York, International Universities Press, 1968, pp 586–602

Freud A: Normality and Pathology of Childhood. New York, International Universities Press, 1965

Freud S: The interpretation of dreams (1900), in The Standard Edition of the Complete Psychological Works of Sigmund Freud, Vols 4 and 5. Translated and edited by Strachey J. London, Hogarth Press, 1963, pp 1–610

Freud S: Three essays on the theory of sexuality (1905), in The Standard Edition of the Complete Psychological Works of Sigmund Freud, Vol 7. Translated and edited by Strachey J. London, Hogarth Press, 1963, pp 135–243

Freud S: Analysis of a phobia in a five-year-old boy (1909), in The Standard Edition of the Complete Psychological Works of Sigmund Freud, Vol 10. Translated and edited by Strachey J. London, Hogarth Press, 1963, pp 5–148

Freud S: Two principles of mental functioning (1911), in The Standard Edition of the Complete Psychological Works of Sigmund Freud, Vol 12. Translated and edited by Strachey J. London, Hogarth Press, 1963, pp 218–226

Freud S: Mourning and melancholia (1917), in The Standard Edition of the Complete Psychological Works of Sigmund Freud, Vol 14. Translated and edited by Strachey J. London, Hogarth Press, 1963, pp 237–258

Freud S: Beyond the pleasure principle (1920), in The Standard Edition of the Complete Psychological Works of Sigmund Freud, Vol 18. Translated and edited by Strachey J. London, Hogarth Press, 1963, pp 7–68

Freud S: The ego and the id (1923), in The Standard Edition of the Complete Psychological Works of Sigmund Freud, Vol 19. Translated and edited by Strachey J. London, Hogarth Press, 1963, pp 12–66

Freud S: Inhibitions, symptoms and anxiety (1926), in The Standard Edition of the Complete Psychological Works of Sigmund Freud, Vol 20. Translated and edited by Strachey J. London, Hogarth Press, 1963, pp 77–178

Frye D, Moore C: Children's Theories of Mind: Mental States and Social Understanding. Hillsdale, NJ, Lawrence Erlbaum, 1991

Gabbard GO: Psychodynamic psychiatry in the "Decade of the Brain." Am J Psychiatry 149:991–998, 1992

Galenson E: Influences on the development of the symbolic function, in Frontiers of Infant Psychiatry, Vol 2. Edited by Call JD, Glenson E, Tyson RL. New York, Basic Books, 1984, pp 30–37

Galenson E: Sexuality in infancy and preschool-aged children, in Child and Adolescent Psychiatric Clinics of North America, Vol 2. Edited by Yates A. Philadelphia, PA, W B Saunders, 1993

Galenson E, Miller R, Roiphe H: The choice of symbols. J Am Acad Child Adolesc Psychiatry 411:83–96, 1976

Gardner MR: Is that a fact? empiricism revisited, or a psychoanalyst at sea. Int J Psychoanal 75:927–939, 1994

Garvey C, Kramer TL: The language of social pretend play. Developmental Review 9:364–382, 1989

Gelman R, Baillargeon R: A review of some Piagetian concepts, in Handbook of Child Psychology, Vol 3. Edited by Mussen P. New York, Wiley, 1983, pp 167–231

Gemelli R: Classification of child stuttering, part I. Child Psychiatry and Human Development 12:220–253, 1982a

Gemelli R: Classification of child stuttering, part II: persistent late onset male stuttering, and treatment issues for persistent stutterers—psychotherapy or speech therapy or both? Child Psychiatry and Human Development 13:3–34, 1982b

Gemelli R: Child stuttering. Pediatric Emergency Casebook 18:1–12, 1985

Gillet E: Levels of description and the unconscious. Psychoanalysis and Contemporary Thought 18:293–316, 1995

Girton M: Infants' attention to intrastimulus motion. J Exp Child Psychol 28:416–423, 1979

Gleitman H: Basic Psychology. New York, WW Norton, 1987

Gless P: The Human Brain. New York, Cambridge University Press, 1988

Gobnik A, Graft P: Knowing how you know: young children's ability to identify and remember the sources of their beliefs. Child Dev 59:1366–1371, 1988

Goldberg SH: The evolution of the patient's theories of pathogenesis. Psychoanal Q 53:54–84, 1994

Goldsmith H: Continuity of personality: a genetic perspective, in Continuities and Discontinuities in Development. Edited by Emde R, Harmon R. New York, Plenum, 1986

Goldsmith HH, Campos JJ: Toward a theory of infant temperament, in The Development of Attachment and Affiliative Systems. Edited by Emde R, Harmond R. New York, Plenum, 1982, pp 161–212

Goldsmith H, Buss A, Plomin R, et al: Roundtable: what is temperament? four approaches. Child Dev 58:505–529, 1987

Graf P: Life-span changes in implicit and explicit memory. Bulletin of the Psychonomic Society 284:353–358, 1990

Graves P: The functioning fetus, in The Course of Life, Vol 1: Infancy. Edited by Greenspan S, Pollack G. Madison, CT, International Universities Press, 1989, pp 433–467

Green R: Childhood cross-gender behavior and subsequent sexual preference. Am J Psychiatry 142:339–341, 1985

Greenberg M, Morris N: Engrossment: the newborn's impact upon the father. Am J Orthopsychiatry 44:520–531, 1974

Greenspan SI: Intelligence and Adaptation: An Integration of Psychoanalytic and Piagetian Developmental Psychology. New York, International Universities Press, 1979

Greenspan S: The Clinical Interview of the Child. New York, McGraw-Hill, 1981

Greenspan S: The development of the ego: biological and environmental specificity in the psychopathological developmental process and the selection and construction of ego defenses. J Am Psycho Assoc 37:605–639, 1989

Greenspan SI, Lieberman AF: Infants, mothers, and their interaction: a quantitative clinical approach to developmental assessment, in The Course of Life, Vol 1: Infancy. Edited by Greenspan SI, Pollock GH. Madison, CT, International Universities Press, 1989, pp 503–561

Grossmann K, Thane K, Grossmann KE: Maternal tactual contact of the newborn after various postpartum conditions of mother-infant contact. Developmental Psychology 17:159–169, 1981

Grotevant H, Cooper C: Patterns of interaction in family relationships and the development of identity exploration in adolescence. Child Dev 56:415–428, 1985

Halford GS: Reflections on 25 years of Piagetian cognitive psychology, 1963–1988. Human Development, Vol 32, 1989

Hamilton NG: Self and Others: Object Relations Theory in Practice. Northvale, NJ, Jason Aronson, 1988

Harlow HF: Primary affectional patterns in primates. Am J Orthopsychiatry 30:676–684, 1960

Harris PL, Donnelly K, Guz GR, et al: Children's understanding of mixed and masked emotions, in Transitional Mechanisms in Child Development. Edited by de Ribaupierre E. Cambridge, England, Cambridge University Press, 1986, pp 125–141

Hartman H: Ego Psychology and the Problem of Adaptation. New York, International Universities Press, 1939

Hartman H, Kris E, Loewenstein R: Comments on the formation of psychic structure. Psychoanal Study Child 2:11–38, 1946

Hauser S, Smith H: The development of experience of affect in adolescence. J Am Psychoanal Assoc 39:131–169, 1991

Havens L: A theoretical basis for the concepts of self and authentic self. J Am Psychoanal Assoc 34:363–378, 1986

Henry J: On Shame, Vulnerability and Other Forms of Self-Destruction. New York, Vantage Books, 1973

Henry J, Stephens P: Stress, Health and the Social Environment. New York, Springer-Verlag New York, 1977

Herzog J: Sleep disturbances and father hunger in 18- to 20-month-old boys: the Erlkoenig Syndrome. Psychoanal Study Child 35:219–236, 1980

Herzog JM: On father hunger: the father's role in the modulation of aggressive drive and fantasy, in Father and Child. Edited by Cath SW, Gurwitt AR, Ross JM. Boston, MA, Little, Brown, 1982, pp 163–174

Herzog JM: Fathers and young children: fathering daughters and fathering sons, in Frontiers of Infant Psychiatry, Vol 2. Edited by Call JD, Galenson E, Tyson RL. New York, Basic Books, 1984, pp 335–342

Hesse H: Beneath the Wheel (1930). New York, Bantam Books, 1972

Hiatt H: Dynamic psychotherapy with the aging patient. Am J Psychotherapy 25:591–600, 1971

Hill JP: Research on adolescents and their families: past and prospect, in Adolescent Social Behavior and Health: New Directions for Child Development. Edited by Irwin CE Jr. San Francisco, CA, Jossey-Bass, 1987, pp 145–163

Hirshfeld DR, Rosenbaum JF, Biederman J, et al: Stable behavioral inhibition and its association with anxiety disorder. J Am Acad Child Adolesc Psychiatry 31:103–112, 1992

Hofferth SJ, Kahn J, Baldwin W: Premarital sexual activity among U.S. teenage women over the past three decades. Family Planning Perspectives 19:46–53, 1987

Hoffman M: Affective and cognitive processes in moral internalization, in Social Cognition and Social Development. Edited by Higgens ET, Ruble DN, Hartnup WW. Cambridge, UK, Cambridge University Press, 1983, pp 236–274

Horner AJ: The Wish for Power and the Fear of Having It. Northvale, NJ, Jason Aronson, 1989

Hudson JA: The emergence of autobiographic memory in mother-child conversations, in Knowing and Remembering in Young Children. Edited by Fivush R, Hudson JA. New York, Cambridge University Press, 1990, pp 166–196

Hudson JA: Understanding events: the development of script knowledge, in The Development of Social Cognition. Edited by Bennett M. New York, Guilford, 1993, pp 142–167

Hutt SJ, Hutt C, Lenard H, et al: Auditory responsivity in the human neonate. Nature 218:888–890, 1968

Inge B, Fritz J, Zahn-Waxler C, et al: Learning to talk about emotions: a functionalist perspective. Child Dev 57:529–548, 1986

Izard CE: The Face of Emotion. New York, Appleton-Century-Crofts, 1971

Izard CE: Patterns of Emotions. New York, Academic Press, 1972

Izard CE: Human Emotions. New York, Plenum, 1977

Izard CE, Hembee EA, Dougherty LM, et al: Changes in 2- to 19-month old infant's facial expressions following acute pain. Developmental Psychology 193:418–426, 1983

Johnson F, Dowling J, Wesner D: Notes on infant psychotherapy. Infant Mental Health Journal 1:19–33, 1980

Johnson W, Emde R, Pannabecker B, et al: Maternal perception of infant emotion from birth through eighteen months. Infant Behavior and Development 5:313–322, 1982

Kagan J: Change and Continuity in Infancy. New York, Wiley, 1971a

Kagan J: A conception of early adolescence, in 12 to 16: Early Adolescence. Edited by Kagan J, Coles R. New York, WW Norton, 1971b, pp 90–105

Kagan J: The form of early development. Arch Gen Psychiatry 36:1047–1054, 1979

Kagan J: The Second Year: The Emergence of Self-Awareness. Cambridge, MA, Harvard University Press, 1981

Kagan J: The Nature of the Child. New York, Basic Books, 1984

Kagan J: Creativity in infancy. Paper presented at symposium on Creativity in Childhood, Baltimore, MD, October 1988

Kagan J: Unstable Ideas: Temperament, Cognition and Self. Cambridge, MA, Harvard University Press, 1989

Kahn M: The concept of cumulative trauma. Psychoanal Study Child 20:239–306, 1963

Kail R, Bisanz J: The information-processing perspective on cognitive development in childhood and adolescence, in Intellectual Development. Edited by Sternberg J, Berg C. New York, Cambridge University Press, 1992, pp 229–261

Kandel E: Genes, nerve cells, and the remembrance of things past. Journal of Neuropsychiatry 1:110–125, 1981

Kandel E: From metapsychology to molecular biology: explorations into the nature of anxiety. Am J Psychiatry 140:1277–1293, 1983

Kandel E, Schwartz J: Molecular biology of learning: modulation of transmitter release. Science 218:433–443, 1982

Kandel E, Schwartz JH, Jessell TM: Principles of Neural Science. New York, Elsevier, 1991

Kanner L: Child Psychiatry. Springfield, IL, Charles C Thomas, 1957

Kaplan EH: Fifteen to eighteen, in The Course of Life, Vol 4: Adolescence. Edited by Greenspan SI, Pollock GH. Madison, CT, International Universities Press, 1991, pp 201–233

Karmiloff-Smith A: Problem solving procedures in the construction and representation of closed railway circuits. Archives de Psychologie 67:37–59, 1979

Katan A: The role of displacement in agoraphobia. Int J Psychoanal 32:41–50, 1951

Kelley HH, Berscheid E, Christensen A, et al: Close Relationships. New York, Freeman, 1983

Kendler KS: Genetic epidemiology in psychiatry: taking both genes and environment seriously. Arch Gen Psychiatry 52:895–899, 1995

Kendler KS: Parenting: a genetic-epidemiologic perspective. Am J Psychiatry 153:11–20, 1996

Kendler K, Eaves L: Models for the joint effect of genotype and environment on liability to psychiatric illness. Am J Psychiatry 143:279–288, 1986

Keniston K: Young Radicals. New York, Harcourt-Brace-World, 1968

Keniston K: Youth as a stage in life. Adolescent Psychiatry 1:161–175, 1971

Kernberg OF: Object Relations Theory and Clinical Psychoanalysis. New York, Jason Aronson, 1976

Kernberg OF: Self, ego, affects and drives. J Am Psychoanal Assoc 30:893–917, 1982

Kernberg OF: An ego psychology-object relations theory approach to the transference. Psychoanal Q 51:197–221, 1987

Kestenbaum CJ: Current sexual attitudes, societal pressure, and the middle-class adolescent girl, in Adolescent Psychiatry, Vol 7. Edited by Feinstein SC, Giovacchini PL. Chicago, IL, University of Chicago Press, 1979, pp 147–157

Kestenberg JS: Outside and inside, male and female. J Am Psychoanal Assoc 16:457–520, 1968

Khatchadourian H: The Biology of Adolescence. San Francisco, CA, Freeman, 1977

Kingston L, Prior M: The development of patterns of stable, transient, and school-age onset aggressive behavior in young children. J Am Acad Child Adolesc Psychiatry 34:348–358, 1995

Klaus MH, Kennell JH: Maternal-Infant Bonding. St. Louis, MO, CV Mosby, 1976

Klein M: The importance of symbol-formation in the development of the ego (1930), in The Writings of Melanie Klein, Vol 1. London, Hogarth Press, 1975, pp 219–232

Klein M: The Psychoanalysis of Children. London, Hogarth Press, 1935

Klinnert MD, Campos JJ, Sorce JF, et al: Emotions as behavior regulators: social referencing in infancy, in Emotion: Theory, Research and Experience, Vol 2. Edited by Plutchik R, Kellerman H. New York, Academic Press, 1983

Knopf IJ: Childhood Psychopathology. Englewood Cliffs, NJ, Prentice-Hall, 1984

Kofsky E: A scalogram study of classificatory development. Child Dev 37:191–204, 1966

Kohlberg LA: The Philosophy of Moral Development, Moral Stages, and the Ideal of Justice: Essays on Moral Development, Vol 1. San Francisco, CA, Harper & Row, 1981

Kohut H: The Analysis of the Self. New York, International Universities Press, 1970

Kohut H: The Analysis of the Self: A Systematic Approach to the Psychoanalytic Treatment of Narcissistic Personality Disorders. New York, International Universities Press, 1971

Kohut H: Restoration of the Self. New Haven, CT, International Universities Press, 1977

Kohut H, Wolf E: The disorders of the self and their treatment: an outline. Int J Psychoanal 59:413–425, 1978

Korn S, Gannon S: Temperament, cultural variation and behavior disorder in preschool children. Child Psychiatry Hum Dev 13:203–212, 1984

Kovacs M, Goldston D, Gatonis C: Suicidal behaviors and childhood-onset depressive disorders: a longitudinal investigation. J Am Acad Child Adolesc Psychiatry 32:8–20, 1993

Kramer S, Rudolf J: The latency stage, in The Course of Life, Vol 3: Middle and Late Childhood. Edited by Greenspan S, Pollack G. Madison, CT, International Universities Press, 1991, pp 319–333

Kupersmidt JD, Dodge KA: The role of poor peer relationships in the development of disorder, in Peer Rejection in Childhood. Edited by Asher SR, Coie JD. New York, Cambridge University Press, 1990, pp 274–305

Lamb ME: Effects of stress and cohort on mother- and father-infant interaction. Developmental Psychology 12:435–443, 1976

Lamb ME: The development of social experiences in the first year of life, in Infant Social Cognition: Empirical and Theoretical Considerations. Edited by Lamb ME, Sherrod LR. Hillsdale, NJ, Lawrence Erlbaum, 1981a, pp 157–172

Lamb ME (ed): The Role of the Father in Child Development, 2nd Edition. New York, Wiley, 1981b

Lane RD, Schwartz GE: Levels of emotional awareness: a cognitive-developmental theory and its application to psychopathology. Am J Psychiatry 144:133–143, 1987

Langer S: Philosophy in a New Key. New York, Mentor, 1962

Laub D, Auerhahn NC: Knowing and not knowing massive psychic trauma: forms of traumatic memory. Int J Psychoanal 74:287–302, 1993

Laufer M, Laufer ME: Adolescence and Developmental Breakdown: A Psychoanalytic View. New Haven, CT, Yale University Press, 1984

Lazarus R: On the primacy of cognition. Am Psychol 392:124–129, 1984

Leekam S: Children's understanding of mind, in The Development of Social Cognition. Edited by Bennett M. New York, Guilford, 1993, pp 26–61

Leigh H, Reiser M: The Patient: Biological, Psychological and Social Dimensions of Clinical Practice. New York, Plenum, 1985

Leslie AM: Pretense and representation:The origins of "theory of mind." Psychol Rev 94:412–426, 1987

Lewis M, Brooks-Gunn J: Social Cognition and the Acquisition of Self. New York, Plenum, 1979

Lewis M, Michalson L: The socialization of emotions, in Emotions and Early Interaction. Edited by Field T, Fogel A. Hillsdale, NJ, Lawrence Erlbaum, 1982, pp 155–185

Lewis M, Michalson L: From emotional state to emotional expression, in Human Development: An Interactional Perspective. New York, Academic Press, 1983

Lewis ML: Clinical Aspects of Child Development. Philadelphia, PA, Lea & Febiger, 1978

Lewis ML: Memory and psychoanalysis: a new look at infantile amnesia and transference. J Am Acad Child Adolesc Psychiatry 34:405–417, 1995

Lewis ML, Volkmar F: Clinical Aspects of Child and Adolescent Development. Philadelphia, PA, Lea & Febiger, 1990

Lichtenberg J: Continuities and transformations between infancy and adolescence, in Adolescent Psychiatry, Vol 10. Edited by Feinstein S, Looney J, Schwartzberg A, et al. Chicago, IL, University of Chicago Press, 1982, pp 182–198

Lichtenberg JD: Psychoanalysis and Motivation. Hillsdale, NJ, Analytic Press, 1989

Lichtenberg JD, Kindler AR: A motivational systems approach. J Am Psychoanal Assoc 42:405–421, 1994

Loewald HW: The waning of the Oedipus complex. J Am Psychoanal Assoc 27:751–775, 1979

Loewald HW: Perspectives on memory, in Papers on Psychoanalysis. New Haven, CT, Yale University Press, 1980, pp 148–174

Loftus E: The malleability of memory. The Advisor: American Professional Society of the Abuse of Children 5:7–9, 1993

Maccoby EE: Social Development. New York, Wiley, 1980

Maccoby EE, Martin J: Socialization in the context of the family: parent-child interaction, in Handbook of Child Psychology, Socialization, Personality and Social Development, 4th Edition, Vol 4. Edited by Mussen PH, Hetherington EM. New York, Wiley, 1983, pp 1–101

MacFarlane A: Olfaction in the development of social preference in the human neonate, in Parent Infant Interaction (Cilia Foundation 33 New Series). New York, Elsevier, 1975, pp 103–117

Magnusson D, Allen V: Human Development: An Interactional Approach. New York, Academic Press, 1983

Mahler MS: Thoughts about development and individualization. Psychoanal Study Child 18:307–324, 1963

Mahler MS: A study of the separation-individualization process, and its possible application to borderline phenomenon in the psychoanalytic situation. Psychoanal Study Child 36:403–424, 1971

Mahler MS: On human symbiosis and the vicissitudes of individualization. J Am Psychoanal Assoc 23:740–763, 1975

Mahler MS, McDevitt J: Thoughts on the emergence of the sense of self, with particular emphasis on the body self. J Am Psychoanal Assoc 30:827–848, 1982

Mahler MS, Pine F, Bergman A: The Psychological Birth of the Human Infant. New York, Basic Books, 1975

Main M: Discourse, prediction, and recent studies in attachment: implications for psychoanalysis. J Am Psychoanal Assoc 41 (suppl):209–245, 1993

Main M, Kaplan N, Cassidy J: Security in infancy, childhood and adulthood: a move to the level of representation, in Growing Points of Attachment Theory and Research. Edited by Bretherton I, Waters W. Monographs of the Society for Research in Child Development 50:1–2, Serial No 209, 1985, pp 66–104

Maletesta C, Haviland J: Learning display rules: the socialization of emotion expression in infancy. Child Development 53:991–1003, 1982

Martinson F: Eroticism in infancy and childhood. The Journal of Sex Research 2:251–262, 1976

Mayer LM: Towards female gender identity. J Am Psychoanal Assoc 43:17–39, 1995

Mayes LC, Cohen DJ: Experiencing self and others: from studies of autism to psychoanalytic theory of social development. J Am Psychoanal Assoc 42:191–219, 1994

Maziade M, Capera P, Laplante B, et al: Value of difficult temperament among seven-year-olds in the general population for predicting psychiatric diagnosis at age 12. Am J Psychiatry 142:943–946, 1985

McCall RB: Issues of continuity and discontinuity in temperament research, in The Study of Temperament: Changes, Continuities, and Challenges. Edited by Plomin R, Dunn J. Hillsdale, NJ, Lawrence Erlbaum, 1986, pp 13–26

McCarthy JB: Adolescent character formation and psychoanalytic theory. Am J Psychoanal 55:245–267, 1995

McDevitt JB: The role of internalization in the development of object relations during the separation-individualization phase. J Am Psychoanal Assoc 27:327–343, 1979

McDevitt JB: The emergence of hostile aggression and its defensive and adaptive modifications during the separation-individualization process. J Am Psychoanal Assoc 31 (suppl):273–300, 1987

McDevitt JB, Mahler MS: Object constancy, individuality, and internalization, in The Course of Life, Vol 2: Early Childhood. Edited by Greenspan SI, Pollock GH. Madison, CT, International Universities Press, 1989, pp 37–61

Meissner W: A note in projective identification. J Am Psychoanal Assoc 28:43–68, 1980

Meissner WW: Can psychoanalysis find its self? J Am Psychoanal Assoc 35:379–401, 1986

Meissner WW: The pathology of belief systems. Psychoanalysis and Contemporary Thought 15:99–129, 1992

Meissner WW: The economic principle in psychoanalysis, I: economics and energetics; II: regulatory principles; III: motivational principles. Psychoanalysis and Contemporary Thought 18:197–293, 1995

Merriam Webster's Collegiate Dictionary, 10th Edition. Springfield, MA, Merriam-Webster, 1993

Meyer A: Collected Papers of Adolf Meyer, 1848–1952, Vols 1–4. Baltimore, MD, Johns Hopkins University Press, 1991

Meyer JK: Body ego, selfness, and gender sense: the development of gender identity. Psychiatr Clin North Am 3:21–36, 1980

Meyer JK: The theory of gender identity disorders. J Am Psychoanal Assoc 30:381–419, 1982

Meyer-Bahlburg HF: Sexuality in early adolescence, in Handbook of Human Sexuality. Edited by Wolman B, Money J. Northvale, NJ, Jason Aronson, 1983, pp 61–77

Miller A: Prisoners of Childhood. New York, Basic Books, 1981

Miller JB: Woman's Growth in Connection: Writings From the Stone Center. New York, Guilford, 1991

Mills M, Melhuish E: Recognition of mother's voice in early infancy. Nature 252:123–124, 1974

Mitchell SA: Aggression and the endangered self. Psychoanal Q 62:351–352, 1993

Modell A: Play and creativity. Paper presented at symposium on Creativity in Childhood, Baltimore, MD, October 1988

Nachman P, Stern D, Best C: Affective reactions to stimuli and infants' preferences for novelty and familiarity. J Am Acad Child Adolesc Psychiatry 25:801–804, 1986

Neimark ED: Current status of formal operations research. Human Development 32:60–67, 1979

Nelson K: Event knowledge and the development of language functions, in Research in Child Language Disorders. Edited by Miller J. New York, Little, Brown, 1990, pp 125–141

Nelson K: Narrative and memory in early childhood. Paper presented at annual meeting of the American Academy of Child and Adolescent Psychiatry, San Antonio, TX, October 1993a

Nelson K: The psychological and social origins of autobiographical memory. Psychological Science 4:7–14, 1993b

Nelson L: Language formulation related to dysfluency and stuttering. Paper presented at the Conference on the Prevention of Stuttering and the Management of Fluency Problems in Children. Evanston, IL, June 1982

Neubauer PB: Preoedipal objects and object primacy. Psychoanal Study Child 40:163–182, 1985

Noshpitz J, King R: Pathways of Growth: Essentials of Child Psychiatry, Vol 1: Normal Development. New York, Wiley, 1991

Noy P: Form creation in art: an ego-psychological approach to creativity. Psychoanal Q 48:229–256, 1979

Offer D: Adolescent development: a normative perspective, in The Course of Life, Vol 4: Adolescence. Edited by Greenspan SI, Pollock GH. Madison, CT, International Universities Press, 1989, pp 181–199

Offer D, Offer JB: From Teenage to Young Manhood: A Psychological Study. New York, Basic Books, 1975

Offer D, Sabshin M: Normality and the Life Cycle. New York, Basic Books, 1984

Offer D, Schonert-Reichl K: Debunking the myths of adolescence: findings from recent research. J Am Acad Child Adolesc Psychiatry 31:1003–1014, 1992

Osofsky J, Cohen G, Drell M: The effects of trauma on young children. Int J Psychoanal 76:595–607, 1995

Overton WF, Steidl JH, Rosenstein D, et al: Formal operations as regulatory context in adolescence, in Adolescent Psychiatry, Vol 18. Edited by Feinstein SC. Chicago, IL, University of Chicago Press, 1992, pp 502–513

Pardes H: Neuroscience and psychiatry: marriage and coexistence. Am J Psychiatry 143:1205–1212, 1986

Parens H: The Development of Aggression in Early Childhood. New York, Jason Aronson, 1979

Parens H: Aggression in Our Children. New York, Jason Aronson, 1987

Parens H, Pollack L, Stern J, et al: On the girl's entry into the oedipus complex. J Am Psychoanal Assoc 24:79–107, 1976

Parke R, Tinsley B: The father's role in infancy: determinants of involvement in caregiving and play, in The Role of the Father in Child Development. Edited by Lamb M. New York, Wiley, 1981, pp 45–76

Parmalee AH: Ontogeny of sleep patterns and associated periodicities in infants, in Pre- and Postnatal Development of the Human Brain, Vol 13. Edited by Berenberg SR, Caniaris M, Masse NP. Basel, S Karger, 1974, pp 115–140

Pavlov I: Conditioned Reflexes. Edited and translated by Anrep GV. New York, Dover, 1927

Peller LE: Libidinal phases, ego development and play. Psychoanal Study Child 9:178–198, 1954

Perry NW: How children remember and why they forget. The Advisor 5:1–16, 1992

Person ES: By Force of Fantasy. New York, Basic Books, 1995

Peterfreund E: Information, systems, and psychoanalysis: an evolutionary biological approach to psychoanalytic theory. Psychol Issues Monograph 25–26, 1971

Piaget J: The Psychology of Intelligence. London, Routledge & Kegan Paul, 1950

Piaget J: The Origins of Intelligence in Children. New York, International Universities Press, 1952

Piaget J: The Construction of Reality in the Child. New York, Basic Books, 1954a

Piaget J: Intelligence and Affectivity: Their Relationship During Child Development (1954b), Revised. Palo Alto, CA, Annual Reviews, 1981

Piaget J: Biologie et Connaissance [Biology and Knowledge]. Paris, Gallimard, 1967

Piaget J: Intellectual evolution from adolescence to adulthood. Human Development 15:1–12, 1972

Piaget J, Inhelder B: The Child's Conception of Space. London, Routledge & Kegan Paul, 1956

Piaget J, Inhelder B: Memory and Intelligence. New York, Basic Books, 1973

Piatelli-Palmarini M (ed): Language and Meaning: The Debate Between Jean Piaget and Noam Chomsky. Cambridge, MA, Harvard University Press, 1980

Pine F: Developmental Theory and Clinical Process. New Haven, CT, Yale University Press, 1985

Pine F: Motivation, personality organization, and the four psychologies of psychoanalysis. J Am Psychoanal Assoc 37:31–64, 1989

Pine F: The era of separation-individuation. Psychoanalytic Inquiry 14:4–25, 1994

Pitcher E, Prelinger E: Children Tell Stories: An Analysis of Fantasy. New Haven, CT, International Universities Press, 1963

Plomin R: Development, Genetics, and Psychology. Hillsdale, NJ, Lawrence Erlbaum, 1986

Plomin R: The role of inheritance in behavior. Science 248:183–188, 1990

Pruett K: Home-based treatment for two infants who witnessed their mother's murder. J Am Acad Child Adolesc Psychiatry 18:647–659, 1979

Pulver S: Psychic structure, function, process, and content: toward a definition. J Am Psychoanal Assoc 36 (suppl):165–188, 1988

Putallaz M, Dunn SE: The importance of peer relations, in Handbook of Developmental Psychopathology. Edited by Lewis M, Miller SM. New York, Plenum, 1990, pp 227–236

Rainer J: Genetics and psychiatry, in Comprehensive Textbook of Psychiatry. Edited by Kaplan H, Freedman A, Sadock B. Baltimore, MD, Williams & Wilkins, 1980, pp 101–121

Rakoff VM: Friendship and adolescence, in Adolescent Psychiatry, Vol 18. Edited by Feinstein SC. Chicago, IL, University of Chicago Press, 1992, pp 104–119

Rapaport D: Introduction: a historical survey of psychoanalytic ego psychology. Psychol Issues 1:5–17, 1959

Reiser M: Mind, Brain, Body: Toward a Convergence of Psychoanalysis and Neurobiology. New York, Basic Books, 1984

Reiser M: Converging sectors of psychoanalysis and neurobiology: mutual challenge and opportunity. J Am Psychoanal Assoc 33:11–34, 1985

Reiss D, Plomin R, Hetherington EM: Genetics and psychiatry: an unheralded window on the environment. Am J Psychiatry 148:283–291, 1991

Richards AK: New views of female development. Paper presented at the annual meeting of the American Psychoanalytic Association, Philadelphia, PA, May 1994

Ritvo S: Adolescent to woman. J Amer Psychoanal Assoc 24:127–138, 1976

Rizzuto A: The adolescent's sartorial dilemmas, in Adolescent Psychiatry, Vol 18. Edited by Feinstein SC. Chicago, IL, University of Chicago Press, 1992, pp 440–448

Rochlin G: The dread of abandonment. Psychoanal Study Child 16:451–470, 1965

Roff JD, Wirt RD: Childhood social adjustment, adolescent status, and young adult mental health. Am J Orthopsychiatry 54:595–602, 1984

Roffwarg H, Muzio J, Dement WC: Ontogenesis of sleep cycles, in Early Human Development. Edited by Hutt SJ, Hutt C. London, Oxford University Press, 1973, pp 113–143

Roiphe H, Galenson E: Infantile Origins of Sexual Identity. New Haven, CT, International Universities Press, 1981

Rosenfeld AA, Wasserman S: Sexual development in the early school-aged child. Child and Adolescent Psychiatric Clinics of North America 2:393–406, 1993

Rosenthal HM: On early alienation from the self. Am J Psychoanal 43:231–243, 1983

Roth S: Psychotherapy: The Art of Wooing Nature. Northvale, NJ, Jason Aronson, 1990

Rothbard JC, Shaver PR: Continuity of attachment across the life span, in Attachment in Adults. Edited by Sperling MB, Berman WH. New York, Guilford, 1994, pp 31–72

Rothstein A: The representational world as a substructure of the ego. J Am Psychoanal Assoc 36:191–208, 1988

Rutter M: Continuities and discontinuities in socioemotional development, in Continuities and Discontinuities in Development. Edited by Emde R, Harmon R. New York, Plenum, 1984, pp 41–63

Rutter M: Meyerian psychobiology, personality development and the role of life experiences. Am J Psychiatry 143:1077–1087, 1986

Rutter M: Nature, nurture and psychopathology: a new look at an old topic. Development and Psychopathology 3:125–136, 1991

Sabatini P: Age and professional specialization in formal reasoning. Unpublished dissertation, Wayne State University, Detroit, MI, 1979

Sabelli HC, Carlson-Sabelli L: Biological priority and psychological supremacy: a new integrative paradigm derived from process theory. Am J Psychiatry 146:1541–1551, 1989

Sameroff AJ: Transactional models in early social relations. Human Development 18:65–79, 1975

Sander LW: Investigation of the infant and its caregiving environment as a biological system, in The Course of Life, Vol 1: Infancy. Edited by Greenspan SI, Pollock GH. Madison, CT, International Universities Press, 1989, pp 359–393

Sandler J: On the concept of the superego. Psychoanal Study Child 15:128–162, 1960

Sandler J, Holder A, Dare C: Frames of reference in psychoanalytic psychology, V: the topographical frame of reference: the organization of the mental apparatus. Br J Med Psychol 46:29–36, 1973

Sarnoff C: Psychotherapeutic Strategies in Late Latency Through Early Adolescence. Northvale, NJ, Jason Aronson, 1987

Scarr S, McCartney K: How people make their own environments: a theory of genotype → environmental effects. Child Dev 54:424–435, 1983

Schacter DL: Understanding implicit memory: a cognitive neuroscience approach. Am Psychol 47:559–569, 1992

Schaffer H: The Child's Entry Into a Social World. New York, Academic Press, 1984

Schecter M, Combrinck-Graham L: The normal development of the seven-to-ten-year-old, in The Course of Life, Vol 3. Edited by Greenspan S, Pollack G. New Haven, CT, International Universities Press, 1991

Schneider S: Impingement of cultural factors on identity formation in adolescence, in Adolescent Psychiatry, Vol 18. Edited by Feinstein SC. Chicago, IL, University of Chicago Press, 1992, pp 407–418

Seigal DJ: Childhood memory. Paper presented at the Meeting of the American Academy of Child and Adolescent Psychiatry. San Antonio, TX, October 1993

Seligman MEP: Helplessness. San Francisco, CA, WH Freeman, 1975

Selman R: The Growth of Interpersonal Understanding. New York, Academic Press, 1980

Shantz CW: Conflicts between children. Child Dev 48:238–305, 1987

Shapiro T: On the quest for the origins of conflict. Psychoanal Q 50:1–21, 1981

Shapiro T: Foreword: The concept of psychic structure in psychoanalysis. J Am Psychoanal Assoc 36 (suppl):iii–vi, 1988

Shapiro T, Hertzig ME: Normal growth and development, in American Psychiatric Press Textbook of Psychiatry. Edited by Talbott JA, Hales RE, Yusofsky SC. Washington, DC, American Psychiatric Press, 1988, pp 91–122

Shapiro T, Perry R: Latency revisited. Psychoanal Study Child 31:79–105, 1976

Sharff J: Projective and Introjective Identification and the Use of the Therapist's Self. Northvale, NJ, Jason Aronson, 1992

Siegel E, Bauman K, Schafer E, et al: Hospital and home support during infancy: impact on maternal attachment, child abuse, and neglect, and health utilization. Pediatrics 66:183–190, 1980

Skinner BF: The Behavior of Organisms. New York, Appleton-Century-Crofts, 1938

Skinner BF: Contingencies of Reinforcement: A Theoretical Analysis. New York, Appleton-Century-Crofts, 1969

Slackman E, Nelson S: Acquisition of an unfamiliar script in story form by young children. Child Dev 55:329–340, 1984

Slobin DI: Cognitive prerequisites for the development of grammar, in Studies of Child Language Development. Edited by Ferguson C, Slobin D. New York, Holt, Rhinehart & Winston, 1973, pp 175–208

Snow C: Mothers' speech to children learning language. Child Dev 43:549–565, 1972

Solnit AJ, Neubauer PB: Object constancy and early triadic relationships. J Am Acad Child Adolesc Psychiatry 25:23–29, 1986

Sommers S: Emotionality reconsidered: the role of cognition in emotional responsiveness. J Pers Soc Psychol 41:553–561, 1981

Sorensen A: Adolescent Sexuality in Contemporary America. New York, World Publishing, 1973

Spence DP: The Freudian Metaphor Toward Paradigm Change in Psychoanalysis. New York, WW Norton, 1987

Spence DP: The special nature of psychoanalytical facts. Int J Psychoanal 75:915–927, 1994

Spitz RA: Hospitalism: an inquiry into the genesis of psychiatric conditions in early childhood. Psychoanal Study Child 1:53–72, 1945

Squire LR: Mechanisms of memory. Science 232:1612–1619, 1986

Squire LR: Memory and Brain. New York, Oxford University Press, 1987

Squire LR: Declarative and non-declarative memory: multiple brain systems supporting learning and memory. Journal of Cognitive Neuroscience 43:232–243, 1992

Sroufe LA: Wariness of strangers and the study of infant development. Child Dev 48:731–746, 1977

Sroufe LA: Infant-caretaker attachment and patterns of attachment in pre-school: the roots of maladaptation and competence, in Minnesota Symposium in Child Psychology. Edited by Perlmutter M. Minneapolis, University of Minnesota Press, 1983, pp 25–42

Sroufe LA: Attachment classification from the perspective of infant-caregiver relationships and infant temperament. Child Dev 56:1–14, 1985

Sroufe LA, Rutter M: The domain of developmental psychopathology. Child Dev 55:17–29, 1984

Stechler G: The dawn of awareness. Psychoanalytical Inquiry 1:503–543, 1982

Stechler G, Halton A: The emergence of assertion and aggression during infancy: a psychoanalytic systems approach. J Am Psychoanal Assoc 35:821–838, 1987

Stechler G, Kaplan S: The development of the self: a psychoanalytic perspective. Psychoanal Study Child 35:85–105, 1980

Steinberg L: Interdependency in the family: autonomy, conflict and harmony in the parent-adolescent relationship, in At the Threshold: The Developing Adolescent. Edited by Feldman S, Elliot G. Cambridge, MA, Harvard University Press, 1991

Stern D: The Interpersonal World of the Infant. New York, Basic Books, 1985

Sternberg RJ: Human intelligence: the model is the message. Science 230:1111–1118, 1985

Stillwell BM, Galvin M, Kopta SM: Conceptualization of conscience in normal children and adolescents, ages 5 to 17. J Am Acad Child Adolesc Psychiatry 30:16–21, 1991

Stoller RJ: Sex and Gender: On the Development of Masculinity and Femininity. New York, Science House, 1968

Stoller RJ: Primary femininity. J Am Psychoanal Assoc 24 (suppl):59–78, 1976

Stoller RJ: Presentations of Gender. New Haven, CT, Yale University Press, 1985

Stolorow R: The concept of psychic structure: its metapsychological and clinical psychoanalytic meanings. International Review of Psychoanalysis 5:313–320, 1978

Sugar M: Late adolescent development and treatment, in Adolescent Psychiatry, Vol 18. Edited by Feinstein SC. Chicago, IL, University of Chicago Press, 1992, pp 131–155

Sugar M: Adolescent sexuality, in Child and Adolescent Psychiatric Clinics of North America, Vol 2: Sexual and Gender Identity Disorders, 1993, pp 407–415

Sullivan HS: The Interpersonal Theory of Psychiatry. New York, W W Norton, 1953

Tanner JM: Physical growth, in Carmichael's Manual of Child Psychology, Vol 1, 3rd Edition. Edited by Mussen PH. New York, Wiley, 1970, pp 77–155

Tanner JM: Foetus Into Man. Cambridge, MA, Harvard University Press, 1978

Tenzer A: Piaget on psychoanalysis. Academy Forum 28:10–11, 1984

Terr L: What happens to early memories of trauma: a study of twenty children under five at the time of documented traumatic events. J Am Acad Child Adolesc Psychiatry 27:96–104, 1988

Terr L: Too Scared to Cry: Psychic Trauma in Childhood. New York, Harper & Row, 1990

Terr L: Childhood traumas: an outline and overview. Am J Psychiatry 148:10–20, 1991

Terr L: Psychological defenses and memories of childhood trauma. Paper presented at annual meeting of American Academy of Child and Adolescent Psychiatry, San Antonio, TX, October 1993

Terr L: Unchained Memories: True Stories of Traumatic Memories, Lost and Found. New York, Basic Books, 1994

Tessler M: Mother-child talk in a museum: the socialization of a memory. Unpublished manuscript, City University of New York Graduate Center, New York, 1986

Tessler M: Making memories together: the influence of mother-child joint encoding on the development of autobiographical memory style. Unpublished doctoral dissertation, City University of New York Graduate Center, New York, 1991

Thomas A, Chess S: Temperament and Development. New York, Brunner/Mazel, 1977

Thomas A, Chess S, Birch H: Temperament and Behavior Disorders in Children. New York, New York University Press, 1968

Thompson MG: How to support our middle schoolers, grades 4 through 9. Paper presented at the Langley School Parent Education Lecture Series, McLean, VA, March 1996

Tizard B, Hodges J: The effect of early institutional rearing on the development of eight-year-old children. J Child Psychol Psychiatry 19:99–118, 1978

Tizard B, Rees J: The effect of early institutional rearing on the behavioral problems and affectional relationships of four-year-old children. J Child Psychol Psychiatry 16:61–74, 1975

Tizard J, Tizard B: The social development of two-year-old children in residential nurseries, in The Origins of Human Social Relations. Edited by Schaffer HR. New York, Academic Press, 1971, pp 125–143

Tolpin M: On the beginnings of a cohesive self: an application of the concept of transmuting internalization to the study of the transitional object and signal anxiety. Psychoanal Study Child 26:316–352, 1971

Tolpin M: Self-objects and oedipal objects. Psychoanal Study Child 33:167–184, 1978

Tomkins SS: Affect, Imagery and Consciousness, Vols 1 and 2: The Positive Affects. New York, Springer, 1962–1963

Tomkins SS: Affect as the primary motivational system, in Feelings and Emotions: The Loyola Symposium. Edited by Arnold MB. New York, Academic Press, 1970, pp 101–110

Trad PV: The Preschool Child: Assessment, Diagnosis, and Treatment. New York, Wiley, 1989

Trad P: Use of developmental principles to decipher the narrative of preschool children. J Am Acad Child Adolesc Psychiatry 31:581–592, 1992

Trevarthan C: The foundations of intersubjectivity: development of interpersonal and cooperative understanding in infants, in The Social Function of Language and Thought: Essays in Honor of Jerome Bruner. Edited by Olson DR. New York, Norton, 1980, pp 152–175

Tyson P: A developmental line of gender identity, gender role and choice of love object. J Am Psychoanal Assoc 30:59–84, 1982a

Tyson P: The role of the father in gender identity, urethral eroticism and phallic narcissism, in On Fathers: Observations and Reflections. Edited by Cath S, Gurwitt A, Ross J. Boston, MA, Little, Brown, 1982b, pp 175–187

Tyson P: Infantile sexuality, gender identity and obstacles to oedipal progression. J Am Psychoanal Assoc 37:1051–1069, 1989

Tyson P: Theories of Female Psychology. J Am Psychoanal Assoc 42:447–469, 1994

Tyson P, Tyson RL: Narcissism and superego development. J Am Psychoanal Assoc 32:75–98, 1984

Tyson P, Tyson R: Psychoanalytic Theories of Development. New Haven, CT, Yale University Press, 1991

Tyson R: The roots of psychopathology and our theories of development. J Am Acad Child Adolesc Psychiatry 25:12–22, 1986

Tyson R, Tyson P: The concept of transference in child psychoanalysis. J Am Acad Child Adolesc Psychiatry 25:30–39, 1986

Valliant GE: Theoretical hierarchy of adaptive ego mechanisms. Arch Gen Psychiatry 24:107–118, 1971

Valliant GE: The natural history of male psychological health, II: some antecedents of healthy adult adjustment. Arch Gen Psychiatry 31:15–22, 1974

Valliant GE: Adaptation to Life. Boston, MA, Little, Brown, 1977

Valliant GE: Empirical studies of ego mechanisms of defense. Am J Psychiatry 48:131–135, 1987

Van Riper C: The Treatment of Stuttering. Princeton, NJ, Prentice-Hall, 1973

Verhulst FC, Koot HM: Longitudinal research in child and adolescent psychiatry. J Am Acad Child Adolesc Psychiatry 30:361–369, 1991

Viorst J: Necessary Losses. New York, Simon & Schuster, 1986

von Bertalanffy L: General System Theory: Foundations, Development, Applications. New York, George Braziller, 1968

Vygotsky LS: Mind in Society: The Development of Higher Psychological Processes. Cambridge, MA, Harvard University Press, 1978

Waelder R: The principle of multiple function: observations on overdetermination (1930), in Psychoanalysis: Observation, Theory, Application. Edited by Guttman SA. New York, International Universities Press, 1976a, pp 68–83

Waelder R: The psychoanalytic theory of play (1932), in Psychoanalysis: Observation, Theory, Application. Edited by Guttman SA. New York, International Universities Press, 1976b, pp 84–100

Walk RD, Gibson EJ: A comparative and analytical study of visual depth perception. Psychological Monographs, Vol 75, No 519, 1961

Wartner VG: Attachment in infancy and at age six, and children's self concept: a follow-up of a German longitudinal study. Ph.D. dissertation, Department of Psychology, University of Virginia, Charlottesville, 1986

Watson JB, Rayner R: Conditioned emotional reaction. J Exp Psychol 3:1–14, 1920

Weiss J: How Psychotherapy Works: Process and Technique. New York, Guilford, 1993

Weiss J, Sampson H, Mt. Zion Psychotherapy Research Group: The Psychoanalytic Process: Theory, Clinical Observations, and Empirical Research. New York, Guilford, 1986

Weissberg-Benchell J: Temperament, Environmental Demands, Adjustment, and Metabolic Control in Children With Insulin Dependent Diabetes Mellitus. Grant Proposal, Children's National Medical Center Intramural Research Program, Washington, DC, 1990

Werman DS: Suppression as a defense, in Defense and Resistance. Edited by Blum HP. New York, International Universities Press, 1985, pp 405–417

Werner H: Comparative Psychology of Mental Development. New York, International Universities Press, 1940

Werner H, Kaplan B: Symbol formation: An Orgasmic-Developmental Approach to Language and the Expression of Thought. New York, Wiley, 1963

Wesley F, Sullivan E: Human Growth and Development: A Psychological Approach. New York, Human Sciences Press, 1980

Winnicott DW: Transitional objects and transitional phenomena (1953), in Playing and Reality. New York, Basic Books, 1971, pp 1–25

Winnicott DW: The capacity to be alone, in The Maturational Processes and the Facilitating Environment. New York, International Universities Press, 1958, pp 29–36

Winnicott DW: The fate of the transitional object (1959), in Psychoanalytic Explorations. Edited by Winnicott C, Shepherd R, Davis M. Cambridge, MA, Harvard University Press, 1989, pp 53–58

Winnicott DW: The Maturational Process and the Facilitating Environment. New York, International Universities Press, 1965

Wolf ES: Disruptions of the therapeutic relationship in psychoanalysis: a view from self psychology. Int J Psychoanal 74:675–688, 1993

Wolff PH: The causes, controls, and organization of behavior in the neonate. Psychol Issues Vol 51, Monograph 17, 1966

Wolff PH: The serial organization of sucking in the young infant. Pediatrics 42:943–956, 1968

Wyatt GE: Changing influences on adolescent sexuality over the past forty years, in Adolescence and Puberty. Edited by Bancroft J, Reinsich JM. New York, Oxford University Press, 1990, pp 782–821

Yorke C, Wiseberg S: A developmental view of anxiety. Psychoanal Study Child 31:107–135, 1976

Yussen S, Santrock J: Child Development. Dubuque, IA, Wm C Brown, 1978

Zajonic R: Feeling and thinking: preferences need no inferences. Am Psychol 35:151–175, 1980

Zeanah CH, Anders TF, Seifer R, et al: Implications of research on infant development for psychodynamic theory and practice. J Am Acad Child Adolesc Psychiatry 28:657–688, 1989

Zelago P, Kotelchuck M, Barber L, et al: Fathers and sons: an experimental facilitation of attachment behaviors. Paper presented to the Society for Research in Child Development. New Orleans, LA, March 1977

Zelnick M, Shah FK: First intercourse among young Americans. Family Planning Perspectives 15:64–70, 1983

Zetzel E, Meissner WW: Basic Concepts of Psychoanalytic Psychiatry. New York, Basic Books, 1973

Index

Schema/schemata, 128
construction, from direct
environmental
experience, 131
new/complex, in knowledge
acquisition, 130–131
Science, organizing principles of,
24
Scripts, in early childhood,
335–337
Secondary process thinking, 41,
42, 121, **122**. *See also*
Fantasy/fantasies
differentiation from primary
process thinking, 398–403
in early childhood, 309–310,
312, 415
in late childhood, 395, **396**
speech in, 415
in toddlerhood, 237–238
Secondary sexual characteristics,
452–454
internal stimulation from,
55–57
maturational emergence of,
55–60
Secrets, 413
Secure attachment, 180
Selective attachments, 201
Selective social smile, 192–193
Self
definition of, 104
development of
in early childhood,
338–365, **347, 358,
359**
in toddlerhood, 267–281,
273
and object interdependence
toddlers and, 259–260
verbal language
development and, 334
organizational structure of, in
infancy, 104–106

true, development of, in early
childhood, 299–302
vs. self-representation, 105
Self-assertion
autonomy and, 257–259
verbal language development
and, 334
Self-autonomy, of adolescent,
468, 469, 516–517. *See also*
Emancipated identity
Self-awareness, 105, 152
in infancy, 91–92
objective, **220**, 220–228
of toddler, 251
toddler behaviors and, **222**
Self-constancy, positive,
278–280
Self-control, in late childhood,
432–439, **435–438**
Self-esteem, 256
development of, 162
in late childhood, 432–439,
435–438
of parent, infant's social smile
and, 193
peer group feedback and, 426
verbal language development
and, 334
Self-image, realistic, in transition
from adolescence to
adulthood, 517
Self-inhibition, of toddlers,
262–263
Selfobject
definition of, 162
experience, 162–163
idealizing, 164
infant as, 192
mirroring, 164–165
mirroring failure, of parents,
167–168
Self-observation, in early
childhood, 297
Self psychology theory, 346–347